MANAGEMENT OF NEUROLOGICAL DISORDERS

Edited by

C M Wiles

Professor of Neurology, Department of Medicine
University of Wales College of Medicine, Cardiff

First published in 1995
by the BMJ Publishing Group, BMA House, Tavistock Square, London WC1H 9JR

British Library Cataloguing in Publication Data

A catalogue record for this book is available
from the British Library

ISBN 0-7279-0903-7

Typeset, printed and bound in Great Britain by
Latimer Trend & Company Ltd., Plymouth

Contents

Introduction

The management of neurological disease and injury touches virtually all practising clinicians, whether in hospital or in general practice. Such have been the advances in understanding, management, and treatment of many disorders over the past decade that it becomes increasingly difficult for the non-specialist, or even the "non-specialist" specialist, to keep up with developments—particularly in the sphere of neurosciences. Patients have increasingly high expectations which are, as yet only slowly, being reflected in the demands of purchasers of health care. While providers of care struggle to meet innumerable quantitative criteria concerning the processes of diagnosis and management (waiting times, waiting lists, etc) it is important not to lose sight of the important related issue, which is the substance and quality of the actual medical care provided. The medical profession must lead from the front in the setting of standards of care based on the traditional but cogent twin pillars of good clinical practice and sound science. Furthermore, physicians (in the broadest sense) have an important role in continuing education for themselves, their patients, and their managerial colleagues.

With the development of a more proactive treatment approach there is an increased requirement for texts and reviews that deal at least as much with clinical management as with diagnosis, the imperative of accurate diagnosis notwithstanding. This book represents a compilation of commissioned articles, many of which have been published recently in the *Journal of Neurology, Neurosurgery, and Psychiatry*, tackling mostly common adult neurological disorders from this perspective: it is by no means comprehensive in coverage but is to some extent complementary to and overlapping with the previous book, *Neurological Emergencies.*[1]

So great has been the impact of genetics on neurological disease, not only in theory but regularly now in practice, that the practising physician cannot afford to ignore this rapidly expanding area of development. Rehabilitation is an integral part of the management of patients with disabilities and handicap arising from neurological disorder and an area too widespread in impact and importance to be left to a few specialists: it involves all who practise clinical neurology, a fact now reflected in accreditation programmes. In the United Kingdom, and many other countries where the number of neurologists and neurosurgeons is relatively low, development of good management for patients must go hand in hand with an awareness of the overall resources, strengths, and deficiencies of the "countrywide" framework in which the specialists are operating. Each of the above topics (the latter of necessity from a United Kingdom perspective) are covered in chapters in this book, in addition to coverage of specific neurological disorders.

Though nowadays no chapter written by a single author can be considered to be the final word on anything, all the authors of this book have extensive clinical and research experience of their subjects sufficient for their contribution to be regarded as authoritative. It is hoped that the chapters will inform general and hospital practitioners, trainees, purchasers of health care, and students in the health sciences who want an up to date account as a starting point for further research. Many authors have incorporated comments on audit into their chapters and have provided material that can indicate to staff and managers some of the questions to be asked in promoting effective audit of medical care. If this book can facilitate the use of standards against which individual institutions can assess the quality of the care they provide for neurological patients it will have achieved its purpose.

C M Wiles
March 1995

1 Hughes RAC. *Neurological Emergencies.* London: BMJ Publishing Group, 1994.

1 Clinical genetics in neurological disease

JOHN C MacMILLAN, PETER S HARPER

Inherited neurological disorders have traditionally engendered feelings of therapeutic nihilism in the medical community: not only are these conditions often difficult to diagnose with any certainty, they are also perceived as "untreatable" whether or not a firm diagnosis has been reached. This negative response is due in part to a lack of knowledge concerning the underlying pathological basis for these disorders.

The 1980s and early 1990s have seen a rapid increase in our understanding of the molecular mechanisms behind many of these debilitating conditions, largely due to advances in recombinant DNA technology. This chapter aims to summarise the role of clinical genetic and molecular genetic practice in the management of the major inherited neurological diseases. We consider diagnostic issues as they pertain to the individual case—that is, the specific disorder affecting the patient and its likely prognosis—and counselling issues for the family, such as the identification of individuals who may develop symptoms in later life (presymptomatic testing) or risks for the inheritance of the disorder by a future family member (prenatal testing and carrier detection). To date there have not been equivalent advances in our therapeutic options in the management of these conditions although experimental protocols have been initiated with this in mind, some of which show promising results in animal models.

The disorders and the relevant molecular genetic analyses under consideration are discussed in two groups: those for which one or more genetic loci have been identified but the gene(s) not yet cloned; and those for which the genes have been isolated and the

1

Table 1.1   Prevalence of major, single-gene neurological disorders in south east Wales

Disorder	Prevalence (/100 000)	95% confidence interval
Hereditary motor and sensory neuropathy types I, II, III, and V	12·9	10·7 to 15·4
Myotonic dystrophy	7·1	5·5 to 9·1
Duchenne muscular dystrophy	9·6*	7·0 to 12·9
Becker muscular dystrophy	5·0*	3·2 to 7·6
Facioscapulohumeral muscular dystrophy	2·9	1·9 to 4·1
Spinal muscular atrophy (all types)	1·3	0·7 to 2·2
Huntington's disease	8·4	6·6 to 10·5
Tuberous sclerosis	1·6	0·9 to 2·6
Von Hippel Lindau disease	0·6	0·2 to 1·4
Hereditary spastic paraplegia	3·4	2·3 to 4·8
Neurofibromatosis type 1	13·3	11·1 to 15·8

* Per 100 000 males.

relevant product characterised. We begin by reviewing the available data from epidemiological and family studies on the frequency of these disorders.

Epidemiology

Individual genetic neurological diseases are not common but as a group they account for a significant burden of disability in a generally younger age group than affected by other neurological diseases. In a review of reports published throughout the world, Emery[1] estimated a population prevalence for the inherited neuromuscular diseases of over 1 in 3000. The authors' study in south east Wales[2] suggests a minimum prevalence for the major inherited neurological disorders of over 58 per 100 000 population (approximately 1 in 1700 population). Table 1.1 shows the disorders and the prevalence of symptomatic individuals in the south east Wales population.

These figures do not take into account asymptomatic gene carriers who may develop clinical disease in the future; nor do they allow for the unaffected but "at risk" family members who are also likely to request information on the disease (this latter group are more likely to seek guidance from a genetics unit but a not insignificant number may be seen initially by the neurologist dealing with the index case).

Linkage analysis

Disorders localised to specific chromosomal sites but not yet cloned

The number of disorders in this group decreases monthly as a result of the continual isolation of new genes for specific diseases. The technology used in "linkage analysis" merits a brief description as it needs to be appreciated that there are limitations to its usefulness in many clinical situations.

Linkage analysis has been the first stage in the localisation of a gene responsible for many genetic disorders. It makes use of restriction fragment length polymorphisms. These are lengths of DNA that have been cut at each end at a specific site recognised by a bacterial restriction endonuclease enzyme. Different enzymes recognise and cleave at different DNA sequence motifs of variable numbers of base pairs. The great variability in human DNA results in differences in the length of sequence between cleavage sites in unrelated individuals. Within a family, however, these anonymous DNA segments (restriction fragment length polymorphisms) are inherited in a mendelian fashion and can be tracked through a family pedigree using standard laboratory techniques. Botstein *et al*[3] first suggested the use of these in the construction of genetic linkage maps for the localisation of disease genes to particular segments of chromosomes and they have superseded the blood group polymorphisms used in early studies.

In a family linkage analysis, each member of the family is assessed for the presence of the disease of interest, and their status (restriction fragment length polymorphism) for the marker locus is ascertained. If the disease locus and the marker locus are close together on the same chromosome (linked) then independent assortment at meiosis will be rare and both traits will be inherited in the offspring. The closer they are to each other the less likely it is that they will separate during the pairing of homologous chromosomes at meiosis—in other words, that a recombination will occur. The recombination fraction, known as theta (θ) gives an indication of the genetic distance between the two loci. Genetic distance is expressed in centiMorgans where 1 cM is defined as a segment of chromosome with a 1% chance of recombination per meiosis[4] and this is equivalent to a θ of 0·01. A recombination fraction of 0·5 means either that the two loci are on different

3

chromosomes or that they are far apart on the same chromosome.

The successful application (accuracy) of linkage analysis in the clinical situation is dependent on several factors: it is crucial that the diagnosis is correct; and the disease must have been localised (mapped to a segment of chromosome) with close polymorphic markers available. Affected individuals should be heterozygous for the marker polymorphisms ("informative"), there should not (ideally) be genetic heterogeneity (more than one disease locus for the clinical phenotype), and the family relationships, especially paternity, must be clearly established. The disease status for each individual typed must be accurate (especially where the disease is of late onset and "unaffected" individuals are crucial to the analysis). Figure 1.1 shows a family typed for a hypothetical two-allele polymorphism known to be linked to the disease of interest. Woman I_2 is affected by the disorder and is heterozygous for the polymorphism (she types 2–1); her unaffected spouse is homozygous (2–2) as is her unaffected son II_1. Son II_3 is clinically affected and has inherited allele 1 from his mother, and has subsequently transmitted this allele to individual III_1. This three-generation situation is ideally suited to linkage analysis as phase is known—that is, the chromosome carrying the mutant gene can be identified—and affected individuals are heterozygous for the polymorphisms of interest. Knowledge of the genotype of individual III_1, who may be too young for the disease to have manifested itself, permits prediction of the likelihood that he or she will develop the disease. In this situation the presence of allele 1 indicates a high risk, the actual value of which would depend on the recombination fraction between the marker and the disease. In general it is unlikely that a marker would be used whose rate of recombination with the disease was greater than 3%. In the example shown the actual value would be 97%, using a marker with 3% recombination, as it is a fully informative situation. This approach can also be used to increase the reproductive options for couples at risk by permitting prenatal diagnosis through linkage analysis and, where affected, termination of an affected pregnancy. Individual III_1 in figure 1.1 could represent a conceptus from which chorionic villus sampling would provide appropriate tissue for analysis in early pregnancy.

Specific disorders

Table 1.2 lists diseases linked to specific chromosomes, but with the gene not yet isolated, for which family linkage studies can play

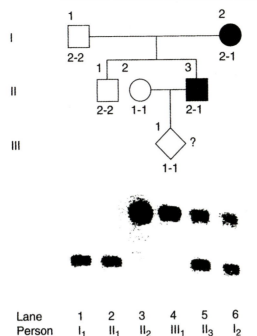

Figure 1.1 *The lanes in the autoradiograph contain DNA from the individuals indicated in the pedigree. The DNA has been digested using a restriction endonuclease enzyme, subjected to electrophoresis on an agarose gel and transferred to a nylon membrane. The DNA probe of interest has been labelled with radioisotope and incubated overnight with the membrane. The membrane has been stored at − 20°C adjacent to radiographic film for seven days. Bands are assigned numbers with the largest band designated 1.*

Table 1.2 Chromosomal localisations for major genetic neurological disorders for which the gene has not yet been cloned

Disorder	Localisation(s)
Facioscapulohumeral* muscular dystrophy	4q35
Familial spastic paraplegia (one dominant type)	14q
Friedreich's ataxia	9q13–21
Limb-girdle muscular dystrophy (dominant)	5q22·3–31·3
Tuberous sclerosis (*see also table 1.3*)	9q34

Gene locations are identified by the chromosome number followed by an indication of which arm (p = short, q = long) and the sub-band.
* But see text for comments on the molecular rearrangement reported in this disorder.

a useful role in patient and family management. It is not intended to be a comprehensive list of all mapped neurogenetic diseases; the interested reader should consult sources such as the bimonthly listings in *Neuromuscular disorders* (Pergamon Press), the summaries of the Human Genome Mapping Project annual meetings, McKusick's *Mendelian inheritance in man* (published and "online" versions), and periodic reviews.[5]

It *may* be possible to provide presymptomatic testing for these disorders for relatives at risk if the family structure is suitable but the presence of genetic heterogeneity, as in tuberous sclerosis, can make even this very difficult in all but the largest families. Various Bayesian approaches have been proposed to take such additional factors into account when counselling individuals in these situations.[6]

Although the gene for facioscapulohumeral muscular dystrophy has not yet been cloned, it is possible to make diagnostic use of molecular DNA analysis where it is thought that an affected person represents a new dominant mutation for the disorder. This paradoxical situation arises as the result of the presence of detectable rearrangements associated with a series of 3·2 kb tandem repeat elements (1 kb = 1000 base pairs) in the subtelomeric region of the long arm of chromosome 4.[7] The DNA probe p13E-11 (locus D4F104S1) detects bands over 50 kb in size after *EcoR1* digestion in normal individuals and a band less than 35 kb in length in individuals with facioscapulohumeral muscular dystrophy. In most cases thought to represent new mutations, it is possible to show that both parents possess two normal-sized alleles whereas the affected individual has one normal-sized and one rearranged fragment.

Some disorders, mostly rare, have not yet been mapped to a specific chromosome(s) and genetic management is confined to counselling families on the inheritance and nature of the disease.

Mutation analysis

Once a gene associated with a particular disease has been isolated it becomes possible to test DNA samples from affected individuals for mutations within that gene. These may take the form of point mutations that substitute alternative nucleic acid bases and result in changes in the amino acid sequence (missense mutations) or introduce stop codons with premature truncation of the translation product (nonsense mutations). Other mutations may involve the insertion or deletion of a number of base pairs (from one to many thousands) resulting in disruption of the normal function of the gene. Occasionally deletions or duplications of whole chromosome segments are found in association with specific disorders. In addition to these "classical" types of mutation, we have seen in the past two years the identification of a new class of mutation that is often unstable in its transmission between generations. This is the trinucleotide repeat, the principal characteristic of which is instability, giving varying molecular and clinical changes in the different affected members of a single kindred, as discussed more fully below.

Mutation analysis has the advantage (over linkage analysis) that it is not dependent on family structure and can therefore be applied to an isolated case of a disorder suspected to be genetic. Various laboratory techniques are used in the detection of mutations[8] and it may take several weeks for a specific defect to be identified, depending on whether the method is in regular service use or still at the research stage.

Disorders for which the responsible gene has been characterised

Table 1.3 lists some disorders for which the gene responsible has been identified and mutation analysis is feasible (the special situation for facioscapulohumeral muscular dystrophy has been mentioned above). The number of disorders in this category is increasing rapidly, and individual genetic units cannot be expected to provide every analysis. In the United Kingdom, the clinician primarily responsible for the individual patient's care should consult their local genetics unit for information about which molecular services are available locally and those which can be obtained elsewhere (usually from other genetic laboratories in the National Health Service). It should be stressed that a comprehensive genetic counselling service should be available to everyone for whom a molecular genetic analysis is undertaken. This is particularly relevant where specific mutation analysis is requested but the individual has not been aware that the disorder may be hereditary. The analyses may have significant implications for siblings or offspring. Examples of these difficulties are given below in respect of specific disorders.

Table 1.3   Cloned genes, their products, functions, and mutations

Disease	Chromosomal localisation	Gene product	Function	Mutation	Mutations identified (%)
CMT disease type 1A	17p11·2	Peripheral myelin protein (PMP)-22	Myelin protein	Duplication / Point mutations	<100 / Few
CMT disease type 1B	1q22–23	Po	Myelin protein	Point mutations	100
CMT disease X linked	Xq13	Connexin 32	Cell contact	Point mutations, deletions	80
DMB/BMD	Xp21	Dystrophin	Cytoskeletal protein	Deletions, duplications, point mutations	50
DRPLA	12p	Unknown	Unknown	Expanded trinucleotide repeat sequence	Unknown
Familial ALS (motor neuron disease)	21q22·1	Cu, Zn-superoxide dismutase (SOD 1)	Free radical removal	Point mutations	Unknown
Familial Alzheimer's disease	21–q21	Amyloid precursor protein	Unknown	Point mutations	14
Fragile X syndrome A	Xq27	Unknown	RNA binding protein	Expanded trinucleotide repeat sequence / Point mutations	<100 / Few
Fragile X syndrome E	Xq29	Unknown	Unknown	Expanded trinucleotide repeat sequence	Unknown
Huntington's disease	4p16·3	Huntingtin	Unknown	Expanded trinucleotide repeat sequence	99
Machado-Joseph disease	14q32·1	Unknown	Unknown	Expanded trinucleotide repeat sequence	Unknown
Myotonic dystrophy	19q13·2	Myotonin	Protein kinase	Expanded trinucleotide repeat sequence	100
Neurofibromatosis type 1	17q11·2	Neurofibromin	Tumour suppressor	Deletions, point mutations	20
Neurofibromatosis type 2	22q11	Merlin	Tumour suppressor	Deletions, point mutations	50
Prion diseases	20pter–p12	Prion protein	Unknown	Point mutations	Unknown
Spinal and bulbar muscular atrophy (Kennedy's disease)	Xq13	Androgen receptor	Unknown on anterior horn cells	Expanded trinucleotide repeat sequence	100
SMA types I, II, and III	5q13	Unknown	Unknown	Deletions, point mutations	100
Spinocerebellar ataxia type 1	6p24-p23	Unknown	Unknown	Expanded trinucleotide repeat sequence	Unknown
Tuberous sclerosis (one type)	16p13	Tuberin	Tumour suppressor	Deletions	Uncertain
Von Hippel Lindau disease	3p25–26	Unknown	Tumour suppressor	Deletions, insertions, point mutations	Unknown

In several disorders listed, a single, or very small number, of distinct mutations in the same gene are responsible for the same phenotype: thus in Leber's hereditary optic neuropathy a point mutation at base pair 11 778 (in the gene for subunit 4 of the reduced nicotinamide adenine dinucleotide (NADH) dehydrogenase (ND4) complex in the respiratory chain) of the mitochondrial genome accounts for 50% of cases, whereas other causative mutations giving an identical clinical picture occur at base pairs 3460 (in ND1), 4160 (ND1), and 15 257 (cytochrome b).[9] Mutation analysis in this situation therefore requires careful planning and interpretation. Recent work has suggested that some mitochondrial mutations may be synergistic—for example, mutations at base pairs 13 708, 15 257, 15 812, and 5244—and the accumulation of these in an individual increases the likelihood that clinical disease will result.[10] Even in Duchenne and Becker muscular dystrophies clustering of mutations (in exons 3, 8, 13, 43, 44, 47, 50, 51, and 52) has allowed the development of practical screening strategies (multiplex polymerase chain reaction) that optimise detection (up to 90% of all deletions) within ever-present financial constraints.[11]

In a number of disorders the situation is less satisfactory: table 1.3 gives, for each disorder, an indication of the proportion of affected individuals in which a mutation in the relevant gene can be identified. It is important to realise, therefore, that failure to identify a mutation does not necessarily mean that the individual does not have the disease in question. It may be possible to use an alternative strategy to confirm the diagnosis and this is the case with Duchenne and Becker muscular dystrophy. The characterisation of dystrophin at the DNA level allows the prediction of structure and function as well as the synthesis of antibodies to several domains of the protein. These can be used histochemically to indicate whether a normal distribution of protein is present in association with the muscle cell membrane—that is, not Duchenne or Becker muscular dystrophy—or the amount is reduced or distribution discontinuous (Becker muscular dystrophy) or the protein is absent (Duchenne muscular dystrophy). This is important in giving a prognosis to the parents of boys with an Xp21 dystrophy identified in screening programmes of neonates[12] if the type of molecular change has not itself suggested the likely phenotype.[11] In cases where no mutation is found in dystrophin, and antibody studies show a normal amount and distribution of protein in muscle, alternative diagnoses need to be considered. Recent work has clarified the situation in the autosomal recessive "Duchenne-like" dystrophy and Fukuyama-type dystrophy, both of which arise as the result of abnormalities of proteins found in association with dystrophin.[13][14] The genes for autosomal recessive and autosomal dominant limb-girdle dystrophy have been localised to specific chromosomes (5 and 15) but not yet identified and a molecular test is not therefore available for these.

Molecular testing may not be of significant clinical help in some situations, as in neurofibromatosis type 1, where only a small proportion of cases (20%) have an identifiable mutation in the neurofibromin gene.[15] Fortunately the disease is clearly identifiable (fully penetrant) by the age of 5 years and a child clinically normal after this will not develop it. Because of the low rate of mutation identification, prenatal testing for this disorder is still largely dependent on linkage analysis although its accuracy has improved with the availability of intragenic markers.

Diseases associated with expansions in trinucleotide repeat sequences

The molecular abnormalities in eight disorders in table 1.3 have been identified as arising from the expansion of a trinucleotide repeat sequence in association with the identified gene. The term *association* is chosen deliberately as the location of these patho-logical sequences differs; in dentatorubropallidoluysian atrophy, Huntington's disease, Machado-Joseph disease, spinocerebellar ataxia, and X linked spinal and bulbar muscular atrophy it lies within the coding sequence, whereas in myotonic dystrophy it is 3′ (downstream) from the coding sequence. In the fragile X mental retardation syndrome associated with a cytogenetically detectable fragile site at Xq27·3 (FRAXA), the expanded sequence lies 5′ (upstream) from the coding sequence. It appears that in this disorder there is a critical degree of expansion beyond which there is silencing of gene expression[16] possibly due to hypermethylation within the gene[17] and it is this deficiency that is responsible for the disease phenotype. In the fragile X syndrome with a fragile site at Xq28 (FRAXE), there is amplification of a GCC repeat wth associated hypermethylation of the neighbouring CpG island (a region associated with an active gene) implying a similar disease mechanism to that seen in FRAXA.[18] In myotonic dystrophy it has been shown that the level of myotonin protein kinase messenger RNA (mRNA) is reduced when the mutant allele has less than 200 repeats and very low when there are 800 repeats.[19] In congenital cases it has been reported that not only is no mutant mRNA detectable but also that there is a reduced level of the normal paternal mRNA.[20] Another group has, however, reported an increase in the level of mutant mRNA in congenital cases.[21]

A specific characteristic of this type of mutation is its instability; the length of the repeat sequence tends to increase as it undergoes successive meiotic passages (as it passes from one generation to the next). In myotonic dystrophy this successive expansion accounts for the long debated phenomenon of anticipation whereby the clinical manifestations (phenotype) become more severe in subsequent generations. It does not, however, account for the observation that congenital cases of myotonic dystrophy are always born of affected mothers.

These trinucleotide repeat amplifications are quantitative mutations and have been the subject of several studies examining correlations between degree of amplification and the age at onset of symptoms.[22] The question arises as to whether it is possible to predict the age at disease onset and severity of the disease phenotype knowing the degree of expansion in the DNA sequence.[23] We would caution against attempting this in a specific clinical situation. Although there is a clear distinction between the degree of expansion in congenital cases of myotonic dystrophy and late onset or minimal manifestations, such as cataract only, there is considerable overlap in other situations, even within the same family.

Phenotype prediction on the basis of degree of sequence expansion in Huntington's disease is fraught with even more difficulties: we have shown that the individual variation in age at onset for a given repeat number can range over a span of 20–30 years[24] and, in addition, that the size of the repeat sequence on the normal paternal allele has an effect in maternally transmitted disease.[25] This may account for the larger variability in age at onset in sibships with disease of maternal compared with paternal origin. As with any inherited disorder, the disease-specific mutation is acting within the individual's unique (with the exception of identical twins) genetic background which may contain several modifying loci. It could well be argued that the lack of a clinically useful correlation has potential benefits to a

11

person requesting presymptomatic testing: the psychological well being of an individual and his or her family would be unlikely to be helped by foreknowledge of a precise age at onset of this devastating disorder.

Hereditary motor and sensory neuropathy type I

In considering the applicability of molecular genetic testing, the case of type I hereditary motor and sensory neuropathy (HMSN I) illustrates some of both the benefits and limitations of using direct mutational analysis in the clinical situation. Hereditary motor and sensory neuropathy type I (also known as Charcot-Marie-Tooth disease type 1, CMT 1) is an autosomal dominant condition with extreme variability in phenotype. The manifestations range from significantly reduced peripheral nerve conduction velocity (median motor conduction velocity <38 m/s) with no clinical signs or symptoms in some gene carriers, to wheelchair dependence in later life in others. The disorder shows genetic heterogeneity with genes on chromosomes 17, 1, and another as yet unidentified locus. In an individual male case it is not possible clinically to distinguish CMT 1 from the X linked form (CMTX).

In over 90% of cases of hereditary motor and sensory neuropathy type I the disorder arises as a result of the duplication of 1·1 million base pairs (1·1 Mb) of DNA on the proximal short arm of chromosome 17 (CMT at this locus is identified as CMT1A).[26] Within this region is a gene coding for peripheral myelin protein-22 (PMP-22), an integral membrane protein that plays an important role in arresting Schwann cell division. Mutations in this gene cause a peripheral neuropathy in the *trembler* mouse model.[27] Individuals with this duplication have three copies of the normal gene and the phenotype probably results from overexpression of the gene. In addition, at least two families have now been identified in which the CMT 1/HMSN I phenotype is associated with a point mutation in the DNA sequence of the PMP-22 gene.[28]

Although this is of great interest to the developmental neurobiologist, it poses the problem of how much molecular analysis should we undertake if the first mutation screen (in this case analysis for the 1·1 Mb duplication) is negative? This may be of crucial importance to patients and their families who will often be concerned about the risk of the same condition arising in either siblings or offspring and to the clinician (geneticist or neurologist) counselling them on those risks.

We are of the opinion that screening for point mutations in duplication-negative HMSN I cases is not practicable as a clinical service (although it may be possible to find a research unit willing to undertake the analysis). One situation that has been clarified with mutation analysis for CMT1/HMSN I is the case of the isolated, affected individual who may be considered to have the autosomal recessive form of HMSN I. Hoogendijk et al[29] have shown that in nine out of 10 isolated cases of HMSN I (in whom both parents were clinically and electrophysiologically normal), the disorder had arisen from a de novo duplication occurring in one of the parental germ cells. The risk to subsequent offspring of such an affected individual is clearly 50% (and not "minimal" as may previously have been counselled) whereas the risk to siblings of such patients would be minimal (this may be modified in some cases by gonadal mosaicism in the parent) rather than the previously counselled 25%. Counselling of a duplication-negative isolated male case remains difficult in view of the possibility that he has the X linked form of CMT. Hayasaka et al[30] have recently reported the identification of point mutations in the gene for Po, another integral membrane protein of peripheral nervous system myelin, in individuals with CMT1b. Where this complexity of situation occurs there is much to be said for the continued application of standard clinical screening protocols (meaurement of motor nerve conduction velocities and sensory nerve action potentials) for individuals at risk in addition to direct molecular analysis.

Considerations when requesting mutation analysis

In myotonic dystrophy, Huntington's disease, and Charcot-Marie-Tooth type 1 (HMSN I) the success of mutation analysis makes it tempting to expand the range of the clinical picture that prompts the dispatch of a blood sample for "DNA analysis". We have already stated our view that, before any sample is taken, the patient should be made aware of the potential genetic implications of a "positive" result. This may not cause undue anxiety if the individual believes other family members show similar signs already, or he or she perceives the disorder not to be unduly serious.

Three disorders merit closer examination in considering the clinical range that should prompt a "DNA analysis": Huntington's disease; Alzheimer's disease; and prion dementia. All may manifest with progressive dementia with or without additional features. Should we therefore screen all cases of dementia for the specific mutations associated with these disorders? Several problems arise in considering this.

Firstly, there is the question of consent. Can the patients be made aware of the implications of a positive result or should their families make the decision on their behalf? After all it is they (the family) who will be most affected by such a result.

Secondly, the sensitivity of the analysis should be considered. In those situations where we believe this to be approaching 100% (Huntington's disease) the family can be reassured by a negative result. In familial Alzheimer's disease, however, there is genetic heterogeneity, and the available molecular analysis (looking for point mutations in the amyloid precursor protein (APP) gene) would screen only one gene accounting for a small proportion of cases.[31] A negative result would not therefore exclude a diagnosis of familial Alzheimer's disease. Screening DNA from patients with dementia for mutations in the prion protein gene associated with Gerstmann-Sträussler syndrome and familial Creutzfeldt-Jakob disease would, superficially, seem reasonable in view of the reported cases where dementia is the only manifestation.[32]

The implications for the siblings and offspring of a patient with an identifiable prion mutation are, however, less clear. Whereas an asymptomatic gene carrier for Huntington's disease has approaching a 100% likelihood of developing clinical manifestations (barring other causes of death), there are currently only limited data with which to counsel an asymptomatic carrier of a prion gene mutation; Collinge et al give an empiric risk of 95%.[33] Any reservations on the application of these mutation analyses in a demented patient would be removed should an effective treatment become available.

There have been no reservations, however, in applying molecular analyses of the dystrophin gene and its product, despite the knowledge that a positive result identifies an untreatable disorder. Hoffman et al[34] have shown that at least 10% of women with a myopathy and raised plasma creatine kinase concentration have an identifiable abnormality in the dystrophin gene or the dystrophin protein, or both. The perceived benefit, that these women and their families can now be counselled on the appropriate risks of recurrences, would appear to have been justification enough for testing.

The availability of analyses for the trinucleotide repeat amplification in the androgen receptor gene in bulbospinal neuronopathy[35] and mutations in the copper/zinc superoxide dismutase gene (SOD1)[36] in some families with autosomal dominant motor neuron disease, makes feasible the screening of isolated individuals (especially males) with motor neuron disease. We are of the opinion that, whereas screening for the androgen receptor gene trinucleotide repeat expansion is valuable (a normal result excludes Kennedy's disease), SOD1 analysis in the absence of a significant family history is not an appropriate use of laboratory services.

Box 1.1 shows the mutation analyses that we consider should be available to neurologists as part of a regional molecular genetic service and the clinical situations in which we feel the request is appropriate. Fragile X (type A) mutation analysis is usually requested by paediatricians when faced with a child with developmental delay and could be added to this list. It would however, add considerably to the workload and would require appropriate additional staff.

The issue of which cases should be referred to a clinical geneticist in conjunction with the request for a specific mutation analysis should be addressed locally, taking into consideration the available staffing levels (see below) and the specific interests of the clinicians. Access to diagnostic molecular services should not be limited by the availability of a clinical geneticist, although it should be a standard of acceptable practice that the appropriateness of the request for mutation analysis should be discussed with a genetics colleague whenever possible.

Once a positive result has been generated the clinician is duty bound to transmit this information to the patient and, with his or her consent, to the family. Clinical neurologists will often find this a most useful time to engage the help of their clinical genetics colleagues, if they were not approached initially to advise on what molecular test may have been applicable. Extended family counselling on the nature and implications of a specific diagnosis is often time consuming and may involve other health professionals such as specialist genetics nurses and clinical psychologists if presymptomatic testing is requested by siblings or offspring.

15

Box 1.1 Clinical indications for specified mutation analyses

Mutation analysis	Clinical indication
Dystrophin gene	"Limb girdle" dystrophy with raised creatine kinase *Raised neonatal creatine kinase
CMT1A duplication	Demyelinating neuropathy
Myotonin-kinase CTG repeat	Muscular dystrophy with myotonia
IT15 CAG repeat	Adult onset chorea Juvenile rigid syndrome
LHON mutations	Acute bilateral optic atrophy
MELAS/MERRF mutations†	Myoclonic epilepsy, proximal myopathy with appropriate histology, young stroke victims

* Ethically approved research protocol.
† On DNA extracted from blood and muscle.
CMT = Charcot-Marie-Tooth; LHON = Leber's hereditory optic neuropathy; MELAS = mitochondrial myopathy, encephalopathy, lactic acidosis, and stroke-like episodes; MERRF = myoclonus epilepsy with ragged-red fibres.

Cases when mutation analysis is inappropriate

We are also aware of the circumstances in which a molecular DNA test should not be undertaken. The most obvious case is when the patient does not want it. This is no different from a person declining a test for HIV carrier status. Most other cases occur where presymptomatic testing is requested and these will usually be directed towards the geneticist. Practising neurologists should be aware of these circumstances, however, as family members may approach them initially, after the diagnosis of a heritable disorder in the patient. Occasionally, an individual at risk for an inherited disorder may approach a neurologist with symptoms unrelated to the genetic disease. In this case it would not be appropriate to offer specific mutation analysis. What is less clear is the merit of mutation analysis in the presence of vague symptoms which may be disease related, such as clumsiness or forgetfulness, where there is a family history of Huntington's disease. The identification of a disease-specific mutation in this state of affairs may not offer a definitive explanation for the individual's symptoms.

Many inherited neurological disorders have onset in mid to later life, and presymptomatic testing of children for these is not appropriate.[37] This would change should effective therapy to prevent clinical disease become available. People should not be under pressure from third parties such as insurance companies to be tested, and those requesting testing should be made aware of the possible interests of such parties in the outcome. It may be useful to consider what impact a positive test result would have on one's own family and social position to gain an appreciation of the possible consequences for the individual in question.

Susceptibility genes

This chapter has focused on those neurological disorders whose aetiology is primarily "single gene" and where advances in our knowledge have followed the isolation of that gene. In many of the most prevalent neurological disorders (multiple sclerosis, idiopathic epilepsy, stroke) there may be an appreciable genetic component, as recognised from familial clustering of cases or from twin studies, but true mendelian inheritance is not seen. Attention is now focusing on the identification of "susceptibility genes" which may predispose an individual to the development of these conditions. Harding et al[38] have proposed that mitochondrial loci may be implicated in the susceptibility to develop multiple sclerosis. It has long been recognised that there is a higher frequency of specific HLA haplotypes in individuals with multiple sclerosis, suggesting additional immunological factors (reviewed in reference 39). It is not known how relevant any single susceptibility locus will turn out to be, nor how amenable to modification this predisposition will be in an individual.

We are in no doubt, however, that individuals with these disorders and their families will in future expect to receive counselling on the genetic contribution to disease susceptibility and advice on strategies for modifying their risks. We are equally convinced that society will require considerable education about the relevance of these factors if individuals who have been identified to be at increased risk are not to be discriminated against in education, employment, and insurance. Legislative intervention may be necessary to avoid the creation of a genetically stigmatised subpopulation.

Applying molecular analysis

Samples

Most analyses are carried out on DNA isolated from peripheral blood lymphocytes collected in containers with EDTA as an anticoagulant. A sample of 20 ml of blood provides sufficient DNA for all analyses. When polymerase chain reaction technology is used, considerably less is required, so that the dried blood spot on a Guthrie card may be adequate. Some mutations may be tissue specific (such as some mitochondrial gene mutations) and the appropriate sample will be required if a false-negative result is to be avoided. Transportation of blood using the fastest available postal service (about two days delay) is adequate provided that arrangements have been made with the recipient laboratory to expect the sample. Tissue such as muscle biopsy specimens may require snap freezing in liquid nitrogen, especially if RNA analysis is required, and again this should be discussed with the unit undertaking the analysis.

Services

The availability of a comprehensive molecular genetic laboratory service is essential if one is to make optimum clinical use of the advances outlined in this review. The pace at which mutation analysis is becoming feasible for genetic disorders in general precludes any single diagnostic unit from providing such a service, and many laboratories have implemented consortium arrangements to enable the widest possible range of services to be available. Single gene neurological disorders do, however, account for 54% of all clinical referrals to regional genetic units[40] and it would seem to be appropriate that a core molecular neurogenetic diagnostic service should be available at a regional level.

We feel that the minimum provision should include molecular analyses for the trinucleotide repeat expansions associated with myotonic dystrophy and Huntington's disease, the CMT1A duplication, a deletion screening protocol for Duchenne and Becker muscular dystrophies, a core mitochondrial mutation screen (see box 1.1), and linkage analysis for the autosomal recessive spinal muscular atrophies of childhood. Direct mutation analysis is just becoming available for deletions of the SMN gene in spinal muscular atrophy.[41] The workload generated at a regional level should be containable by two trained laboratory scientific officers working alongside colleagues carrying out other analyses. Additional analyses will generally be available by negotiation with other units. The Laboratory and National Consortium Directory, compiled by the Clinical Molecular Genetics Society, lists by disease and centre the services available throughout the United Kingdom. This publication also indicates the target times by which a result should be available (these vary by disease and centre).

The provision of a clinical service to complement the molecular analyses is essential. As we discussed above, it will often be necessary to undertake extended family counselling when a genetic diagnosis is made. Most districts will have access to the services of a clinical geneticist and a specialist genetic nurse, who will be able to provide such a service. We feel that, in addition, there should be, at a regional level, the provision of a clinical specialist with training in both clinical neurology and clinical and molecular genetics. This individual would be able to offer an optimal clinical service for patients and colleagues and provide informed interpretation of relevant molecular DNA analyses.

Conclusions

Molecular genetic studies have begun to elucidate the pathobiological mechanisms underlying many of the inherited neurological disorders. Improved diagnostic accuracy enables a more accurate prognosis to be given to the patient and facilitates appropriate genetic counselling for the family unit. It is likely that more effective therapy will follow for some of these disorders but the prospect of a "cure", as perceived by the patient, remains a matter of speculation. This should not prevent individuals and their families benefiting from the advances made to date.

Clinical genetics in neurological disease

- Consider genetic aetiology as an explanation of the symptoms or signs in all cases, irrespective of the age of the patient
- Take a detailed family history and be suspicious when an apparently separate neurological disorder is present, or when a relevant parent or relative died at a younger age than one at which the disease in question might have been manifested—for example, a cardiovascular death at age 40 when Huntington's disease is a possible diagnosis
- Request an opinion from a genetics colleague early in your investigations. They can not only advise you on the availability of specific molecular analyses but will also often have extensive local pedigree registers that are relevant to the disorder under consideration, especially for the X linked muscular dystrophies and Huntington's disease
- Beware of requesting specific mutation analysis where an individual from a known affected family presents with only non-specific symptoms—for example, clumsiness in an individual at 50% risk of Huntington's disease. Avoid an unintentional "predictive" result
- Be aware of the family implications of a positive genetic diagnosis. Keep the patient and family informed of any requests for specific molecular analyses. Consider whether the patient or family should be counselled before requesting such an analysis

We wish to thank Dr M Upadhyaya for useful discussions on the molecular genetics of facioscapulohumeral muscular dystrophy, S Cochran for unpublished data on CMTX, Dr L Lazarou for the autoradiograph used in the figure, and Mr P Davies for discussions on the feasibility of the estimated laboratory workload. JC MacMillan holds an MRC clinician scientist fellowship.

1 Emery AEH. Population frequencies of inherited neuromuscular diseases—a world survey. *Neuromusc Disord* 1991;**1**:19–30.
2 MacMillan JC, Harper PS. Single gene neurological disorders in South Wales; an epidemiological study. *Ann Neurol* 1991;**30**:411–4.
3 Botstein D, White RL, Skolnick M, Davis RW. Construction of a genetic linkage map in man using restriction fragment length polymorphisms. *Am J Hum Genet* 1980;**32**:314–31.
4 Haldane JBS. The combination of linkage values and the calculation of distances between loci of linked factors. *J Genet* 1919;**8**:299–309.
5 Martin JB. Molecular genetics in neurology. *Ann Neurol* 1993;**34**:757–73.
6 Daniels RJ, Suthers GK, Morrison KE, *et al.* Prenatal prediction of spinal muscular atrophy. *J Med Genet* 1992;**29**:165–70.

7 Upadhyaya M, Jardine P, Maynard J, et al. Molecular analysis of British facioscapulohumeral dystrophy families for 4q rearrangements. Hum Mol Genet 1993;2:981–7.

8 Rossiter BJF, Caskey CT. Molecular studies of human genetic disease. FASEB J 1991;5: 21–7.

9 Shoffner JM, Wallace DC. Mitochondrial genetics: principles and practice. Am J Hum Genet 1992;51:1179–86.

10 Brown MD, Voljavec AS, Lott MT, MacDonald I, Wallace DC. Leber's hereditary optic neuropathy: a model for mitochondrial neurodegenerative disease. FASEB J 1992;6:2791–9.

11 Koenig M, Beggs AH, Moyer M, et al. The molecular basis for Duchenne versus Becker muscular dystrophy: correlation of severity with type of deletion. Am J Hum Genet 1989; 45:498–506.

12 Bradley DM, Parsons EP, Clarke AJ. Experience with screening newborns for Duchenne muscular dystrophy in Wales. BMJ 1993;306:357–60.

13 Matsumura K, Tome FMS, Collin H, et al. Deficiency of the 50K dystrophin-associated glycoprotein in severe childhood autosomal recessive muscular dystrophy. Nature 1992; 359:320–2.

14 Matsumura K, Nonaka I, Campbell KP. Abnormal expression of dystrophin-associated proteins in Fukuyama-type congenital muscular dystrophy. Lancet 1993;341:521–1.

15 Upadhyaya M, Shen M, Cherryson A, et al. Analysis of mutations at the neurofibromatosis 1 (NF1) locus. Hum Mol Genet 1993;1:735–40.

16 Pieretti M, Zhang F, Fu YH, et al. Absence of expression of the FMR-1 gene in fragile X syndrome. Cell 1991;66:817–22.

17 Scott Hansen R, Gartler SM, Scott CR, Chen S, Laird CD. Methylation analysis of CGG sites in the CpG island of the human FMR1 gene. Hum Mol Genet 1992;1:571–8.

18 Knight SJL, Flannery AV, Hirst MC, et al. Trinucleotide repeat amplification and hypermethylation of a CpG island in FRAXE mental retardation. Cell 1993;74:127–34.

19 Fu YH, Friedman DL, Richards S, et al. Decreased expression of myotonin-protein kinase messenger RNA and protein in adult form of myotonic dystrophy. Science 1993;260:235–8.

20 Hofmann-Radvanyi H, Lavedan C, Rabès J-P, et al. Myotonic dystrophy: absence of CTG enlarged transcript in congenital forms, and low expression of the normal allele. Hum Mol Genet 1993;2:1263–6.

21 Sabouri LA, Mahadevan MS, Narang M, Lee DSC, Surh LC, Korneluk RG. Effect of the myotonic dystrophy (DM) mutation on mRNA levels of the DM gene. Nature Genet 1993; 4:233–8.

22 Harley HG, Rundle SA, MacMillan JC, et al. Size of the unstable CTG repeat sequence in relation to phenotype and parental transmission in myotonic dystrophy. Am J Hum Genet 1993;52:1164–74.

23 Suthers GK, Huson SM, Davies K. Instability versus predictability: the molecular diagnosis of myotonic dystrophy. J Med Genet 1992;29:761–5.

24 MacMillan JC, Snell RG, Tyler A, et al. Molecular analysis and clinical correlations of the Huntington's disease mutation. Lancet 1993;342:954–8.

25 Snell R, MacMillan JC, Cheadle JP, et al. Relationship between trinucleotide repeat expansion and phenotypic variation in Huntington's disease. Nature Genet 1993;4:393–7.

26 MacMillan JC, Upadhyaya M, Harper PS. Charcot-Marie-Tooth disease type 1a (CMT1A): evidence for trisomy of the region p11·2 of chromosome 17 in south Wales families. J Med Genet 1992;29:12–3.

27 Suter U, Welcher AA, Ozcelik T, et al. Trembler mouse carries a point mutation in a myelin gene. Nature 1992;356:241–4.

28 Valentijn LJ, Baas F, Wolterman RA, et al. Identical point mutations of PMP-22 in trembler-J mouse and Charcot-Marie-Tooth disease type 1A. Nature Genet 1992;2: 288–91.

29 Hoogendijk JE, Hensels GW, Gabreels-Festen AAWM, et al. De-novo mutation in hereditary motor and sensory neuropathy type I. Lancet 1992;339:1081–2.

30 Hyasaka K, Takada G, Ionasescu V. Mutation of the myelin Po gene in Charcot-Marie-Tooth neuropathy type 1B. Hum Mol Genet 1993;2:1369–72.

31 Fidani L, Rooke K, Chartier-Harlin M-C, et al. Screening for mutations in the open reading frame and promoter of the β-amyloid precursor protein gene in familial Alzheimer's disease: identification of a further family with APP717 Val-Ile. Hum Mol Genet 1992;1:165–8.

32 Collinge J, Harding AE, Owen F, et al. Diagnosis of Gerstmann-Sträussler syndrome in familial dementia with prion protein gene analysis. Lancet 1989;334:15–7.

33 Collinge J, Poulter M, Davis MB, et al. Presymptomatic detection or exclusion of prion protein gene defects in families with inherited prion diseases. Am J Hum Genet 1991;49: 1351–4.

34 Hoffman EP, Arahata K, Minetti C, *et al.* Dystrophinopathy in isolated cases of myopathy in females. *Neurology* 1992;**42**:967–75.

35 La Spada AR, Wilson M, Lubahn DB, Harding AE, Fischbeck KH. Androgen receptor gene mutations in X-linked spinal and bulbar muscular atrophy. *Nature* 1991;**352**:77–9.

36 Rosen DR, Siddique T, Patterson D, *et al.* Mutations in Cu/Zn superoxide dismutase gene are associated with familial amyotrophic lateral sclerosis. *Nature* 1993;**362**:59–62.

37 Harper PS, Clarke A. Should we test children for "adult" genetic diseases? *Lancet* 1990; **335**:1205–6.

38 Harding AE, Sweeny MG, Miller DH, *et al.* Occurrence of a multiple sclerosis-like illness in women who have a Leber's hereditary optic neuropathy mitochondrial DNA mutation. *Brain* 1992;**115**:979–89.

39 Jersild C, Grunnet N. Demyelinating disease. In King RA, Rotter JI, Motulsky AG, eds. *The genetic basis of common diseases.* Oxford: Oxford University Press, 1992;753–74.

40 Rona RJ, Swan AV, Wilson OM, *et al.* DNA probe technology: implications for service planning in Britain. *Clin Genet* 1992;**42**:186–95.

41 Lefebvre S, Bürglen L, Reboullet S, *et al.* Identification and characterisation of a spinal muscular atrophy-determining gene. *Cell* 1995;**80**:155–65.

2 Headache

J M S PEARCE

Current issues: general management

Morbidity: the burden of headache to patient and society

Morbidity due to headaches is a major problem. Tension headaches outnumber migraine by 5:1. Box 2.1 compares the more common causes of chronic or recurrent headaches in different age groups.

A recent study from Minnesota, United States, confirms the overall incidence of migraine to be about 10% in the population, with a pronounced variation related to age and a higher incidence in women in a defined population.[1] From 6400 patient records, 629 residents fulfilled the International Headache Society's 1988 criteria[2] for migraine between 1979 and 1981. The overall age-adjusted incidence per 100 000 person years was 137 for males and 294 for females. The highest incidence was in women aged 20–24 years (689 per 100 000 person years), whereas in boys aged 10–14 years the incidence was 246 per 100 000 person years.

Based on a study of 1000 people using the International Headache Society's criteria, the overall lifetime prevalence of classic migraine was 5%, with a female to male ratio of 2:1.[3] The overall lifetime prevalence of common migraine was 8%, with a female to male ratio of 7:1. Women were more likely to have common than classic migraine. Neither classic nor common varieties correlated with age, but in both types the most conspicuous precipitating factor was stress and mental tension.

The rate of consultation is a concern for those planning medical resources. Among subjects with classic and common migraine, 50% and 62%, respectively, consult their general practitioner because of migraine at some time in their lives. Patients frequently attend for medical help, and lose much time from work which is often

---

Box 2.1   Common headaches at different ages

3–16 (years)	17–60 (years)	60+ (years)
Migraine	Migraine	Referred from neck
Tension	Tension	Cranial arteritis
Psychogenic or fatigue	Cluster	Paget's disease of the skull
Post-traumatic	Post-traumatic	Glaucoma
Occasional	Cranial and dural tumours	Cranial and dural tumours
Tumours: posterior fossa, intraventricular	Cerebral tumours including abscess and subdural haematoma	Cerebral tumours including abscess and subdural haematoma
	Depression	Rare cluster headache
	Referred from neck	Paget's disease of the skull
	Paget's disease of the skull	Post-herpetic and cranial neuralgias
	Post-herpetic* and cranial neuralgias	Post-traumatic
		Continuing tension headache
		Continuing migraine

* Uncommon presentation at this age

---

unrecorded. In a random sample of 740 subjects aged 25–64 years living in the Copenhagen County, Denmark, 119 had migraine and 578 had tension headache (1:5).[4] Among subjects with migraine 56% had consulted their general practitioner in the previous year for migraine; among subjects with tension headache 16% had had consultations. Specialists had been consulted by 16% of migraine sufferers and by 4% of subjects with tension-type headache. Less than 3% of all patients studied had required hospital admission and laboratory investigations for headache. Half the migraine sufferers and 83% of subjects with tension-type headache in the previous year had taken drug therapy. Thus migraine and tension headaches can be seen as potent sources of demand for medical attention and for the consumption of drugs.

In the Danish study, 43% of employed migraine sufferers and 12% of employed subjects with tension-type headache had lost working time in the preceding year. The total loss of work days due to migraine was estimated at 270 per 1000 persons per year; for tension headache the corresponding figure was 820. Women consulted a doctor more often than men, but there was no sex difference in absenteeism.

Principal objectives and instruments of management

If a patient with headache has cranial arteritis or a brain tumour, then all sociological intervention must take second place to prompt diagnosis and treatment. Over 95% of patients seen in a general practitioner's surgery or hospital clinic, however, have tension headache, migraine, or atypical headache without a structural lesion. For such patients whose symptoms are strongly influenced by social, personal, and family problems, several therapeutic commodities are needed.

For effective therapy doctors need to be accurate in diagnosis, clear in the direction of treatment, honest when they do not know how or why a symptom has developed or changed—yet reassuring. They should be understanding but not dismissive; and they should be prepared to see patients repeatedly until the headaches are controlled, and especially to continue to comfort and support when they are not cured. Such paragons are not ubiquitous. Painstaking efforts to communicate with patients from the start save many subsequent consultations.

Political and financial constraints have failed to provide for the necessary number of doctor hours to cater for this ideal. In reality, this has been matched by the never-ending expectations of patients for the latest technical facilities, for a specialist's personal attentions (no longer is a neurologist adequate; it has to be a "headache expert"), and for clinical infallibility—or else litigation may result.

Such issues of time and expertise have, by default, produced the notion that nurses, social workers, osteopaths, homeopaths, and psychologists, among others, might provide for these patients. Regrettably, they cannot. Although, under medical direction, they can help, they are no substitute for a doctor's training and knowledge. Physicians are unwise to abrogate their traditional role by delegating patients' management to let themselves off the hook. Such fashionable trends denigrate the physicians' role, but much more importantly, diminish their therapeutic effectiveness.

25

The armamentarium is, however, limited. The frustration of implacable patients is reflected in their search for "alternative therapies". Medical science assesses its tools by rigorous analysis and scientific trials. Medicine should not be daunted by practitioners of alternative medicine since, with rare exceptions, they have so far failed to subject their unbounded claims of therapeutic triumphs to scientific scrutiny. When they do so, and when their methods produce validated benefit, physicians should welcome and use them.

General practitioners provide primary diagnostic facilities which essentially serve to separate those with major pathology (tumours, glaucoma, arteritis) from functional headaches. Many of the latter group are dealt with adequately by history taking, examination, reassurance, and selected analgesics and antimigraine drugs. Patients posing diagnostic problems and those with refractory headaches should be referred to a neurologist.

"Headache clinics" are convenient, and well suited to trials and research; but, to be of benefit to patients they should, ideally, be available on a daily basis, staffed by one or more experienced physicians to provide continuity of service: these ideals are not generally practicable.

Audit

This concept, woolly in definition and often inadequate in application, is not easy to impose on the management of patients with headaches. Patients and their general practitioners can be questioned about their satisfaction with the service; improvement in headache scores would need several applications per patient over a long period of time to demonstrate efficacy above the substantial placebo effect of seeing a new doctor, receiving the investigations that patients perceive as reassuring, and being offered new treatments. Without implementation of results of audit ("closing the loop") and further appraisal, the exercise is meaningless. To instigate standards of good practice, yardsticks need to be established and agreed.

In a district or regional service, the assessment of wrong diagnoses—for example, missed tumours, subarachnoid haemorrhage, or missed cranial arteritis, is feasible. Similarly, errors of diagnosis, choice of first-line treatment, and patterns of secondary referral can be appraised in casualty departments and in general practitioner referrals.

Box 2.2   Indications for specialist referral and investigations

- Sudden onset, new headache
- Atypical symptoms or signs suggesting organic pathology
- Abnormal signs—for example, papilloedema to suggest raised intracranial pressure; a red, tender scalp vessel to indicate cranial arteritis
- An unremitting course, unresponsive to conventional treatment
- The advent of progressive physical signs

The headache patient

This account is restricted to headache and excludes the related but separate facial pains and neuralgias. The clinical approach rests heavily on a detailed analysis of symptoms and a thorough general and neurological examination. Selective investigations are applicable to only a small number of patients who require neurological referral (box 2.2). Headaches may be acute (usually signifying meningeal irritation or, rarely, raised intracranial pressure (ICP)), recurrent as in migraine, or chronic as in tension headaches.

Headache as a symptom of intracranial disease

Few headaches fail to evoke some anxiety, which can distort, disguise, or magnify the primary clinical features. Confronted by a patient with headaches, the first clinical responsibility is to exclude a structural or dynamic cause. Any expanding mass—tumour, abscess, or haematoma—can cause raised pressure.

Headaches of abrupt onset may signify trauma, spontaneous intracranial haemorrhage, hydrocephalus, or acute meningeal irritation at any age; the elderly are not immune. The most common cause is acute meningeal irritation due to subarachnoid haemorrhage or to meningitis—bacterial or viral, (rarely HIV, fungal, or malignant). An abrupt onset, fever, neck stiffness, and Kernig's sign accompany the obvious severe pain, vomiting, and photophobia. Hospital referral for CSF examination is mandatory if haemorrhage or infection is considered. Computed tomography (or magnetic resonance imaging) should be the first investigation to exclude a mass lesion, haematoma, or hydrocephalus, each of which contraindicates lumbar puncture. Subarachnoid haemorrhage may be shown, but can be missed by computed tomography in up to 20% of patients on admission.

When a mass lesion is excluded, lumbar puncture may be necessary to examine the CSF for subarachnoid bleeding and meningitis. Acute migraine and tension headache uncommonly produce a meningitic picture, diagnosable only by exclusion. Acute headache should be distinguished from the common and totally benign "exploding head syndrome" in which patients are alarmed by a sudden, momentary, very loud noise in the twilight stage of sleep.[5]

Raised-pressure headache

This is an aching, throbbing headache aggravated by alcohol, exertion, and by coughing or straining. These features suggest a vascular or hydrodynamic mechanism that may be caused by a tumour or hydrocephalus. Similar symptoms, however, are also common in migraine and other vascular pains. The location is non-specific, although when a progressive headache radiates to the neck, tonsillar coning is imminent. The headache is: (*a*) worse in the morning and may waken the patient from sleep; (*b*) aggravated by sitting up or standing and relieved by lying down; (*c*) aggravated by coughing, straining, and vomiting; (*d*) relieved by aspirin or paracetamol in the early stages (in contrast to psychogenic headache); (*e*) associated with vomiting and eventually by papilloedema and progressing focal signs. By the stage of stupor and hemiplegia with a dilated (Hutchinson's) pupil, diagnosis has been delayed too long.

Chronic and recurrent headaches

Referred pain

The orbits, paranasal sinuses, cervical spine, mediastinum, and teeth can cause pain referred via branches of the trigeminal nerve to the forehead and temple. Sinusitis and toothache are commonplace examples, but otitis media, glaucoma, orbital cellulitis, and cavernous sinus thrombosis may produce referred frontotemporal pain. Secondary involuntary contraction of scalp and facial muscles further complicate the picture, causing a secondary generalised "tension headache" which may obscure the primary source. Primary care physicians can treat acute infection by antibiotics but, when cranial spread is suspected, patients should be referred to the neurological/neurosurgical centre immediately.

Tension headache

Tension headache is the most common of human complaints, constituting 70% of referrals to a "headache clinic". It is often a short-lived complaint with an obvious preceding cause: overwork, lack of sleep, or an emotional crisis. This is benign and often designated by patients as "my normal headaches".

Current systems classify the most common recurring headaches as either migraine or tension type. This traditional approach can be questioned. Some suggest that these two headache patterns are different expressions of the same pathophysiological process, having overlapping symptomatic presentations with certain features emphasised to a greater or lesser extent. Additionally, the same therapies have been shown to be effective for patients in either headache group.[6] An alternative continuum classification model has been suggested, as there is an undoubted overlap between common migraine and tension headache, although their common co-existence has added to the confusion.

By contrast, Solomon and Lipton propose that the diagnosis of migraine without aura (common migraine) is warranted if any two of the following symptoms are present: unilateral site, throbbing quality, nausea, photophobia, or phonophobia.[7] These criteria are derived from a study comparing the features of 100 patients with migraine without aura and 100 patients with chronic daily ("tension") headache. The authors' proposed criteria for the diagnosis of migraine without aura were highly sensitive and adequately specific in discriminating the two groups. There are also differences in laboratory data. Binding of ^{3}H-labelled imipramine to platelets was measured and significantly less was found in patients with migraine compared with controls, but no less in tension headache. In migraine, there was no significant relation between imipramine binding and depression or anxiety score, suggesting that the reduction in platelet imipramine binding is a concomitant of migraine itself.[8] A significant reduction in peripheral blood mononuclear cell β endorphin concentrations was observed in migraine patients with and without aura, but not in patients with tension-type headache.[9] Adult and childhood migraineurs without aura have an increased amplitude of the contingent negative variation between attacks.[10] Likewise vascular phenomena, well described in migraine, contrast with the transcranial Doppler ultrasound of blood flow velocities in chronic tension headache, which show no significant differences from controls.

The case for classic migraine as a separate entity is even more persuasive. The teenager with infrequent but prostrating attacks of photopsia, dysphasia, vomiting, and hemicrania, is at least clinically distinct from the angst-ridden 40 year old patient with a continuous, daily, vertex, pressure headache for 20 years which does not prevent remunerative work.

Acute tension headache

This type of headache rarely presents as an emergency. When it does, the headache has increased over a few hours, but has become very severe, simulating subarachnoid bleeding. Lumbar puncture may be necessary to exclude meningeal irritation by blood or infection. More often the emotional basis is obvious and recovery ensues quickly after reassurance, analgesia, and sedation. Liaison with the general practitioner should lead to continued support and prompt return to work.

Chronic tension headache (chronic daily headache)

More common than the acute syndrome, pain is diffusely felt all over the head, often located on the vertex, or may start in the forehead or in the neck. Primary tension headache is psychogenic; its mechanisms are not wholly understood.[11] It is commonly bilateral, but may be unilateral. Patients characteristically complain of pressure, a feeling of tightness, or a heavy weight pressing on the crown. "A tight band like a skullcap" or "as if a clamp or vice was squeezing my head" are common descriptions. Many say "it is not really a pain, but a pressure". The symptoms may also seem to derive from inside the cranium: "as if my head is bursting" or "about to explode". A "creeping" sensation (formication) may be felt under the scalp, or a sense of sharp knives or burning hot needles driven in, may be related.

Tension headache occurs daily, worse in the evenings. Visual disturbance, photophobia, and vomiting seldom occur. Most patients continue their normal work. Symptoms continue for years without evident deterioration of general health. Symptoms are worse when the patient is tired or under pressure of work or domestic stresses.[12] Most sufferers have insight, so that a carefully taken history clarifies both the diagnosis and the aggravating circumstances; many sufferers are emotional and anxious, with fears of brain tumours, hypertension, or "clots in the brain". I enquire specifically about fears of serious brain disease, whether the fears are voiced by the patient or not. Illnesses seen on television programmes, like maladies of relatives and acquaintances, are often "contagious"; these too need careful appraisal. Thorough clinical examination is of the utmost therapeutic value and provides a rational basis for effective reassurance that is denied to the psychologist or counsellor.

Treatment is most effective when the history is short. To cure such headaches after many years is a daunting and often unsuccessful task.[13] An important step is to enquire about the events that determined the onset. These are often forgotten, or perhaps suppressed, yet repeated enquiry at subsequent consultations will often unravel the apparent mystery, the consequent knowledge being sufficient to explain the cause to the patient. Sensitive patients with fragile personalities may be unable to cope with life's stresses and unconsciously use headaches to escape responsibilities with which they can't cope. Sedatives, tranquilizers, and tension-relieving drugs are of limited value unless the psychological issues are adequately handled. Glib reassurance will not eradicate headache if fundamental psychological problems are unresolved. When the history is short and if a cause is exposed, explanation and reassurance may suffice.

Patients often misuse analgesics, which aggravates the situation, but with persuasion the misuse can be reversed with dramatic benefit (see below). More often, when daily pain has persisted for years, the prognosis is poor, but short courses of benzodiazepines or amitriptyline may be helpful. Supportive psychotherapy in liaison with a practice nurse or psychotherapist may help: much depends on the quality, experience, and good sense of the staff available.

Latent depression presenting as tension headache is easily overlooked. Early morning insomnia, negativism, anhedonia, guilt, and diurnal mood swings are suggestive. The headache is worse in the morning (resembling that of raised pressure), and a cause for the misery is not always apparent. Full doses of tricyclic antidepressants or fluoxetine are needed.[46] The prognosis for depression is often good.

Migraine

Classic migraine

Classic migraine is synonymous with migraine with aura and occurs in 20% of migraineurs. It is a paroxysmal disorder with headaches, often unilateral at the onset, associated with nausea, anorexia, and often vomiting; it is preceded or accompanied by visual, sensory, motor, and mood disturbances; and it is often familial.

Common migraine

This is synonymous with migraine without aura and occurs in 75% of patients. The term refers to similar paroxysmal headaches without the aura. Both types of attack may occur at various times in the same patient. It is common for migraineurs to have tension headaches between their migraines: these should be identified to prevent misdirected treatment. Daily headaches are never migrainous.

Migraine variants

These are hemiplegic, basilar, and ophthalmoplegic, *migraine sine cephalgia*, etc, and occur in less than 5% of patients, usually requiring a neurologist's appraisal and sometimes brain imaging.

Natural course and management

In childhood, attacks begin before the age of 10 years in a third of patients. They may be overlooked if the child is unable to describe headaches and strange visual or sensory experiences clearly. They are also concealed by labels of "bilious attacks" or "periodic syndrome". Diagnosis can be difficult as affected children may simply appear pale, ill, limp, and inert, complaining of poorly localised abdominal pain. Headache is usually present, vomiting is common, and there may be a fever of up to 38·5°C so that the suspicion of appendicitis or mesenteric adenitis often arises. It should be remembered that over 80% of migraineurs have their first attacks before the age of 30 years, and the diagnosis should therefore be viewed with suspicion if onset is after the age of 40, although an increased frequency of attacks at the menopause is common. Some subjects have only a few attacks in a lifetime but most have several attacks each year. Promises of remission at the menopause are often ill-founded, though attacks tend to lessen after the age of 50 years. Remission occurs in 70% of pregnancies. It is well recognised that exacerbation, or complicated migraine with infarction, may result from oestrogen-containing contraceptives.[14]

Many attacks in adults end gradually after 24 to 48 hours but attacks in children often last only two to six hours. In later life headaches may disappear completely, attacks presenting with teichopsiae and no headache (*migraine sine cephalgia*). The mechanism is uncertain. Indeed, the apparent onset of migraine in the elderly implies atherosclerotic, thromboembolic disease. Food idiosyncrasies, food allergies, red wines, specific dietary amines, and omission of food are occasional precipitants. Emotional stress and fatigue is the principal aggravating factor but is not causal.

Migraine is caused by a primarily cerebral (neural) mechanism with a fluctuating threshold, which determines the timing and pattern of attacks.[15] A neural trigger activates the trigeminovascular reflex, releasing vasogenic amines from blood vessel walls accompanied by their painful, pulsatile distension. The cerebral mechanism responds to mood, emotions, tiredness, relaxation, hormonal changes, bright lights, and noise. Its threshold is susceptible to hypothalamic function which, in turn, is modulated by seasonal patterns, diurnal and biological clocks, and by hormonal factors and coitus.[16] Personality and variations of mood and behaviour also influence the pattern of attacks, remissions, and treatment.

Symptomatic treatment

Assessment of the patient's habits, work, personality, and stresses is important. Suitably trained clinic nurses can assist in the time-consuming elucidation of these factors in selected cases. Known precipitants should be sought, with the aid of a diary and should, when possible, be eliminated (box 2.3). The patient's recognition of stressful patterns and the acceptance of a benign disorder will achieve some benefit. Good rapport enhances reassurance and facilitates the notable placebo effect of all therapy which often confounds the analysis of drug trials.

The aims of treatment are the control of symptoms and the prevention or reduction of attacks. Many prophylactic drugs act

---

Box 2.3   Common precipitants of migraine

- Fatigue, overwork, travel
- Relaxation after stress—holiday and Saturday morning headache
- Bright lights, discos
- Sleep excess or shortage—Sunday morning headache
- Missing meals
- Rare dietary sensitivity
- Alcohol, red wines
- Menstruation
- Exercise—vascular headaches such as footballer's migraine, coital cephalgia

---

by central serotonin ($5HT_2$) antagonism,[17] whereas control of an attack relies on constriction of cranial vessels mediated by α adrenergic or $5HT_1$ receptors.[18]

Analgesics

Rest, dark, and quiet, where practicable, are supplemented by simple analgesics (paracetamol 1 g or soluble aspirin 0·6 g) or nonsteroidal anti-inflammatory drugs such as naproxen 500 mg. The addition of caffeine and spasmolytics add to expense but not to benefit. Codeine 15–30 mg may enhance pain relief. Analgesics should be taken immediately the attack begins, then repeated every four to six hours as needed. Absorption is improved by ingestion with metoclopramide 10 mg or domperidone 10–20 mg. If vomiting is severe, suppositories of domperidone, prochlorperazine, or chlorpromazine are valuable. Analgesic misuse can cause headaches.

Ergotamine

Ergotamine (or dihydroergotamine[19]) is an effective remedy for acute attacks in about 50% of cases and should be tried before more expensive agents. Ergotamine has no place as a prophylactic, however, and, when overused, can lead to habituation with ergotamine-dependent headache, similar to chronic analgesic-dependent headaches which mimic migraine. When suspected, the drugs should be withdrawn, often in hospital under short term sedation.

Ergotamine is an α adrenergic agonist with potent $5HT_1$ receptor affinity, a potent vasoconstrictor. Absorption is erratic, oral doses often producing sub-therapeutic blood levels. Suppositories (1–2 mg), inhalation (0·36 mg), or sublingual (1–2 mg) are the most effective acceptable routes, but injections are not generally tolerated. If two doses at intervals of two to six hours are ineffective, no more should be given for that attack. If a patient is taking ergotamine more than twice each week, there is a major risk of habituation. Many patients experience vague malaise, nausea, and cramps with ergotamine, but coronary, cerebral, and limb (St Anthony's fire) ischaemia are rare but well proved hazards. Vascular claudication, angina, and pregnancy are contraindications.

Sumatriptan

Sumatriptan is a specific and selective agonist of $5HT_1$ receptors on cranial blood vessels that causes vasoconstriction.[20] It has negligible effects on other receptors. Sumatriptan does not penetrate the blood–brain barrier and has no CNS effects. Intravenous sumatriptan does not change regional cerebral blood flow; it constricts the carotid vascular bed, but has no effect on pial vessels in cats. It has a plasma half life of two hours.

The subcutaneous preparation (6 mg) gives relief of headache in 77% patients at 60 minutes, and in 83% at two hours, with corresponding reduction in nausea, vomiting, and photophobia.[21] It is also effective in cluster headache, with relief of symptoms at 15 minutes in 74% compared with 26% of those given placebo.[22]

Oral medication (100 mg) provides relief in about 70% of attacks within two hours.[23] Second and third attacks respond as well as the first. Comparative trials have shown slight but appreciable superiority to aspirin 900 mg plus metoclopramide 10 mg. Recurrence of headache occurs within 48 hours in 42% of patients.[24] In comparisons of sumatriptan and Cafergot, oral sumatriptan 100 mg relieved headache after two hours in 66% compared with 48% of those given oral Cafergot.[25] The poor oral absorption of ergotamine, however, was a serious limitation of this study.

Another study showed a good response to oral sumatriptan in 51% of patients at two hours compared with 9% given placebo; rescue medication was needed in 41% of the sumatriptan group, but in 88% of the placebo group.[26] A total of 39%, however, had recurrent headache within 24 hours—a significant "rebound effect" which may relate to the natural course of migraine, or to a pharmacological effect.

In over 100 000 treated attacks, toxicity has not been a problem.[27] There are now proved cardiovascular ischaemic sequelae of angina, infarction[28] and ventricular arrhythmias, but these are rare if established ischaemic heart disease, Prinzmetal's angina, and arrhythmias are respected as contraindications. Vague non-ischaemic chest discomfort occurs in some patients. Nausea, vomiting, and tingling, deemed mild and transient, occur in 38% of patients within four hours. Rebound in a third of patients responds well to further doses, but compounds the pressing issue of cost. Sumatriptan is an effective, safe, and prompt remedy, suppressing all the symptoms, not headache alone.[29] It works in 70% of sufferers, however—not in every patient. The present high cost limits its use.

Good communication with family doctors, and advice by clinic or practice nurses on the use of self-injectors and inhalers and the frequency of tablets are important. Audit of the results of treatment by completing headache charts can be invaluable, but patients should not overuse diary cards which can engender excessive introspection and neurosis.

Prophylaxis

Prophylaxis should be considered if attacks occur more often than twice each month. Non-pharmacological techniques are successful in certain subjects, but claims for their general application should be viewed with scepticism. Current data support no significant difference in the efficacy of hypnosis, biofeedback, and relaxation training. Prophylactics aim to reduce the frequency, but none is a panacea. They should be given for three to six months, then reassessed. In patients with exacerbations related to stress, amitriptyline 100–150 mg at night, introduced gradually, is often effective. Which of its actions—sedative, antidepressant, anti-serotoninergic, or calcium channel blockade—is implicated, is not known. β blockers without intrinsic sympathomimetic activity—propranol,[30] atenolol, and metoprolol—reduce the frequency in about 60% of cases and are most effective in the tense or hypertensive subject with tachycardia and overt physical signs of autonomic "overdrive". Their action is probably central.

Serotonin inhibitors are valuable in 60–70% of patients. Cyproheptadine 4 mg three times a day inhibits calcium channels and serotonin and histaminergic activity. Pizotifen 0·5 mg three times a day or 1·5 mg at night is moderately effective and free of hazards other than sedation and weight gain.[31] Methysergide 1–2 mg three times a day is the most effective drug in this group but should be used under hospital supervision in courses not exceeding three to four months. Pleural, pericardial, and retroperitoneal fibrosis are rare but serious side effects that result from prolonged use; they usually regress when the drug is stopped. Myocardial and peripheral vascular ischaemia are uncommon complications. Although calcium antagonists can cause a vasodilator-type headache, some—for example, flunarizine and verapamil—have been established as useful prophylactic drugs.[32]

Menstrual migraine

Menstrual migraine, defined as occurring exclusively within 48 hours of menstruation, is uncommon but may be relieved by sumatriptan or by oestrogen patches or implants. Migraine between periods, but worse with menstruation, is common (35%) but resistant to diuretics and hormonal manipulation.

Cluster headache

Synonyms are migrainous neuralgia, Harris's syndrome, and Horton's syndrome.

Often misdiagnosed, this is a distinct syndrome separable from migraine; it predominantly affects men (male:female ratio 10:1). It begins at any age, most often 20 to 50 years, and is manifested as daily bouts of unilateral headache of great severity lasting 30–120 minutes. The brevity, severity, lack of aura, and vomiting occurring daily in clusters, lasting usually for 4–16 weeks, clearly separate it from migraine. The pain is boring, aching, or stabbing and is centred on one orbit with radiation to the forehead, temple, or cheek and jaw ("lower-half headache"). It characteristically strikes at night, an hour or so after sleep, and may recur during the day, often at the same time ("alarm-clock headache"). In many cases the ipsilateral eye becomes red and bloodshot, watering profusely. The nostril may be blocked or run. A transient Horner's syndrome is seen in 25% of cases and occasionally persists.

Box 2.4   Diagnostic criteria for cluster headaches

Episodic
(a) At least five attacks fulfilling (b)–(d)
(b) Severe unilateral orbital or supraorbital pain, with or without temporal pain, lasting 15–180 minutes untreated
(c) Headache is associated with at least one of the following signs which have to be present on the painful side
   - Conjunctival infection
   - Lacrimation
   - Nasal congestion
   - Rhinorrhoea
   - Forehead and facial sweating
   - Miosis
   - Ptosis
   - Eyelid oedema
(d) Frequency of attacks: from one every other day to eight a day
(e) History or physical and neurological examinations, or both, do not suggest other disorders associated with head trauma

Chronic
Attacks occur for more than one year without remission, or with remission lasting less than 14 days. The attacks are clinically indistinguishable from episodic cluster headache

---

Restlessness, crying, and head banging betray the frightening severity of the pain and, in contrast to migraine, most patients get out of bed and pace the floor, even taking nocturnal walks. Alcohol and other vasodilators precipitate attacks: nitroglycerine is useful as a provocative test—a typical attack following within an hour of a sublingual 0·5 mg tablet. "Acute episodic cluster" lasts for one to four months, although occasionally they continue for a year or more, when it is known as "chronic migrainous neuralgia". Remissions are complete but the clusters recur every year or two. The quality, timing, duration, and distribution of pain separate it from trigeminal neuralgia, migraine, and other cephalgias. There is no family history, and it is uncommon for a patient to have both migraine and cluster headache. There is an unexplained high incidence of peptic ulcer.[33]

The International Headache Society's diagnostic criteria are summarised in box 2.4.

Treatment

The aim is prevention of attacks.[34] During clusters, alcohol is prohibited. Ergotamine is given one hour *in anticipation* of daytime attacks, and at bedtime for nocturnal attacks. Suppositories are the most useful preparation. Control is good in 75% of patients and the drug is stopped each Sunday to see if the cluster re-emerges; if so, ergotamine is continued for a further week, until the cluster ends. If ergot is unsuccessful, sumatriptan 6 mg subcutaneously or 100 mg orally,[22] methysergide 1–2 mg three times a day or verapamil 40–80 mg three times a day are useful alternatives. Oxygen 5–10 litres a minute for 10 minutes at the onset is often effective[29] but β blockers and pizotifen are not. Lithium is useful in the chronic variant if other methods fail. In intractable cases, a short course of steroids often provides relief. Surgery is seldom indicated, but trigeminal lesions meet with occasional success in refractory patients.

Chronic paroxysmal hemicrania

This is a rare variant[35] of cluster headache, occurring predominantly in females, with identical attacks, often five to 20 a day, which last from three to 15 minutes; they respond almost invariably to indomethacin, 75–150 mg daily.

Cervicogenic headache

Head pain referred from cervical spondylosis is undoubtedly common, with pain on one or both sides of the neck radiating not only to the occiput but also to the temples and frontal region. It may be a dull "toothache" pain, worse in the morning when the neck has been kinked on high pillows during sleep; it can initiate migraine. It can last throughout the day, aggravated by neck movement and tension and is a nondescript pain, without accompanying vomiting or physical signs other than restriction of lateral flexion and rotation of the neck. Such signs are common, however, in those without headache. Vague and intermittent symptoms of tinnitus, dizziness, and visual disturbance are sometimes attributed to compression of the vertebral arteries, but this is unproved. Pain arises from the posterior zygapophyseal joints and related ligaments as the result of osteophytes with irritation of the C_2 root or greater occipital nerves.[36] Manipulation

---

Box 2.5   Diagnostic criteria for cranial arteritis[38]

- Age $\geqslant 50$ years at onset
- New onset of localised headache
- Temporal artery tenderness or decreased temporal artery pulse
- Erythrocyte sedimentation rate ($\geqslant 50$ mm in the first hour)
- Biopsy specimen showing necrotising arteritis

The presence of three or more of these five criteria provides a sensitivity of 93·5% and a specificity of 91·2%. Scalp tenderness and claudication of the jaw or tongue or on deglutition increases sensitivity to 95·3%.

---

endangers the vertebral arteries and is contraindicated. Collars are comforting but of little value. Injections of the facet joint region anatomically related to the pain will induce useful temporary remission in about 70% of subjects.[37] Hydrocortisone 25 mg or methylprednisolone are used, with 1 ml of 2% lignocaine on three occasions at weekly intervals. The benefit may wane in a few months, when the injections can be repeated.

Giant cell arteritis

Synonyms of giant cell arteritis are cranial or temporal arteritis.

This condition is crucially important as a treatable cause of headache, it is also a preventable cause of blindness and strokes. The diagnostic features are shown in box 2.5.

Pain is generalised or may be sited over the classic, but rare, reddened, tender, superficial temporal or occipital artery. The history is of a few weeks' duration. The patient is unwell with aches and pains in the shoulder and pelvic girdle muscles (polymyalgia rheumatica) and there may be fever, sweats, and masseter claudication. Visual involvement (in 50% of patients) is due to ischaemic optic neuropathy that presents with unilateral blindness, or due to a branch retinal or ciliary occlusion, and is irreversible. Posterior cerebral artery lesions cause hemianopia.

Ophthalmoplegia and diplopia may be the presenting sign, based on ischaemic lesions in the third, fourth, or sixth cranial nerves, before the onset of headache and malaise: hence the importance of early diagnosis. It affects the vertebral, and less often the carotid, arteries and may present as a stroke or transient ischaemic attack.

Every elderly subject with recent headaches or unilateral visual loss should be suspected of having this condition. Serial erythrocyte sedimentation rates (usually 70–120 mm in the first hour), sometimes supplemented by an adequate biopsy specimen of the clinically affected scalp vessel, which should be serially sectioned, will prove the diagnosis. Cranial arteritis may spontaneously remit and the erythrocyte sedimentation rate then falls; thus a single, normal erythrocyte sedimentation rate does not exclude arteritis. Biopsy is indicated in clinically borderline cases.

Atypical presentations that should prompt assiduous investigation include: (a) patients with minimal headache; (b) headache in an appropriately aged patient with, initially, a normal erythrocyte sedimentation rate; (c) fever of unknown origin; (d) psychiatric symptoms of hallucinations, depression, and "confusional state"; (e) isolated third or sixth nerve palsy; rarely internuclear ophthalmoplegia.

Steroids will avert blindness in almost every case, and should be started immediately the patient is seen and the blood sample for an erythrocyte sedimentation rate taken. They do not affect the biopsy changes for at least 48 hours. Headaches often abate within 24 hours of treatment.

The initial dose of 60 mg prednisolone a day is quickly reduced as symptoms abate and the erythrocyte sedimentation rate falls. The maintenance dose of 5–10 mg a day is usually reached within a month or two and is governed by clinical progress and erythrocyte sedimentation rate measurements. Late relapses are common[39] and treatment may be required for many years, with gradual reductions by 1 mg a month only when the patient and the erythrocyte sedimentation rate have been normal for over two years. In many, small doses are necessary for life, as proved by serious relapses months after the dose of prednisolone is reduced.[39]

Hypnic headache (Solomon's syndrome)

This is a curious headache, seen mainly in those over 60 years. Patients are woken by pulsating headache, sometimes accompanied by nausea, at the same time, one to three times each night.[40] This occurs most nights, lasts about 30 minutes and may coincide with rapid eye movement sleep. It is uncommon and differs from chronic cluster headache in age, generalised location, and absence of

41

autonomic features. There are no physical signs and the disorder is benign. The response to lithium carbonate 300 mg at night is often spectacular.

Post-traumatic headache and its management

Headache after head injury is a common complaint. In most circumstances a knock on the head will cause local bruising and abrasions no different from those resulting from a kick on the shin; local pain subsides in three to 10 days without sequelae. The emotional vulnerability of the head and the easy recourse to medicolegal compensation complicate both symptoms and mechanisms. Many victims of severe head injury, with post-traumatic amnesia of 24 hours or more, waken with no headache. Similarly, the headache of patients after major craniotomy seldom lasts more than three to seven days. The commonest complaints are heard from those with minor injury (loss of consciousness less than 20 minutes; Glasgow coma score 13–15; stay in hospital less than 48 hours). Despite minor cognitive deficits, most patients leave hospital within a few days, have no organic signs, recover quickly, and return to work without further complaints. This is particularly true of those suffering injury during contact sports. Attributable, post-traumatic headaches persist for a few weeks, and seldom more than six months, unless complicated by other issues.

The main concern of physicians is the assessment of symptoms in those with headaches without accompanying neurological signs, but often with a collection of intrinsically subjective symptoms often called the "post-traumatic syndrome".[41] The complaints are: forgetfulness, irritability, slowness, poor concentration, fatigue, dizziness (usually not vertigo), somnolence, intolerance of alcohol, light, and noise, loss of initiative, depression, anxiety, loss of interests, and impaired libido. The number of complaints is often inversely related to the severity of the injury.

In 2493 individuals examined as part of a nationwide general population survey, post-traumatic stress disorder was found in 1% of the total population, about 3·5% in civilians exposed to physical attack and in Vietnam veterans who were not wounded, and 20% in veterans wounded in Vietnam.[42] Although hyperalertness and sleep disturbances occurred commonly in the general population, the full syndrome (DSM-III-R) was common only among veterans wounded in Vietnam. This argues against the validity of the widespread use of this label in those subjected to minor injuries.

Trauma probably never causes migraine, but pre-existing migraine may be temporarily worse, usually for up to three to six months, probably as a non-specific reaction to stress or to disabilities.[43]

The failure of doctors to provide complete reassurance soon after injury is important in determining patients' fears of brain damage or subdural haematoma; it also delays return to work and induces iatrogenic morbid anxiety. Headaches are at the site of trauma, often with scalp tenderness, or more often—like tension headaches—are diffuse, aching, tight, or heavy. They resist analgesics, and investigations in most patients are both unrevealing and unwarranted. Headaches sometimes improve when the patient is counselled and returns to work, but do not invariably disappear even when satisfactory settlement is attained. Anxieties, phobias, loss of self esteem, resentment, and depression are genuine accompanying features in some cases, and serve to induce or to aggravate headache. Deliberate exaggeration, or malingering in occasional cases, are motivated by quest for attention and financial gain. In litigants there is great pressure from trades union officials and lawyers which, together with the common delay in settlement, serve to prolong and exaggerate the symptoms.

Post-herpetic neuralgia

This dreaded complication of trigeminal herpes zoster, particularly common in the elderly (occurring in 50% of over 70s) and rare under the age of 60, is defined by pain persisting for more than one month after the eruption. Two-thirds spontaneously recover in one year, leaving a minority with prolonged and intractable pain. Healed post-herpetic hyperpigmented or depigmented areas, or both, in a segmental distribution are necessary for a correct diagnosis. An underlying neoplasm of the affected roots and systemic immunosuppression should be excluded by judicious investigation.

The mechanism of pain is uncertain. The preferential loss of large diameter neurons, according to the "gate theory" of Melzack and Wall, permits increased transmission of nociceptive information through the dorsal horn, thus evoking pain. There can be no general recommendation for acyclovir or steroids in the acute stages, but in the frail and elderly who are highly vulnerable it may be justifiable to employ both drugs[44] at the onset of herpes zoster infection in an attempt to avert this potentially grave affliction, in which suicide is well known. In the established case, symptomatic improvement is disappointing. It is worth trying tricyclics building slowly up to high doses (such as imipramine or amitryptiline 125 to 200 mg a day). Additional regular non-opiate analgesics by day and, in severe cases, oral morphine or heroin at night will often be justifiable. Local counterirritants, now called "neuroaugmentation", in the form of freezing sprays or topical capsaicin 0·025% cream, can be helpful. Transcutaneous electrical nerve stimulators find occasional success.

Box 2.6 Simplified plan of management for headache

Patient presents with headaches of abrupt onset

- Exclude trauma. If signs of meningeal irritation, suspect intracranial haemorrhage or meningitis and admit to hospital. Perform computed tomography or magnetic resonance imaging and, if no tumour, haematoma, or hydrocephalus found, perform lumbar puncture
  NB: lumbar puncture within six hours of the ictus may miss an early bleed
- If no signs of meningeal irritation, consider a mass lesion, arrange computed tomography or magnetic resonance imaging and refer to neurosurgery if necessary

Patient presents with increasing headache, short history

- Exclude local cranial pathology, such as glaucoma, sinusitis, dental disease; look for signs of raised intracranial pressure, suspect mass, or hydrocephalus. Arrange computed tomography or magnetic resonance imaging. Do not lumbar puncture

Patient presents with chronic or intermittent headache with no neurological signs

- Exclude local cranial pathology: glaucoma, sinusitis, dental disease. If continuous, suspect tension headache; if paroxysmal, suspect migraine with or without aura. Look for features of cluster headache, other headache syndromes, and cranial neuralgias

Conclusion

Most headaches presenting to the general practitioner and hospital physician have no ominous intracranial cause, but are a source of suffering and loss of working time. Many headaches are infrequent and self limiting. A painstaking clinical approach by a good listener will resolve many problems and will prevent the refractory course in some of those in whom a cursory initial examination fails to secure reassurance. Patients presenting problems in diagnosis, and those unresponsive to appropriate treatment will benefit by referral to a neurologist.

Box 2.6 shows a simplified plan of management.

Management of headache

- Of all people presenting with headache to GPs or hospital clinic, 95% have no structural lesion
- A few need selective investigations to exclude a structural or dynamic cause
- Patients posing diagnostic problems or with refractory headaches should be referred to neurologists
- Abrupt onset headache may signify trauma, spontaneous intracranial haemorrhage, hydrocephalus, or acute meningeal irritation at any age—most commonly the last (caused by subarachnoid haemorrhage or meningitis); the first investigation should be computed tomogram or magnetic resonance imaging to exclude a mass lesion, haematoma, or hydrocephalus (which contraindicate lumbar puncture); a tomogram can miss 20% of subarachnoid haemorrhages, however, so if no mass lesion is found lumber puncture may be needed to examine the CSF for subarachnoid bleeding and meningitis
- Aching throbbing headache (aggravated by alcohol, exertion, coughing, or straining) may signify a tumour or hydrocephalus, though migraine may have similar symptoms
- Pain referred from orbits, paranasal sinuses, cervical spine, mediastinum, or teeth via the trigeminal nerve may cause secondary involuntary contractions of scalp and facial muscles that lead to apparent tension headache, which can mask the true cause of headaches
- Tension headache (daily and continuous, caused by muscle contraction) is the most common type of headache; sedatives, tranquilisers, and tension-relieving drugs are of limited value

Management of headache—*continued*

- In over 80% of patients with migraine it starts when they are under 30, so onset at over 40 may show an incorrect diagnosis; treatment of acute attacks is with analgesics, antiemetics, and 5-HT$_1$ agonists (ergotamine and sumatriptan); serotonin (5-HT$_2$) inhibitors help to prevent attacks in 60–70% of patients; and β blockers without intrinsic sympathomimetic activity (propranolol, atenolol, and metoprolol) reduce the frequency of attacks in about 60%
- Episodic cluster headache (severe, daily, and unilateral—mainly in men) is treated symptomatically with ergotamine, sumatriptan, and (in chronic cases) lithium and verapamil
- Headache in middle aged and elderly people may be cervicogenic (relieved often by local facet joint injections of lignocaine and steroids) or (in the over 60s) caused by giant cell arteritis, which requires early diagnosis and steroid treatment to prevent blindness and stroke
- Post-traumatic headache is part of an ill-defined syndrome; it resists analgesics and is treated by support
- Other cranial neuralgias need rational investigation and management to find distinctive features

1 Stang PE, Yanagihara T, Swanson JW, *et al.* Incidence of migraine headache: a population based study in Olmsted County, Minnesota. *Neurology* 1992;**42**:1657–62.
2 International Headache Society. Classification. Diagnostic criteria. *Cephalalgia* 1988; **8**(suppl 7):19–45.
3 Rasmussen BK. Migraine with aura and migraine without aura: an epidemiological study. *Cephalalgia* 1992;**12**:221–8.
4 Rasmussen BK, Jensen R, Olesen J. Impact of headache on sickness absence and utilisation of medical services: a Danish population study. *J Epidemiol Community Health* 1992;**46**: 443–6.
5 Pearce JMS. Clinical features of the exploding head syndrome. *J Neurol Neurosurg Psychiatry* 1989;**52**:907–10.
6 Marcus DA. Migraine and tension-type headaches. The questionable validity of current classification systems. *Clin J Pain* 1992;**8**:28–36.
7 Solomon S, Lipton RB. Criteria for the diagnosis of migraine in clinical practice. *Headache* 1991;**31**:384–7.
8 Jarman J, Davies PTG, Fernandez M, *et al.* Platelet [^{3}H]-imipramine binding in migraine and tension headache in relation to depression. *J Psychiatr Res* 1991;**25**:205–11.
9 Leone M, Sacerdote P, D'Amico D, Panerai AE, Bussone G. Beta-endorphin concentrations in the peripheral blood mononuclear cells of migraine and tension-type headache patients. *Cephalalgia* 1992;**12**:155–7.
10 Besken E, Pothmann R, Sartory G. Contingent negative variation in childhood migraine. *Cephalalgia* 1993;**13**:42–3.
11 Pearce JMS. Tension headaches: clinical features and mechanisms. In: AV Holden, W Winlow, eds. *The neurobiology of pain.* Manchester University Press 1984:235–43.
12 Ehde DM, Holm JE. Stress and headache: comparisons of migraine, tension, and headache-free subjects. *Headache Q* 1992;**3**:54–60.
13 Kunkel RS. Muscle contraction (tension) headache. *Clin J Pain* 1989;**5**:39–44.

14 Silberstein SD, Merriam GR. Estrogens, progestins and headache. *Neurology* 1991;**41**: 786–93.

15 Pearce JMS. Is migraine explained by Leao's spreading depression? *Lancet* 1985;ii:76.

16 Silbert PL, Edjs RH, Stewart Wynne EG, Gubbay SS. Benign vascular sexual headache and exertional headache: interrelationships and long term prognosis. *J Neurol Neurosurg Psychiatry* 1991;**54**:417–21.

17 Lance JW. A concept of migraine and the search for the ideal headache drugs. *Headache* 1990;Jan:17–23.

18 Lance JW. 5-Hydroxytryptamine and its role in migraine. *Eur Neurol* 1991;**31**:279–81.

19 Scott AK. Dihydroergotamine: a review of its use in the treatment of migraine and other headaches. *Clin Neuropharmacol* 1992;**15**:289–96.

20 Humphrey PPA, Feniuk W. Mode of action of the anti-migraine drug sumatriptan. *Trends Pharmacol Sci* 1991;**12**:444–6.

21 The Sumatriptan Auto-injector Study Group. Self-treatment of acute migraine with subcutaneous sumatriptan using an auto-injector device. *Eur Neurol* 1991;**31**:323–31.

22 Ekbom K, Waldenlind E, Levi R, *et al.* Treatment of acute cluster headache with sumatriptan. *N Engl J Med* 1991;**325**:322–6.

23 Pearce JMS. Sumatriptan: efficacy and contribution to migraine mechanisms. *J Neurol Neurosurg Psychiatry* 1992;**55**:1103–6.

24 The Oral Sumatriptan and Aspirin plus Metoclopramide Comparative Study Group. A study to compare oral sumatriptan with aspirin plus metoclopramide in the acute treatment of migraine. *Eur Neurol* 1992;**32**:177–84.

25 The Multinational Oral Sumatriptan and Cafergot Comparative Study Group. A randomized double-blind comparison of sumatriptan and Cafergot in the acute treatment of migraine. *Eur Neurol* 1991;**31**:314–22.

26 Goadsby PJ, Zagami AS, Donnan GA, *et al.* Oral sumatriptan in acute migraine. *Lancet* 1991;**338**:782–3.

27 Glaxo Holdings plc cited in: *Sumatriptan in clinical practice.* Ninth Migraine Trust International Symposium, London, 8 September 1992.

28 Ottervanger JP, Paalman HJA, Boxma GL, Stricker BHC. Transmural myocardial infarction with Sumatriptan. *Lancet* 1993;**341**:861–2.

29 Pearce JMS. Sumatriptan in migraine. *BMJ* 1991;**303**:1491.

30 Ludin HP. Flunarizine and propranolol in the treatment of migraine. *Headache* 1989;**29**: 219–24.

31 Saxena PR, Den-Boer MO. Pharmacology of antimigraine drugs. *J Neurol* 1991; **238**(suppl)S28–35.

32 Igarashi M, May WN, Golden GS. Pharmacologic treatment of childhood migraine. *J Pediatr* 1992;**120**:653–7.

33 Kudrow L. Diagnosis and treatment of cluster headache. *Med Clin North Am* 1991;**75**: 579–94.

34 Pearce JMS. Cluster headache and its variants. Festschrift for Lord Walton. *Postgrad Med J* 1992;**68**:517–21.

35 Sjaastad O, Dale I. A new (?) headache entity "chronic paroxysmal hemicrania". *Acta Neurol Scand* 1976;**54**:140–59.

36 Sjaastad O. Cervicogenic headache: the controversial headache. *Clin Neurol Neurosurg* 1992; **94**(suppl):S147–9.

37 Bovim G, Sand T. Cervicogenic headache, migraine without aura and tension-type headache. Diagnostic blockade of greater occipital and supra-orbital nerves. *Pain* 1992;**51**:43–8.

38 Hunder GG, Bloch DA, Michel BA, *et al.* The American College of Rheumatology 1990 criteria for the classification of giant cell arteritis. *Arthritis Rheum* 1990;**33**:1122–8.

39 Bengtsson BA, Malmvall BE. Prognosis of giant cell arteritis including temporal arteritis and polymyalgia rheumatica. A follow-up study on ninety patients treated with corticosteroids. *Acta Med Scand* 1981;**209**:337–45.

40 Newman LC, Lipton RB, Solomon S. The hypnic headache syndrome: a benign headache disorder of the elderly. *Neurology* 1990;**40**:1904–5.

41 Pearce JMS. The post-traumatic syndrome and whiplash injury. In: Kennard C, ed. Edinburgh: Churchill Livingstone, 1995:133–49 (ch 7). *Recent advances in clinical neurology*, Vol 8.

42 Helzer JE, Robins LN, McEvoy L. Post-traumatic stress disorder in the general population: findings of the epidemiologic catchment area survey. *N Engl J Med* 1987;**317**:1630–4.

43 Weiss HD, Stern BJ, Goldberg J. Post-traumatic migraine: chronic migraine precipitated by minor head or neck trauma. *Headache* 1991;**31**:451–6.

44 Watson CPN. Postherpetic neuralgia. *Neurol Clin* 1989;**7**:231–48.

3 Epilepsy

DAVID CHADWICK

Epilepsy is the most common of chronic neurological disorders and it imposes the biggest burden on health care systems. It varies greatly in its clinical features, aetiology, severity, and prognosis and its association with other neurological disabilities. For this reason practitioners of many different disciplines may be responsible for supplying care, including neurologists, paediatricians, geriatricians, psychiatrists, and specialists in mental handicap, and in all spheres the professions allied to medicine have an important input.

Unfortunately, services for people with epilepsy in the United Kingdom are poorly developed and vary considerably from region to region. The quality of care they offer is varied but often quite poor. A number of reasons are apparent for this, the prime being that British neurology has remained a small specialty and one in which few British neurologists have epilepsy as a major interest. This has meant that many patients with epilepsy are managed by clinicians without appreciable neurological training.

Definition

Epilepsy is most easily defined in physiological terms, being "the name for occasional sudden, excessive, rapid and local discharges of grey matter".[1] An epileptic *seizure* can be defined clinically as an intermittent stereotyped disturbance of consciousness, behaviour, emotion, motor function, or sensation that on clinical grounds is believed to result from cortical neuronal discharge. *Epilepsy* can then be defined as a condition in which seizures recur, usually spontaneously. Two major types are recognised—namely, epilepsy with focal or generalised seizures.

The international classification of epileptic seizures (ICES) was proposed in 1981[2] and box 3.1 summarises this. It makes use

Box 3.1 Classification of seizures

Partial seizures (seizures beginning locally):
    Simple (consciousness not impaired)
        With motor symptoms
        With somatosensory or special sensory symptoms
        With autonomic symptoms
        With psychic symptoms

    Complex (with impairment of consciousness):
        Beginning as simple partial seizures (progressing to complex
            seizure)
        Impairment of consciousness at onset
    Partial seizures becoming secondarily generalised

Generalised seizures:
    Absence seizures
        Typical (petit mal)
        Atypical
    Myoclonic seizures
    Clonic seizures
    Tonic seizures
    Tonic–clonic seizures
    Atonic seizures

of both clinical and electroencephalographic information. Similar seizures may occur at different ages and have very different implications. Conversely, patients may experience differing seizures during the course of their lives so that a classification of different epileptic syndromes based on seizure types occurring within the syndrome, age at onset, and aetiology will also be of vital importance in the management of patients with epilepsy. Box 3.2 presents a proposed classification of epilepsy.[3]

Epilepsy must be regarded as a symptom complex rather than a disease entity. The causes of epilepsy are many and varied and include purely genetic disorders (for example, the idiopathic generalised epilepsies) as well as those that result from any type of acquired cerebral insult.

Epidemiology

Despite problems with differing definitions of epilepsy and case ascertainment methods, there is remarkable agreement about the

Box 3.2 International classification of epilepsies, epileptic syndromes, and related seizure disorders (ICE) (adapted from ref[5])

Localisation-related (focal, local, partial)

Idiopathic (primary)
Benign childhood epilepsy with centrotemporal spike
Childhood epilepsy with occipital paroxysms
Primary reading epilepsy

Cryptogenic
Defined by:
seizure type (see ICES),
clinical features,
aetiology,
anatomical localisation

Symptomatic (secondary)
Temporal lobe epilepsies
Frontal lobe epilepsies
Parietal lobe epilepsies

Generalised

Benign neonatal familial convulsions
Benign neonatal convulsions
Benign myoclonic epilepsy in infancy
Childhood absence epilepsy (pyknolepsy)
Juvenile absence epilepsy
Juvenile myoclonic epilepsy (impulsive petit mal)
Epilepsies with grand mal seizures on awakening
Other generalised idiopathic epilepsies
Epilepsies with seizures precipitated by specific modes of activation

Cryptogenic or symptomatic
West's syndrome (infantile spasms, Blitz–Nick–Salaam Krämpfe)
Lennox–Gastaut syndrome
Epilepsy with myoclonic–astatic seizures
Epilepsy with myoclonic absences

Non-specific aetiology
Early myoclonic encephalopathy
Early infantile epileptic encephalopathy with suppression bursts

[Continued opposite

Box 3.2 International classification of epilepsies, epileptic syndromes, and related seizure disorders (ICE) (adapted from ref[3])—*continued*

Localisation-related (focal, local, partial)

Occipital lobe epilepsies
Chronic progressive epilepsia partialis continua of childhood
Syndromes characterised by seizures with specific modes of precipitation

Undetermined epilepsies

With both generalised and focal seizures
Neonatal seizures
Severe myoclonic epilepsy in infancy
Epilepsy with continuous spike-wave during slow-wave sleep
Acquired epileptic aphasia (Landau-Kleffner syndrome)
Other undetermined epilepsies
Without unequivocal generalised or focal features

Generalised

Other symptomatic generalised epilepsies
Specific syndromes
Epileptic seizures may complicate many disease states

Special syndromes
Situation-related seizures
Febrile convulsions
Isolated seizures or isolated status epilepticus
Seizures occurring only when there is an acute or toxic event due to factors such as alcohol, drugs, eclampsia, non-ketotic hyperglycaemia

ICES = International classification of epileptic seizures

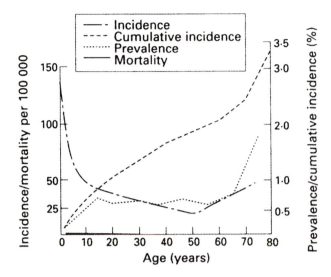

Figure 3.1 *Incidence, prevalence, and cumulative incidence rates for epilepsy in Rochester, Minnesota 1935–74 (reproduced from Anderson et al[5a] with permission).*

epidemiology of epilepsy in different populations.[4] Incidence rates vary in an age specific way between about 20 and 70 per 100 000 a year, whereas the prevalence for active epilepsy is in the range of 4–10 per 1000. Figure 3.1 gives age specific incidence, prevalence, and cumulative incidence for a population in Rochester, Minnesota. It can be seen that the incidence of epilepsy is highest at the extremes of life but there are significant differences between the cumulative incidence and prevalence of epilepsy, indicating that most patients who develop epilepsy do not have a chronic disorder.

Most seizures and epilepsies developing in adult life will be regarded as symptomatic but significant numbers of patients may be investigated without a cause becoming apparent. In the National General Practice Study of Epilepsy, 60% of all patients had no identifiable cause of epilepsy, although a proportion of these will have had a specific (genetically determined) epilepsy syndrome.[5]

It may be useful to differentiate causes of seizures and epilepsy into acute symptomatic seizures occurring in response to metabolic or cerebral insult, and remote symptomatic epilepsies in which epilepsy develops in relation to a persisting cerebral lesion or damage. Some aetiologies—for example, head injury, stroke, and intracranial infections—may cause both acute symptomatic seizures and remote symptomatic epilepsy. The presence of the first does not necessarily result in the second.

Sander et al[5] found that the commonest remote symptomatic causes of epilepsy were vascular disease (15%) and tumour (6%).[5] Remote symptomatic epilepsy was commonest in the elderly patients, in whom vascular disease accounted for 49% of cases. Tumour was a rare cause of epilepsy below the age of 30 (1%), but accounted for 19% of cases aged between 50 and 59. Trauma caused 3% of cases and infection 2%. Acute symptomatic seizures occurred in 15%, and alcohol was the commonest single cause (6%), the incidence being highest between 30 and 39 years of age (27%).

The cost of epilepsy to the NHS was around £110 million in 1988.[6] In a recent pilot survey of five general practices in the Mersey Region the overall prevalence for active epilepsy was 0·8% (225 adults and 48 children) of the population, of whom about a third had attended hospital services on at least one occasion within the previous 12 months; 57% had been free of seizures since the previous year; 14% had more than one seizure a month; 8% had some additional neurological, mental, or psychiatric handicaps; 60% of children and 11% of adults had had at least one electroencephalogram during the previous 12 months, 26% and 8% some form of scanning, and 82% and 94% respectively were receiving at least one antiepileptic drug.

Diagnosis

The diagnosis of epilepsy is clinical, and is based on a detailed description of events experienced by the patient before, during, and after a seizure and, more importantly, on an eye witness account. In view of the social and economic implications diagnostic errors need to be avoided at all costs. Thus the first basic rule about diagnosing epilepsy is never to make the diagnosis without incontrovertible clinical evidence. If there is any doubt, the clinician should resist the temptation to attach a label and should rely on the passage of time and the further description of symptomatic events to reach a firm conclusion. Hardly anyone with epilepsy will come to any harm from a delay in diagnosis whereas a false positive diagnosis is gravely damaging.

53

Box 3.3   Differential diagnosis of epilepsy

Syncope
  Reflex syncope:
    Postural
    Psychogenic
    Carotid sinus syncope
    Micturition syncope
    Valsalva
  Cardiac syncope:
    Dysrhythmias (heart block, tachycardias, etc)
    Valvular disease (especially aortic stenosis)
    Cardiomyopathies
    Shunts
  Perfusion failure:
    Hypovolaemia
    Syndrome of autonomic failure
Psychogenic attacks:
  Pseudoseizures
  Panic attacks
  Hyperventilation
  Night terrors
  Breath holding
Transient ischaemic attacks
Migraine
Narcolepsy
Hypoglycaemia

Is it epilepsy?

The first test will be to differentiate *seizures* from other transient symptoms (box 3.3). Syncope and pseudoseizures are most often mistaken for epilepsy. Both are common in young adults. Pseudoseizures may account for anything up to 20% of apparently intractable epilepsies in this age group.[7] Once it is accepted that seizures have occurred, it is important to determine whether they are acute symptomatic events (not necessarily requiring antiepileptic drug treatment) or spontaneously occurring seizures indicating a truly epileptic disorder. Causes of acute symptomatic seizures include alcohol and other drugs, fever in children aged between 1 and 5 years, and metabolic disturbance. The hallmark of almost all of these types of seizures is that they usually occur in patients with acute encephalopathy who have an associated confusional state or systemic disturbance that often outlasts the seizures themselves. Other associated symptoms and signs commonly indicate the correct diagnosis, for which specific treatment will be required.

What kind of epilepsy?

Although the diagnosis of a specific epileptic syndrome may require confirmation from interictal or ictal electroencephalograms, clinical information will often be sufficient to allow a presumptive diagnosis. Thus a history of occasional nocturnal focal motor seizures involving face or arm in children below the age of 12 may strongly suggest benign Rolandic epilepsy, whereas in an adolescent the development of myoclonic jerking on awakening with occasional tonic–clonic seizures points to juvenile myoclonic epilepsy. Seizures associated with a specific epileptic aura indicate a localised onset and therefore imply a greater likelihood of symptomatic epilepsy caused by a localised cerebral lesion.

What is the aetiology of the epilepsy?

The cause may be readily apparent from clinical information alone. A previous neurological disorder may often be the cause of the seizures. Thus the history must include direct questions about early perinatal events and development, severe head injury (especially those that are complicated by longlasting post-traumatic amnesia, depressed skull fracture, or intracerebral haematoma), and infection of the CNS. A family history of epilepsy may suggest a genetic cause when seizure disorders develop in people aged 5 to about 25 years.

The electroencephalogram

The electroencephalogram provides valuable information that may (a) add weight to the clinical diagnosis; (b) aid the classification of epilepsy; and (c) show changes that may increase the suspicion of an underlying structural lesion.

Electroencephalography as a diagnostic aid

Routine interictal electroencephalography is one of the most abused investigations in clinical medicine and is unquestionably responsible for great human suffering. The diagnostic value of an interictal electroencephalogram is widely misunderstood. Electroencephalograms are often requested either to exclude or to prove a diagnosis of epilepsy—something that can seldom, if ever, be done. Between 10 and 15% of the population may have an "abnormal" electroencephalogram; most such abnormalities are mild and of no diagnostic importance. More rigid definitions are focal or generalised spike or polyspike and slow wave abnormality in the electroencephalogram, and probably only 1% of a non-epileptic population have such abnormalities. Waking interictal electroencephalograms of patients with epilepsy show that about 35% consistently have specific epileptiform discharges and 50% do so on some occasion with repeated recording; about 15% never do. A single routine electroencephalogram is likely to show an epileptic abnormality in about 50% of patients with epilepsy.

Continuous ambulatory electroencephalographic monitoring or videotelemetry may be helpful in the diagnosis of frequent events that can be captured. Such facilities will only be available in specialist centres.

Classification of epilepsy

The electroencephalogram is especially important in two clinical settings. In patients whose seizures occur without an aura and are characterised by a brief period of absence with or without automatism, it may be difficult to differentiate absence seizures from complex partial seizures. The finding of generalised spike wave or focal spike activity, respectively, will clarify the diagnosis. The differentiation has important implications for treatment and prognosis. In patients with tonic–clonic seizures without an aura, especially when these occur during sleep, the electroencephalogram can again differentiate between primary generalised epilepsies characterised by generalised spike wave activity and seizures with a focal onset in which there may be localised abnormalities.

Detection of structural brain lesions

Electroencephalography may, by showing the presence of focal slow wave abnormalities, suggest the presence of a structural lesion as a cause for a patient's epilepsy. This use of electroen-cephalography is of diminishing value with the increasing availability of imaging.

Neurological imaging in the diagnosis of epilepsy

In practical terms imaging means computed tomography or magnetic resonance imaging. The frequency of abnormalities in computed tomograms of patients with epilepsy varies greatly. In surveys of patients with established epilepsy from specialist centres, 60%–80% may have abnormal tomograms but most of these abnormalities are atrophic in nature. Tumours may be identified in about 10% of patients. In patients who present with either a first seizure or early epilepsy the frequency is lower—abnormalities are detected in less than 20% of cases—but again atrophic abnormalities predominate. Tomographic abnormalities are very strongly predicted by the presence of focal rather than generalised seizures, focal neurological signs, and focal electroencephalographic abnormalities. When all three are present, abnormalities on tomography may be found in up to 70% or 80% of cases.[8] Computed tomography is most clearly indicated in patients with onset of epilepsy after the age of 20 who have focal seizures.

Magnetic resonance imaging is increasingly important in epilepsy. In particular it is sensitive in detecting hippocampal and medial temporal atrophy and sclerosis, which are important causes of drug resistant temporal lobe epilepsy. It can also show dysplastic and developmental extratemporal lesions. It may be more important to offer magnetic resonance imaging to patients whose epilepsy is unresponsive to antiepileptic drug treatment than to pursue a policy of indiscriminate imaging for all patients at the presentation of their epilepsy.

Prevention

A role for primary prevention in epilepsy has yet to be clearly identified. Inevitably the incidence of some of the causes of epilepsy in the community may be reduced. Stroke is a common cause of epilepsy in later life and a reduction in its incidence should be accompanied by a decline in the incidence of epilepsy (see earlier). Road traffic accidents represent a major cause of head trauma, some of which will be complicated by post-traumatic epilepsy. Reduced perinatal morbidity and an improved genetic understanding of rare genetic disorders that can be associated with epilepsy could reduce the incidence of epilepsy in early life.

Secondary prevention is of much greater importance in epilepsy. For many patients the aim of medical or surgical management is a complete cure or control of seizures. It remains controversial whether early intervention with antiepileptic drugs is able to influence the longer term outcome of epilepsy, and clinical trials to establish this are of considerable importance. It is important that adequate counselling concerning provocative factors is given to patients and their families. This is particularly the case with febrile seizures for which the main arm of management may well be early intervention to control temperature during episodes of infection. Equally, many tonic–clonic seizures occurring in the idiopathic generalised epilepsies may be avoided if subjects are aware of the importance of sleep deprivation and alcohol in provoking seizures. Counselling about alcohol and drug abuse may reduce the recurrence of acute symptomatic seizures.

Seizures contribute to disability by interrupting normal activities of everyday life and by producing forms of behaviour that may be hazardous or be misinterpreted by observers. Of greatest concern to patients and their families is the risk of accidental injury or even death.[9] Information needs to include sensible counselling to reduce the risks to people with epilepsy from accidental injury from seizures.

Mortality from epilepsy

All available studies show an increased mortality ratio for epilepsy of between two and three times that expected.[10] A number of factors seem to contribute to this. The greatest excess seems to occur in the first decade of life[11] or follows soon after diagnosis and is more obvious in males: the risk is highest for patients with tonic–clonic seizures and seizures that recur often.

Considerable controversy surrounds the contribution of sudden unexpected death in people with epilepsy. Some studies have highlighted cases in which people with epilepsy are found dead, usually in bed.[12 13] It is assumed that deaths are related to seizures and possibly to associated cardiac dysrhythmias. Accidental death is more common in epilepsy than would be expected, drowning being the commonest cause. Whereas status epilepticus continues to be associated with mortality its rarity means that it does not contribute significantly to the excess mortality associated with epilepsy.

Accidental injury

Injuries caused by falling are not uncommon in people with epilepsy but most injuries are not severe. Presumably, they are more likely to occur in patients whose epilepsy involves frequent loss of consciousness with or without falls. Unfortunately, very few systematic analyses have been performed.

Hauser *et al*[14] have shown that patients with epilepsy were overrepresented (× 3) in a study of non-fatal head trauma, accounting for 7·4% of admissions with such trauma to five New York hospitals. Injuries were significantly more likely to be caused by falls and less likely to be sustained in road traffic accidents in epileptic than in non-epileptic trauma victims. Russell-Jones and Shorvon[15] found that 2·7% of seizures at the Chalfont Centre for Epilepsy resulted in a head injury requiring some medical intervention, but only one in over 9000 seizures was complicated by skull fracture or intracranial haematoma.

There have been no studies of the incidence of burns in unselected populations of patients with epilepsy. It is suggested, however, that epilepsy is overrepresented as a cause of burns. Bhatnagar[16] in a retrospective review of presentations to an Indian burns unit, identified epilepsy as the cause of 2·6% of all burns, and 8·4% of those requiring admission. In a study of patients attending an epilepsy clinic 38% of patients had a history of burns with 13% seeking hospital treatment, 4% requiring admission, and 1% needing skin grafts. Those who sustained burns were older, had a longer history of epilepsy, and were more likely to have complex partial seizures than those who had no history of burns.[17]

Epilepsy and psychosocial handicap

The social, psychological, and emotional problems encountered with epilepsy are considerable and may be complicated by the effects of associated neurological impairments and the effects of anticonvulsant therapy.[18-20] Psychosocial problems may be the result of the unpredictability and the severity of seizures, rather than their frequency.[21] The fear evoked by the unpredictable nature of the seizures may lead to social withdrawal, with loss of existing friendships and an inability to form new relationships. Loss of employment or inability to compete in the job market may lead to loss of self esteem and financial hardship. These factors often result in anxiety, depression, and a loss of sense of control. This loss of control may have serious psychological consequences, including feelings of helplessness and low self esteem.[20 22]

Epilepsy and psychiatric disorders

The relation between epilepsy and psychiatric disorders has evoked much discussion. Studies on unselected populations of patients have shown an increased incidence of psychiatric illness in patients with epilepsy.[23 24] These show that, in both adults and children, having epilepsy rather than other chronic conditions is associated with increased psychopathology. A recent general practice survey[25] has shown that psychiatric morbidity (especially anxiety and non-psychiatric depression) occurs more commonly in people with epilepsy than would be expected by chance and is particularly common in patients with focal epilepsy as opposed to primary generalised epilepsy.

There have been some conflicting studies investigating the incidence and prevalence of interictal as opposed to postictal psychosis in patients with epilepsy. Pond and Bidwell found that 29% of a general practice population of people with epilepsy had a history of psychiatric illness but none of psychosis.[23] By contrast, studies on outpatients have reported a prevalence of psychosis between 2% and 5%.[26 27] In an earlier study of 69 patients with schizophrenia-like psychosis, 80% were found to have focal temporal lobe electroencephalographic abnormalities,[28] leading the authors to conclude that the characteristics of the psychoses accompanying epilepsy were distinct from functional psychosis. This finding has not, however, been confirmed in subsequent prospective studies.[29]

A review of studies of mortality and suicide in people with epilepsy by Barraclough[30] confirmed that they had an increased risk of suicide. Barraclough estimated a fivefold increase in incidence in those with temporal lobe epilepsy. Feelings of helplessness, lack of control, low self esteem, and anxiety were important risk factors in the aetiology of suicide.

Prognosis

Most studies have been hospital based; this has an adverse effect on apparent outcome because patients with refractory epilepsy are

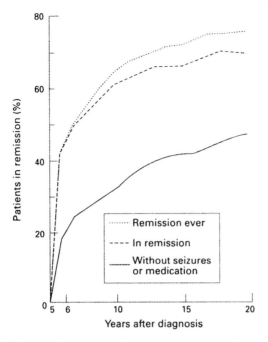

Figure 3.2 *Actuarial percentage of patients in remission after a diagnosis of epilepsy (reproduced from Annegers et al[31] with permission).*

more likely to be referred to specialist centres. In this respect the study of Annegers *et al*[31] is of particular importance in being community rather than hospital based. In Rochester, United States, 457 patients with a history of two or more non-febrile seizures were followed up for at least five years, and in the case of 141 for 20 years. The probability of being in a remission lasting for five years or more was 61% at 10 years, and as high as 70% at 20 years (fig 3.2). Results of this large study are supported by those of a smaller one of 122 patients drawn from a general practice population.[32] By 15 years after the onset of seizures, 80% of these patients had achieved a two year remission, and only 38% were still taking antiepileptic drugs. Further support for such high rates of remission has been obtained from studies of patients followed up prospectively from diagnosis and the start of treatment, which show that between 50% and 77% of such patients are "controlled", depending on how control is defined.[33 34]

61

Factors influencing prognosis

Age of onset of epilepsy seems to be the most important factor. Seizures beginning within the first year of life (when they are usually symptomatic of cerebral pathology) carry an adverse prognosis,[35 35a] but this aside, Annegers et al[31] found that both partial and generalised epilepsies had a better prognosis if they started before the age of 20.

Whatever the age of onset, the duration of the epilepsy before treatment seems to be an important prognostic factor. Annegers et al[31] showed that most patients who achieve remission do so early during the course of treatment. With continuing seizures it becomes progressively less likely that an individual patient will enter remission.[34] Thus there is a plateau in the proportion of patients in remission 15–20 years after the onset of epilepsy. Similar findings have been reported with shorter term follow up in children.[35]

Seizure classification is of importance in assessing outcome. Remission rates range from around 60% to 80% for patients with only tonic–clonic seizures, to between 20% and 60% in patients with complex partial seizures.[33 36] The combination of complex partial seizures with secondary generalised tonic–clonic seizures coming under good control with anticonvulsant therapy, whereas partial seizures remain resistant to drug treatment.[33 37] Generalised epilepsies of childhood carry varying prognoses. Between 70% and 80% of patients with simple absences (petit mal) are likely to enter remission.[35 35a] Complex absences show a lower remission rate (33%–65%), and in patients with the West or Lennox-Gastaut syndromes remission rates may be as low as 35% to 65%.

Epilepsy of unknown aetiology has a better prognosis than symptomatic epilepsy.[31 36] In keeping with this, epilepsy complicated by associated neurological or psychiatric deficit carries an adverse prognosis.[35]

There is no clear indication that any specific abnormalities on electroencephalography, either historically or at the particular time when prognosis is to be predicted, are of any great value.[37 38]

The evidence about the factors affecting the prognosis of epilepsy does not allow any satisfactory measurement and assessment of the varying weights that prognostic factors carry. The prognosis of 306 patients diagnosed between 1935 and 1978 was studied[39] using Cox's proportional hazards model to investigate those factors determining the likelihood of achieving a five year seizure-free

Table 3.1   Factors affecting prognosis of epilepsy (from Shaffer *et al*[39])

Factor	Five years seizure free Relative risk (95% CL)*	Five years seizure free and not taking medication Relative risk (95% CL)
Age <16 at first fit	1·09 (0·82 to 1·44)	1·88 (1·23 to 2·8)
No early brain damage	2·15 (1·22 to 3·78)	4·27 (1·35 to 13·47)
No known aetiology	1·50 (1·05 to 2·13)	2·64 (1·45 to 2·84)
Never had a tonic-clonic fit	1·37 (1·03 to 1·82)	2·19 (1·48 to 3·24)
No generalised spike wave in third year EEG	3·47 (1·37 to 8·8)	2·36 (0·56 to 10·16)

* Univariate Cox regression estimate of relative risk from 298 patients.
CL = Confidence limits.

period and a five year seizure-free period while not taking drugs. It can be seen (table 3.1) that no single factor is strongly predictive of remission, but those that are include the absence of early brain damage, never having had a tonic–clonic seizure, and the absence of generalised spike wave activity from a number of electroencephalograms. Similar factors were also predictive of five year seizure-free periods while not taking antiepileptic drugs.

Communication and counselling

Diagnosis

The diagnosis of epilepsy is often frightening and disconcerting for patients and their families. There remains a considerable misunderstanding of the nature of epilepsy and it is one of the few organic neurological diagnoses associated with considerable stigma. For this reason patients need a careful explanation of the basis of epilepsy; an emphasis that it is an organic disorder and that it is not a primary psychiatric disorder or stroke. Patients and their families need time to assimilate this information and to ask any relevant questions. Supplementary written information is extremely valuable, and the epilepsy associations are good sources of this. Doctors are often poor information givers, and patients may feel unable to ask the questions that they want answered. As clinical time is often limited, intervention by knowledgeable counsellors or specialist nurse services probably represents a better way of addressing these issues.

63

Effects of prognosis and treatment

At the time of diagnosis patients need to be given a clear indication of the likely outcome of their epilepsy and in particular whether treatment with antiepileptic drugs is necessary, and if so for how long it may need to be maintained. Failure to provide satisfactory information is bound to complicate the problems of poor compliance.

Implications of epilepsy and limitation of social disadvantage

The unpredictable nature of epileptic seizures and the stigmatisation and concealment that often comes with the diagnosis creates particular problems that must be considered at an early stage. There can be a considerable fear of accidental injury or death as a result of seizures. Any counselling about these risks needs to be put clearly in context. Although sensible avoidance of higher risk situations needs to be emphasised, overprotection and limitation should be avoided except in the most severe of the epilepsies.

For most, reassurance about the low risks of serious injury by accident seems appropriate, perhaps with advice to avoid climbing to appreciable heights, to use microwave cooking in preference to gas or electric hobs, and to ensure that fires are adequately guarded. Showers are to be preferred to baths, and swimming in open water best avoided. For most people a full range of leisure activities should be possible although perhaps with some accompanying supervision when appropriate (for instance, swimming in a pool or cycling on a busy road).

For patients with frequent seizures complicated by falls, more supervision and attendance may be necessary; occasionally protective helmets may be worn, although these can be regarded as unduly stigmatising by some.

For children, liaison with schools concerning the diagnosis of epilepsy is important, and teaching staff need to be reassured and advised about the child usually being able to fulfil a full pattern of school activity with the probable exception of climbing. Epilepsy itself is rarely a reason for special education and most children will be in mainstream schooling. Special education is usually necessary for children with associated mental and neurological handicap.

One of the most important implications of the diagnosis of epilepsy in adults is the effect on driving. In the United Kingdom the diagnosis results in an immediate disqualification from all forms of driving, which will continue until a seizure-free period lasting one year has been attained, or until only seizures beginning during sleep have occurred for at least three years. Where a single seizure has occurred, a seizure-free period of one year is also required. Drivers with epilepsy must be informed of the legal requirement to inform the Driver and Vehicle Licensing Agency of recent seizures.

Employment issues also demand discussion. It is unwise for people with a recent history of epilepsy to work at heights or close to large volumes of water that might present a risk. The risks of working with machinery require more selective evaluation as now most factory machinery should be adequately protected. Unfortunately, the diagnosis of epilepsy inevitably leads to significant employment problems. There are statutory limitations that affect the driving of public service or heavy goods vehicles and employment as an airline pilot, taxi driver, train driver, etc. People with epilepsy also experience considerable unwarranted job discrimination and they need careful counselling about how and when to declare a history of epilepsy to a prospective employer.

For women it is important to explain the relevance of epilepsy and its drug treatment to contraception (interaction with oral contraceptives), pregnancy (risks of teratogenicity), and the genetic risk of epilepsy in offspring.

Sharing care

Because of the variable nature and severity of epilepsy no single system of care is appropriate for all patients, and many different agencies will come into contact with many people with epilepsy. For this reason effective systems of liaison should exist between the agencies that may be involved, and the primary aim must be to offer continuity of care with a single clearly identified clinician having the prime responsibility for the medical management of the individual patient.

The diagnosis and initiation of treatment of the epilepsy will usually require specialist skills. Most patients with newly diagnosed epilepsy, however, quickly enter a remission and at this stage the patient's general practitioner can usually assume responsibility.

After two to three years of remission referral back to specialist services may be required for counselling about withdrawal of antiepileptic drugs. Patients with poorly controlled seizures may also benefit from specialist referral for reconsideration of the diagnosis, second line or newer drug treatment, or, when appropriate, consideration of surgical treatment. There is no doubt that standards of care could often be improved by better liaison between primary care and specialist services. The use of liaison cards for epilepsy is poorly developed and would seem to be highly appropriate. Shared care systems for people with diabetes have made extensive use of nurse practitioners as "key workers". This model would also be of particular benefit in epilepsy; a specialist liaison nurse working between specialist services and general practice could improve communication, not only with general practitioners but also with other community teams dealing with learning disability and psychiatric disorder.

One subject about which communications often break down is that of the transfer of people with epilepsy from paediatric to adult services. This is a particularly traumatic time in that the state guarantees the individual patient a place in society with his or her peer group up until the age of 16, but after leaving school no such guarantee is extended to further education, training, or employment. At the same time the young person with epilepsy is often discharged from the well integrated paediatric services and has to cope with forming relations with a new clinician dealing with adults and less well equipped to provide a comprehensive system of clinical and social support. Here there seems to be a clear role for joint specialist clinics run by paediatricians and neurologists who work with adults to facilitate the process of the handing over of care.

Management

Starting treatment

Antiepileptic treatment has, in the past, been advocated before seizures occur. Such prophylactic treatment has been given to patients with a high prospective risk of epilepsy after head injury and craniotomy for various neurosurgical conditions.[40] Because no clear evidence exists that antiepileptic treatment is effective in preventing late epilepsy,[41 42] it seems better to delay treatment until seizures have occurred rather than to adopt a policy of treating all those at risk—particularly as there may be a high incidence of side effects with prophylactic treatment[43] and poor compliance.[44]

When two or more unprovoked seizures have occurred within a short interval, antiepileptic treatment is usually indicated. Problems do, however, arise in defining a short interval. Most would include periods of six months to one year within the definition. Even when seizures occur in a close temporal relation, the identification of specific precipitating factors may make it more important to counsel patients than to start drug treatment. The most common examples are febrile convulsions in children and alcohol withdrawal seizures in adults. Less commonly, seizures may be precipitated in photosensitive subjects by television, visual display units, or other photic stimuli.

Choice of drug

There is now considerable evidence[45] that patients with newly diagnosed epilepsy should be treated with a single drug. The major factors that influence the choice of antiepileptic drug are comparative efficacy and toxicity.

Although many clinicians have been persuaded that one drug is likely to be most effective against particular seizure types and epileptic syndromes, it is difficult to identify satisfactory clinical trials that support this contention.[46] Table 3.2 summarises conventional practice. In children the differences in efficacy between sodium valproate and ethosuximide on one hand, and phenytoin and carbamazepine on the other for treating absence seizures seem too obvious to demand confirmation in a prospective clinical study. Studies do not, however, differentiate between the efficacy of sodium valproate and ethosuximide in absence epilepsy.[47 48] Similarly, the preferential response of juvenile myoclonic epilepsy to sodium valproate seems to identify this as the drug of choice in this syndrome.[49] It is much more doubtful whether there are major differences in efficacy between carbamazepine, phenytoin, barbiturates, lamotrigine and sodium valproate in treating partial epilepsies.[46 50–52]

When differences in efficacy are marginal, the importance of comparative drug toxicity becomes a major consideration in the

Table 3.2 Choice of antiepileptic drugs (adapted from Chadwick[46a])

	First line drugs	Second line drugs
Generalised epilepsy		
Idiopathic		
Simple absence	Sodium valproate, ethosuximide	Benzodiazepines, lamotrigine
Juvenile myoclonic	Sodium valproate	Lamotrigine
Awakening tonic–clonic	Sodium valproate	Carbamazepine, phenytoin. lamotrigine
Symptomatic	Sodium valproate, benzodiazepines	Carbamazipine, phenytoin, lamotrigine
Partial epilepsy	Carbamazepine, lamotrigine	Gabapentin, phenytoin, sodium valproate, vigabatrin
Unclassified epilepsy	Sodium valproate	Lamotrigine

choice of antiepileptic agent. Antiepileptic drugs possess four distinct types of toxicity: acute dose-related toxicity, acute idiosyncratic toxicity, chronic toxicity, and teratogenicity.

Acute dose-related toxicity

Most antiepileptic drugs, including phenytoin, carbamazepine, barbiturates, and benzodiazepines, give rise to a non-specific encephalopathy associated with high blood concentrations. Patients exhibit sedation and nystagmus and, with increasing blood concentration, ataxia, dysarthria, and ultimately confusion and drowsiness.[53] In some instances frequency of seizures may increase with high blood concentrations and occasionally involuntary movements are seen, particularly with phenytoin.[54] Phenytoin is especially likely to result in dose-related toxicity because of its unusual pharmacokinetics (see later). Carbamazepine may cause similar symptoms if the dose is not built up slowly. This is probably related to autoinduction of liver microsomal enzymes. Sodium valproate does not seem to be associated with this typical syndrome of neurotoxicity, but some patients with high blood concentrations may exhibit restlessness and irritability (sometimes with a frank confusion state). Postural tremor is a common accompaniment.[55]

All antiepileptic drugs have adverse effects on cognitive function of behaviour at therapeutic concentrations that become more apparent both with polytherapy and with increasing blood concentrations. Agents such as carbamazepine and sodium valproate have fewer adverse effects in this respect, and this is one argument for preferring these agents to longer established antiepileptic drugs.

Toxicity may occur because of drug interactions. Thus valproate may potentiate the sedative effects of phenobarbitone and greatly prolong the half life of lamotrigine, making dosage reduction necessary during concurrent medication.

Acute idiosyncratic toxicity

Most antiepileptic drugs, particularly phenytoin, carbamazepine, and lamotrigine, may cause a maculopapular erythematous eruption which, in more severe cases, may be associated with fever, lymphadenopathy, and hepatitis.[53] The incidence of allergic skin reaction with phenytoin may be as high as 10% and with carbamazepine up to 15%.[43] It may be possible to avoid such reactions with a cautious build up of initial doses. Marrow aplasia is a rare complication of carbamazepine. Reports of fatal liver failure in association with sodium valproate treatment largely concern children under the age of 2 years who often have multiple handicaps and receive many different antiepileptic drugs. It may be that they have an underlying error of metabolism that predisposes them to liver failure.[56] Vigabatrin has been associated with behaviour disorders and psychosis, particularly in patients with a psychiatric history.[57] The potential for rare idiosyncratic side effects of lamotrigine and gabapentin is currently uncertain.

Chronic toxicity

Antiepileptic drugs are unusual in that they may be given to patients over long periods as treatment for chronic epilepsy. This may lead to the development of a wide variety of syndromes of chronic toxicity (box 3.4). Several factors seem to predispose to the development of these disorders—namely, the use of polypharmacy, the dosage, and the duration of treatment. Although it seems that sodium valproate and carbamazepine may have fewer chronic toxic effects than barbiturates and phenytoin, the delay in recognising common chronic toxic effects of the older agents should warn us that continued vigilance is needed in the use of the newer antiepileptic drugs.

Teratogenicity

All antiepileptic drugs must be regarded as potentially teratogenic. Phenytoin, and probably barbiturate antiepileptic drugs, seem to increase the risk of major fetal malformation by two to three times: the most common malformations are harelip, cleft palate, and cardiovascular anomalies. The risks are higher with polytherapy than with monotherapy. There seems to be an association between neural tube defects and exposure to sodium valproate or carbamazepine. Estimates of this risk suggest it is 1% to 2% of pregnancies in women taking these drugs.[58 59] Patients should be advised to take folate supplements. Early screening for neural tube defects, by ultrasound and amniocentesis, and testing for α-fetoprotein, therefore, seem to be indicated in women becoming pregnant while taking these drugs.

Box 3.4 Chronic toxicity of anticonvulsant drugs (adapted from ref[57a])

Nervous system:
Memory and cognitive impairment
Hyperactivity and behavioural disturbance
Pseudodementia
Cerebellar atrophy
Peripheral neuropathy

Skin:
Acne
Hirsutism
Alopecia
Chloasma

Liver:
Enzyme induction

Blood:
Megaloblastic anaemia
Thrombocytopenia
Lymphoma

Immune system:
IgA deficiency
Drug-induced systemic lupus erythematosus

Endocrine system:
Decreased thyroxine concentrations
Increased cortisol and sex hormone metabolism

Bone:
Osteomalacia

Connective tissue:
Gum hypertrophy
Coarsened facial features
Dupuytren's contracture

Pregnancy:
Obstetric complications
Teratogenicity
Fetal hydantoin syndrome

Long term management of drug treatment

Most patients developing epilepsy achieve a longlasting remission soon after the start of treatment. For these patients drug withdrawal may be considered after two, three, or more years (see later). Some 20% of patients developing epilepsy have a chronic disorder uncontrolled by drugs. In patients receiving, and complying with, optimum doses of a single antiepileptic drug, the addition of further agents is likely to result in a significant (>75%) improvement in seizure control in only about 10% of patients.[60] Such a policy, however, inevitably increases the risks of dose-related, idiosyncratic, and chronic toxicity. In essence, a law of diminishing returns applies. Thus for this group of patients an appropriate aim may not be complete remission of seizures but a compromise of reduced seizure frequency with less severe seizures, to be achieved with one, or at most two, drugs.

Some patients may continue to have seizures but are not disabled by them; they may have very infrequent seizures or seizures that are minor in their symptomatology or confined to sleep. In such patients, assuming that a single drug appropriate to the seizure type and epilepsy syndrome has been used, there is usually little to be gained from alternative or additional drugs.

Patients who continue to be disabled by the occurrence of seizures despite treatment with a single drug at optimum dosage demand further careful consideration. In particular it is important to consider whether there are factors that would explain an unsatisfactory response to treatment—for example, unidentified structural pathology, the presence of complex partial seizures, poor compliance, or pseudoseizures. If this is not the case, then it is important to review the diagnosis: a common reason for failure of treatment is that the patient does not have epilepsy.

Where none of these conditions apply, it may be reasonable to try alternative drugs as monotherapy, and in some instances to undertake a trial of the addition of a second drug. This demands careful discussion with the patient, however, and the understanding that the second drug will be withdrawn in the absence of a satisfactory sustained response. Patients with intractable partial seizures despite adequate drug treatment may benefit from surgical treatment (see later).

Administering and monitoring drug treatment

Pharmacokinetic data (table 3.3) defines drug absorption, distribution, metabolism, and elimination, but it does not describe the mode of action of drugs in the CNS. One clinical application

Table 3.3 Pharmacokinetics of anticonvulsant drugs (adapted from ref [57a])

Drug	Absorption (time (h) to peak serum concentration after oral dose)	Protein binding (%)	Active metabolites	Metabolism	
				Half life (h)	Doses/day
Carbamazepine	4–24	75	10,11-Epoxide	8–30	2 or 3
Ethosuximide	1–4	—	—	40–70	2 or 3
Gabopentin	2–3	—	—	5–7	3
Lamotrigine	2–3	50	—	12–48	2
Phenobarbitone	1–6	45	—	50–160	2
Phenytoin	4–12	90	—	9–140	1
Primidone	2–5	20	Phenobarbitone: phenylethyl-malonamide	4–12	2
Valproate	1–4	90	—	8–20	2 or 3
Vigabatrin	1–2	—	—	5–7	1 or 2

of pharmacokinetics is therapeutic drug monitoring in serum or plasma, but this technique samples a physiological pool that can be remote from the site of drug action.

Phenytoin has a non-linear relation between the dose and the serum concentration.[61] This results in a narrow therapeutic window, and monitoring is necessary to avoid neurotoxicity in patients whose dosage is being increased. The concept of the "therapeutic" or "optimum" range for phenytoin has been extended to other antiepileptic drugs, and many laboratories now routinely estimate serum concentrations of drugs other than phenytoin. This is seen increasingly as a questionable practice.

A single measurement will give a good approximation of the steady state concentration for drugs with long half lives (phenytoin and phenobarbitone) but not for drugs with short half lives. Measurements of sodium valproate concentrations from specimens taken at random during the day are virtually uninterpretable as they may represent unpredictable peak, trough, or intermediate concentrations. Collecting early morning specimens for measuring troughs is, however, rarely practicable.

It is important to be aware of what is measured during routine estimations of blood concentrations of antiepileptic drugs and, perhaps more importantly, what is not measured. Some drugs have metabolites that contribute to the therapeutic effect but which are not routinely assayed. These include the 10,11-epoxide of carbamazepine and phenylethylmalonamide derived from primidone. Most laboratories in the United Kingdom measure the drug concentration in whole plasma or serum. Phenytoin, carbamazepine, and sodium valproate are heavily protein-bound, but only the free drug fraction is in equilibrium with the brain and pharmacologically active. Measuring free drug concentrations by equilibrium dialysis or ultrafiltration techniques is expensive and not readily available.

Even when concentrations of free drugs and their metabolites in the blood are known, important pharmacodynamic considerations may alter the relation between the blood concentration and the therapeutic effect. Thus for sodium valproate the onset of action is slower and longer lasting than can be explained by the pharmacokinetics of the drug.[62] Similarly, tolerance to the neurotoxicity and therapeutic effects of benzodiazepines and barbiturate drugs is unexplained by pharmacokinetic changes and must be due to drug and receptor interaction.

74

There are further fundamental biological reasons for doubting the value of routine monitoring of blood concentrations of antiepileptic drugs. The upper limit of a therapeutic range may be defined as the concentration of the drug at which toxic effects are likely to appear. The most consistent relation between the serum concentration and toxic effect is for phenytoin, but even with this drug some patients may tolerate, and indeed require, serum concentrations above 20 μg/ml.[63] For sodium valproate, phenobarbitone, and carbamazepine there is a wide variation in individual tolerance of serum concentrations.

The lower limit of the therapeutic range is even more difficult to define, and most patients have epilepsy that is controlled by antiepileptic serum concentrations well below the optimum range.[33] Unquestioning acceptance of therapeutic ranges creates problems: patients with satisfactory control of seizures and low blood concentrations of drugs may have their doses increased needlessly, and patients who tolerate and need high blood concentrations may have their doses reduced. Treating patients is much more important than treating blood concentrations.

Routine monitoring should increasingly be restricted to certain categories of patients: firstly, those receiving phenytoin or multiple drug treatment in whom dosage adjustment is necessary because of dose-related toxicity and poor seizure control; secondly, mentally retarded patients in whom the assessment of toxicity may be difficult; thirdly, patients with renal or hepatic disease; fourthly, perhaps pregnant patients[64] in whom monitoring of free drug concentrations may be indicated; and, finally, patients who may not be complying with treatment.

Antiepileptic drug withdrawal

The fact that antiepileptic drugs have been associated with many adverse reactions is a potent argument for exploring the possibility of withdrawing drugs from patients who achieve remissions lasting two or more years. Against this are the dangers of a recurrence of seizures, which may have important consequences for driving and employment as well as self esteem.

Advice offered to patients on this subject varies widely. Paediatricians and paediatric neurologists suggest a trial withdrawal of antiepileptic drugs in most children attaining remission, as they are concerned about the impact of drugs on cognitive function and learning and are impressed by the high expectation of success. Neurologists tend to be much more circumspect when dealing with adults, expressing concern over the possible effects of further seizures on driving and employment. In the United Kingdom, if not elsewhere, most patients attaining prolonged remission are unlikely to receive any advice from a neurologist or other physician with an interest in the treatment of epilepsy because they will have been discharged from regular follow up. Of 122 patients with a history of epilepsy drawn from general practice, 49 had stopped treatment, most of them on their own initiative.[32]

The few studies that have been undertaken to investigate the success of withdrawing drugs and the factors that identify patients likely to remain free of seizures have been reviewed.[65 66] Comparison of the available studies is difficult because there is often little information about the patients, a lack of uniformity in the duration of remission before withdrawal of the antiepileptic drugs, and no information about the period over which withdrawal occurred or for how long patients were subsequently followed up.

One question that has not been widely considered is the relative risk of recurrence on withdrawal of antiepileptic drugs compared with continued treatment. The Medical Research Council's Antiepileptic Drug Withdrawal Group[67] studied this in a randomised clinical trial. The risk of relapse on continued treatment was about 10% a year, but was two to three times greater in the group withdrawn from treatment for up to two years after withdrawal had started.

A more detailed assessment of prognostic factors has also been undertaken in the Medical Research Council antiepileptic drug withdrawal study. Relatively few clinical factors influenced the risk of recurrence. A Cox's proportional hazard model selected seven prognostic factors for increased risk of seizures recurring: age 16 years and over (relative risk 1·75); taking more than one antiepileptic drug (1·83); a history of seizures after starting antiepileptic drug treatment (1·56); a history of tonic–clonic seizures (primarily or secondarily generalised) (1·56); a history of myoclonic seizures (1·84); and an abnormal electroencephalogram in the previous year (1·32). The risk of recurrence also declined as the period without seizures increased, but in a complex way.

These factors have been used to generate a statistical model for everyday practical use (table 3.4).[68] The index can be used to obtain estimates of the probabilities of seizures recurring within

Table 3.4 Prognostic index for seizure recurrence by one and two years under policies of continued antiepileptic drug (AED) treatment and slow withdrawal

1	Starting score (all patients)	—	−175
2	Age 16 years or older	Add	45
3	Taking more than one AED	Add	50
4	Seizures after the start of AED treatment	Add	35
5	History of primary or secondarily generalised tonic–clonic seizures	Add	35
6	History of myoclonic seizures	Add	50
7	EEG in past year		
	Not available	Add	15
	Abnormal	Add	20
8	Period seizure-free in years(t)	Add	200/t
9	Total score		T
10	Divide total score by 100 and exponentiate (e^x) $z = e^{T/100}$		

Probability of seizure recurrence

	By one year	By two years
After continued treatment	$1-0.89^z$	$1-0.79^z$
After slow withdrawal	$1-0.69^z$	$1-0.60^z$

one or two years of starting slow withdrawal of antiepileptic drugs or of continuing treatment. The estimates can easily be made on a pocket calculator.

This model, derived from the only randomised study of withdrawal of antiepileptic drugs from patients in remission, provides the best available information for patients considering drug withdrawal. It should be emphasised that the decisions to be made about stopping antiepileptic drugs lie with the patient, because social factors such as the possession of a driving licence are often as important or more important than the risk of recurrence of seizures.

Surgical treatment of epilepsy

Although the surgical treatment of epilepsy was pioneered in the United Kingdom over 100 years ago, it has never been made widely available to patients with epilepsy. The increasing sophistication of electroencephalogram investigation, neurological imaging, and neuropsychology, however, means that this form of treatment can be highly successful in large numbers of patients. It has been estimated that at least 75 000 patients in the United States may be suitable for surgical treatment[69] and in the United Kingdom there may be well over 12 000 patients who would benefit.

The philosophy of surgical treatment requires either the accurate identification and excision of the localised site of onset of seizures or the disconnection of epileptogenic zones, so as to interrupt seizure spread in a palliative procedure (callosotomy or multiple sub-pial resections).

Engel[70] reviewed the varying procedures undertaken at centres worldwide: 68% of operations involved some form of temporal lobe surgery, extratemporal cortical excisions accounted for 24%, 2% were hemispherectomies, and 6% corpus callosotomies. To be considered for any of these procedures, patients need to have a history of medically refractory epilepsy and be sufficiently disabled by their epilepsy to warrant the risks of surgical treatment and the necessary presurgical evaluation. There should be a high probability that an improvement in seizure control will lead to a significant improvement in the patient's quality of life. The evaluation of patients for surgical treatment requires a multidisciplinary specialist team (box 3.5).

Temporal lobe surgery

There is no doubt that patients with medial temporal lesions experience the best results from epilepsy surgery. The ideal candidate for temporal lobe surgery has a history of seizures typical of a medial temporal onset, an initial epigastric aura being the most common mode of onset.[71] The two pathological conditions with the best outcome are medial temporal sclerosis (Ammon's horn sclerosis) and an indolent glioma of the medial temporal region,[72] both of which may be defined by magnetic resonance imaging. In the first a history of a prolonged febrile seizure before the age of 4 or 5 years is a particularly strong clinical indicator. Patients should usually be aged between 12 and 30, as psychosocial adjustment may be more difficult in patients having resective surgery after the age of 30.[73] Patients will show a unilateral anterior temporal interictal spike, and sphenoidal or other ictal surface recordings will confirm a temporal onset of seizures.

It must be recognised that many patients who do not conform to these criteria will, nevertheless, have a significant chance of benefiting from temporal lobe surgery, although they may require more detailed presurgical evaluation. All adolescents and young adults with refractory temporal lobe epilepsy should be offered appropriate presurgical evaluation.

Box 3.5 Requirements for surgery for epilepsy

Expertise	Investigation/interview	Role
Neurologist/epileptologist	Trial of antiepileptic drugs	Selection of suitable patients
Neurophysiologist	Interictal electroencephalography	
	Ictal electroencephalography	
	Surface electrodes	
	Sphenoidal electrodes	
	Foramen ovale*	Lateralisation and localisation
	Subdural electrodes*	of seizure onset
	Depth electrodes*	
Neuroradiologist	Magnetic resonance imaging and volumetry	Identification of foreign tissue lesions, dysplasia, and medial temporal sclerosis
	Positron emission tomography*	Identification of interictal hypoperfusion and hypometabolism
Neuropsychologist	Cognitive assessment	Lateralisation of functional deficits and
	Intracarotid amytal	predictive testing of effects of
Neuropsychiatrist	Preoperative assessment	surgery
	Postoperative support and treatment	Identification of high risk patients
Neurosurgeon	Appropriate surgical treatment	

* May not be essential in all centres.

The outcome of temporal lobe surgery and other operations is summarised in table 3.5. The most common surgical procedure is the en bloc anterior temporal lobectomy pioneered by Falconer *et al.*[74] More recently, amygdalohippocampectomy has been pioneered for patients in whom it can be shown that there is a definite medical temporal onset to seizures.[75] Potentially, this procedure may offer results as good as classical en bloc resection with, it is hoped, a reduced morbidity.

Extratemporal cortical excisions

The outcome of such procedures is somewhat less satisfactory than temporal lobe surgery but extratemporal resections can reasonably be considered in patients with localised extratemporal lesions defined by imaging techniques and in patients where neurophysiological investigation shows a consistent focal onset of seizures outside the temporal lobe. Complex partial seizures arising from frontal-orbital areas may be particularly helped by surgery.[76]

Hemispherectomy

This procedure may be suitable for patients with intractable epilepsy and infantile hemiplegia[77] with a useless hand and also in children with rare chronic progressive focal encephalitis (Rasmussen's syndrome). Overall, 70% to 80% of patients become free of seizures after this operation, and behavioural abnormalities can also improve.

Callosotomy

Section of the corpus callosum and hippocampal commissure is an accepted palliative procedure for uncontrolled secondary generalised seizures.[78] The selection criteria for corpus callosotomy are more poorly defined than for other surgical procedures. The operation is most commonly considered in children and adolescents with very severe epilepsy, with a multifocal origin of seizures, or with seizures of sudden onset resulting in falls.

Clinical audit in epilepsy

It is generally accepted that health care systems should provide not only treatments of confirmed efficacy but that the provision should take place with the maximum effectiveness and efficiency.

Table 3.5 Survey results: outcome with respect to epileptic seizures (reproduced from Engel[70])

Classification	Hemispherectomy	Anterior temporal lobectomy	Extratemporal resection	Corpus callosum section
Total patients	88	2336	825	197
Total centres	17	40	32	16
No seizure-free	68	1296	356	10
Percentage	77·3	55·5	43·2	5·0
(range)	(0–100)	(26–80)	(0–73)	(0–13)
No improved	16	648	229	140
Percentage	18·2	27·7	27·8	71·0
No not improved	4	392	240	47
Percentage	4·5	16·8	29·1	23·9
(range)	(0–33)	(6–29)	(17–89)	(10–38)

Donabedian[79] has defined three constituents of the quality of care: structure (the instruments of care of their organisation); process (the activities of care); and outcome (the end results of care). In the United Kingdom as elsewhere there has been increasing emphasis in recent years on the need for medical audit, defined as "the systematic critical analysis of the quality of medical care...". Kessner *et al*[80] have listed several criteria that should be met if a condition is to be a useful tracer for an audit:

(1) It should have a definite functional impact (so conditions that are self limiting and for which there is no specific treatment are not useful).
(2) It should have a prevalence sufficiently high to allow collection of adequate data.
(3) It should be well defined and easy to diagnose.
(4) Its clinical course should vary with the use and effectiveness of medical care.
(5) Techniques of medical management should be well defined for at least one of prevention, diagnosis, treatment, or rehabilitation.
(6) The effect on the condition of non-medical factors should be understood.

Epilepsy represents an appropriate condition for audit as it fulfils the first two of these criteria wholly and the next three partially. We know little about the last criterion in relation to epilepsy, but can assume that it is considerable.

There has been little systematic work in developing comprehensive means of assessing quality of care in epilepsy. In the UK, government reports on services for people with epilepsy have emphasised the importance of the primary health care services, specialist epilepsy clinics, and assessment centres in the management of epilepsy, in both its medical and psychosocial dimensions. The report of the working group on services for people with epilepsy[81] stated that whereas general practitioners should normally refer all their patients with seizures to a hospital consultant for diagnosis, initial assessment, and recommendations for treatment, patients should thereafter be cared for by the general practitioner, except in specific cases where problems persist, recur, or develop.

Assessments of the process of care in epilepsy should particularly focus on issues of communications and the interpersonal aspects of care. In this respect patients' satisfaction may be seen as

---

Box 3.6   Audit of care

Process measures	*Outcome measures*
Diagnosis	
Is classification of seizures, epilepsy syndrome, and aetiology documented?	
Who made diagnosis?	What is misdiagnosis rate?
Was electroencephalography or computed tomography done?	
Are results available?	
Treatment	
Use of drugs appropriate?	
Monotherapy	
Blood level monitoring	Remission rates
Starting and stopping	
Are suitable patients considered for surgery?	Quality of life
Is there a system for shared care?	
Is there continuity of care?	
Information and support	
Counselling services available?	Patient satisfaction
Written informational materials?	Patient knowledge
Appropriate referrals	Adjustment
Education	Compliance
Employment	
Social services	
Patient organisations	

---

representing one important outcome of care, and it also speaks to the measurement of the process of care. Previous research suggests that patients' satisfaction makes a direct contribution to other important outcomes.[82] Thus patients who are less satisfied with care are less likely to comply with treatment regimens and are less likely to reattend for treatment—both factors that are important in achieving good management and control of epilepsy. With this in mind a model for the audit of care in epilepsy can be proposed, particularly examining adequacy of diagnosis, ongoing care, information provision, and psychosocial adjustment. A structure should exist that provides primary care services with the specialist expertise, investigational, and treatment facilities necessary for the population in question. Assessment of the process and outcome of care may use some of the criteria in box 3.6.

Management of epilepsy

- Stroke, cerebral tumour, and alcohol are the commonest causes of epileptic seizures but a third of cases may be genetically determined
- Diagnosis requires differentiation of epileptic seizures from non-epileptic causes of loss of consciousness, particularly syncope and pseudoseizures. Seizure type and epilepsy syndrome should be diagnosed, and any underlying cause identified and treated appropriately
- Routine interictal electroencephalography will rarely, if ever, prove or disprove a diagnosis of epilepsy
- The diagnosis is associated with increased mortality, accidental injury, psychosocial handicap, and psychiatric disorder
- Because of the profound psychosocial implications patients need to be fully informed at diagnosis
- The overall prognosis for remission is good, but 20–30% of people who develop epilepsy have a chronic intractable disorder
- Most patients respond quickly to monotherapy with an antiepileptic drug if this is appropriate for the seizure type and epilepsy syndrome
- Patients with medically refractable epilepsy should be reviewed periodically; newer drugs may benefit them and an operation may treat some satisfactorily
- Adequate care will demand contributions from and satisfactory communication between primary care and specialist services

1 Jackson JH. On the anatomical, physiological and pathological investigation of epilepsies. *West Riding Lunatic Asylum Medical Reports* 1873;**3**:3–5. Reprinted in: Taylor J, ed. *Selected writings of John Hughlings Jackson.* London: Hodder and Stoughton 1958:90–111.
2 Commission on classification and terminology of the International League Against Epilepsy. Proposal for revised clinical and electro-encephalographic classification of epileptic seizures. *Epilepsia* 1981;**22**:489–501.
3 Commission on classification and terminology of the International League Against Epilepsy. Proposal for revised classification of epilepsies and epileptic syndromes. *Epilepsia* 1989;**30**: 389–99.
4 Sander JWAS, Shorvon SD. Incidence and prevalence studies in epilepsy and their methodological problems: a review. *J Neurol Neurosurg Psychiatry* 1987;**50**:829–39.
5 Sander JWA, Hart YM, Johnson AL, Shorvon SD. National general practice study of epilepsy: newly diagnosed epileptic seizures in a general population. *Lancet* 1990;**336**: 1267–71.
5a Anderson VE, Hauser WA, Rich SS. Genetic heterogeneity in the epilepsies. *Adv Neurol* 1986;**44**:59.
6 Griffin J, Wyles M. *Epilepsy towards tomorrow.* London: Office of Health Economics, 1991.
7 Howell SJL, Owen L, Chadwick DW. Pseudostatus epilepticus. *Q J Med* 1989;**266**:507–19.
8 Young AC, Bog Costanzi J, Mohr PD, Forbes W. Is routine computerised axial tomography in epilepsy worthwhile? *Lancet* 1982;**ii**:1446–7.
9 Mittan R, Locke G. Fear of seizures: epilepsy's forgotten problem. *Urban Health* 1982;Jan/Feb:40–1.

10 Hauser WA, Hesdorffer DC. *Epilepsy: frequency, causes and consequences.* New York: Demos Publications, 1990.

11 Hauser WA, Annegers JF, Elverback LR. Mortality of patients with epilepsy. *Epilepsy* 1980; **21**:339–412.

12 Neuspiel DR, Kuller LH. Sudden and unexpected natural death in childhood and adolescence. *JAMA* 1985;**254**:1321–5.

13 Leestma JE, Kalelkar MB, Teas SS, *et al.* Sudden unexpected death associated with seizures: analysis of 66 cases. *Epilepsia* 1984;**25**:84–8.

14 Hauser WA, Rich SS, Jacobs MP, Anderson VE. Patterns of seizure occurrence and recurrent risks in patients with newly diagnosed epilepsy. *Abstracts of 15th Epilepsy International Symposium.* Hartford, CT: American Epilepsy Society, 1983:16.

15 Russell-Jones DL, Shorvon SD. The frequency and consequences of head injury in epileptic seizures. *J Neurol Neurosurg Psychiatry* 1989;**52**:659–62.

16 Bhatnagar SK, Srivastava JL, Gupta JL. Burns: a complication of epilepsy. *Burns* 1977;**3**: 93–5.

17 Hampton KK, Peatfield RC, Pullar T, Bodansky HJK, Walton C, Feely M. Burns because of epilepsy. *BMJ* 1988;**296**:1659–60.

18 Dodrill CB, Batzel L, Queisser HR, Temkin NR. An objective method for the assessment of psychological and social problems among epileptics. *Epilepsia* 1980;**21**:123–35.

19 Masland RL. Psychosocial aspects of epilepsy. In: Porter EJ, Morselli PL, eds. *The epilepsies.* London: Butterworths, 1988:356–77.

20 Betts TA. Depression, anxiety and epilepsy. In: Reynolds EH, Trimble MR, eds. *Epilepsy and psychiatry.* Edinburgh: Churchill Livingstone, 1981: 60–71.

21 Lechtenberg R. *Epilepsy and the family.* Cambridge, MA: Harvard University Press, 1984.

22 Garber J, Seligman M, eds. *Human helplessness: theory and application.* New York: Academic Press, 1980.

23 Pond D, Bidwell BH. A survey of epilepsy in fourteen general practices. *Epilepsia* 1959;**1**: 285–99.

24 Gudmundsson G. Epilepsy in Iceland. *Acta Neurol Scand* 1966;**43**(suppl 25):1–124.

25 Edeh J, Toone B. Relationship between interictal psychopathology and type of epilepsy: results of a survey in general practice. *Br J Psychiatry* 1987;**151**:95–101.

26 Currie S, Heathfield KWG, Henson RA, Scott DF. Clinical course and prognosis of temporal lobe epilepsy: a survey of 666 patients. *Brain* 1971;**94**:173–90.

27 Bruens JH. Psychoses in epilepsy. In: Vinkin PL, Bruyn LW, eds. *Handbook of clinical neurology.* Amsterdam: North Holland, 1974;**15**:593–610.

28 Slater E, Beard AW, Glithero E. The schizophrenia-like psychoses of epilepsy. *Br J Psychiatry* 1963;**109**:5–150.

29 Perez MM, Trimble MR. Epileptic psychosis—diagnostic comparison with process schizophrenia. *Br J Psychiatry* 1980;**146**:155–64.

30 Barraclough B. Suicide and epilepsy. In: Reynolds E, Trimble M, eds. *Epilepsy and psychiatry.* Edinburgh: Churchill Livingstone, 1980:72–6.

31 Annegers JF, Hauser WA, Elverback LR. Remission of seizures and relapse in patients with epilepsy. *Epilepsia* 1979;**20**:729–37.

32 Goodridge DMG, Shorvon SD. Epileptic seizures in a population of 6000: II—treatment and prognosis. *BMJ* 1983;**287**:645–7.

33 Turnbull DM, Howell D, Rawlins MD, Chadwick DW. Which drug for the adult epileptic patient: phenytoin or valproate? *BMJ* 1985;**290**:815–9.

34 Reynolds EH. Early treatment and prognosis of epilepsy. *Epilepsia* 1987;**28**:97–106.

35 Sofijanov NG. Clinical evolution and prognosis of childhood epilepsies. *Epilepsia* 1982;**23**: 61–9.

35a Group for the study of the prognosis of epilepsy in Japan. Natural history and prognosis of epilepsy: report of a multi-institutional study in Japan. *Epilepsia* 1981;**22**:35–53.

36 Juul-Jensen P. Epilepsy. A clinical and social analysis of 1020 adult patients with epileptic seizures. *Acta Neurol Scand* 1964;**40**(suppl 5):1–285.

37 Rodin EA. *The prognosis of patients with epilepsy.* Springfield, IL: Charles C Thomas, 1968.

38 Rowan AJ, French JA. The role of the electroencephalogram in the diagnosis and management of epilepsy. *Recent Advances in Epilepsy* 1988;**4**:63–92.

39 Shafer SQ, Hauser WA, Annegers JF, Klass DW. EEG and other early predictors of epilepsy remission: a community study. *Epilepsia* 1988;**29**:590–600.

40 Foy PM, Copeland GP, Shaw MDM. The incidence of postoperative seizures. *Acta Neurochir (Wein)* 1981;**55**:253–264.

41 Temkin NR, Dikmen SS, Wilesnky AJ, *et al*. A randomized, double-blind study of phenytoin for the prevention of post-traumatic seizures. *N Engl J Med* 1990;**323**:497–502.

42 Foy PM, Chadwick DW, Rajgopalan N, *et al*. Do prophylactic anticonvulsant drugs alter the pattern of seizures following craniotomy. *J Neurol Neurosurg Psychiatry* 1992;**55**:753–7.

43 Chadwick D, Shaw MDM, Foy P, Rawlins MD, Turnbull DM. Serum anticonvulsant concentrations and the risk of drug induced skin eruptions. *J Neurol Neurosurg Psychiatry* 1984;**47**:642–4.

44 McQueen JK, Blackwood DH, Harris P, *et al*. Low risk of late post-traumatic seizures following severe head injury: implications for clinical trials of prophylaxis. *J Neurol Neurosurg Psychiatry* 1983;**46**:899–904.

45 Reynolds EH, Shorvon SD, Galbraith AW, *et al*. Phenytoin monotherapy for epilepsy: a long-term prospective study, assisted by serum level monitoring, in previously untreated patients. *Epilepsia* 1981;**22**:475–88.

46 Chadwick D, Turnbull EH. The comparative efficacy of antiepileptic drugs for partial and tonic-clonic seizures. *J Neurol Neurosurg Psychiatry* 1985;**48**:1073–7.

47 Suzuki M, Maruyama H, Ishibashi Y, *et al*. A double-blind comparative trial of sodium dipropylacetate and ethosuximide in epilepsy in children with special emphasis on pure petit mal seizures. *Medical Progress* 1972;**82**:470–488. (In Japanese.)

48 Callaghan N, O'Hare J, O'Driscoll D, *et al*. Comparative study of ethosuximide and sodium valproate in the treatment of typical absence seizures (petit mal). *Dev Med Child Neurol* 1982;**24**:830–6.

49 Delgado-Escueta AV, Enrile-Bascal F. Juvenile myoclonic epilepsy of Janz. *Neurology* 1984;**34**:285–94.

50 Mattson RH, Cramer JA, Collins JF, *et al*. Comparison of carbamazepine, phenobarbital, phenytoin and primidone in partial and secondary generalised tonic-clonic seizures. *N Engl J Med* 1985;**313**:145–51.

51 Mattson RH, Cramer JA, Collins JF, *et al*. A comparison of valproate with carbamazepine for the treatment of complex partial seizures with secondarily generalized tonic-clonic seizures in adults. *N Engl J Med* 1992;**327**:765–71.

51a Brodie M, Richens A, Yuen AWC. Double blind comparison of lamotrigine and carbamazepine in newly diagnosed epilepsy. *Lancet* 1995;**345**:476–9.

52 Heller AJ, Chesterman P, Elwes RDC, *et al*. Phenobarbitone, phenytoin, carbamazepine, or sodium valproate for newly diagnosed adult epilepsy. *J Neurol Neurosurg Psychiatry* 1995;**58**:44–50.

53 Schmidt D. *Adverse effects of antiepileptic drugs*. New York: Raven Press, 1982.

54 Chadwick D, Reynods EH, Marsden CD. Anticonvulsant induced dyskinesias: a comparison with dyskinesias induced by neuroleptics. *J Neurol Neurosurg Psychiatry* 1976;**39**:1210–8.

55 Turnbull DM, Rawlins MD, Weightman D, Chadwick DW. Plasma concentrations of sodium valproate: their clinical value. *Ann Neurol* 1983;**14**:38–42.

56 Dreifuss FE, Santilli N, Langer DH, *et al*. Valproic acid fatalities: a retrospective review. *Neurology* 1987;**37**:379–85.

57 Sander JWAS, Trevisol-Bittencourt PC, Hart YM, Shorvon SD. Evaluation of vigabatrin as an add-on drug in the management of severe epilepsy. *J Neurol Neurosurg Psychiatry* 1990;**53**:1008–10.

57a Chadwick D, Cartlidge A, Bates D. *Medical neurology*. Edinburgh: Churchill Livingstone, 1989.

58 Lindhout D, Schmidt D. In-utero exposure to valproate and neural tube defects. *Lancet* 1986;**i**:392–3.

59 Rosa FH. Spina bifida in maternal carbamazepine exposure cohort data. *Teratology* 1990;**41**:587–8.

60 Crawford PM, Chadwick D. A comparative study of progabide, valproate and placebo as add-on therapy in patients with refractory epilepsy. *J Neurol Neurosurg Psychiatry* 1986;**49**:1251–7.

61 Richens A, Dunlop A. Serum phenytoin levels in the management of epilepsy. *Lancet* 1975;**ii**:247–9.

62 Rowan AJ, Binnie CD, Warfield CA, *et al*. The delayed effect of sodium valproate on the photoconvulsive response in man. *Epilepsia* 1979;**20**:61–8.

63 Gannaway DJ, Mawer GE. Serum phenytoin concentrations and clinical response in patients with epilepsy. *Br J Clin Pharmacol* 1981;**12**:833–9.

64 Knott C, Williams CP, Reynolds F. Phenytoin kinetics during pregnancy and the puerperium. *Br J Obstet Gynaecol* 1986;**93**:1030–70.

65 Chadwick D. Concentration effect relationships of valproate. *Clin Pharmacokinet* 1985;**10**: 155–63.

66 Pedley TA. Discontinuing antiepileptic drugs. *N Engl J Med* 1988;**318**:982–4.

67 Medical Research Council Antiepileptic Drug Withdrawal Study Group. (Chadwick D, clinical co-ordinator). Randomized study of antiepileptic drug withdrawal in patients in remission. *Lancet* 1991;**337**:1175–80.

68 Medical Research Council Antiepileptic Drug Withdrawal Study Group. (Chadwick D, clinical co-ordinator). Prognostic index for recurrence of seizures after remission of epilepsy. *BMJ* 1993;**306**:1374–8.

69 Dreifuss FE. Goals of surgery for epilepsy. In: Engel J, ed. *Surgical treatment of the epilepsies.* New York: Raven Press, 1987:31–50.

70 Engel J. Outcome with respect to epileptic seizures. In: Engel J, ed. *Surgical treatment of the epilepsies.* New York: Raven Press, 1987:553–72.

71 Duncan JS, Sagar HJ. Characteristics, pathology and outcome after temporal lobectomy. *Neurology* 1987;**37**:405–9.

72 Oxbury JM, Adams CBT. Neurosurgery for epilepsy. *Br J Hosp Med* 1989;**41**:372–7.

73 Crandall PH. Cortical resections. In: Engel J, ed. *Surgical treatment of epilepsies.* New York: Raven Press, 1987:377–404.

74 Falconer MA, Hill D, Meyer A, *et al.* Treatment of temporal lobe epilepsy by temporal lobectomy. A survey of findings and results. *Lancet* 1955;**1**:827–35.

75 Yasargil MG, Wieser HG. Selective amygdalohippocampectomy at the University Hospital, Zurich. In: Engel J, ed. *Surgical treatment of the epilepsies.* New York: Raven Press, 1987: 653–8.

76 Quesney LF. Seizures of frontal lobe origin. In: Pedley TA, Meldrum BS, eds. *Recent advances in epilepsy.* Edinburgh: Churchill Livingstone, 1986;**3**:81–110.

77 Adams CBT. Hemispherectomy—a modification. *J Neurol Neurosurg Psychiatry* 1983;**46**: 617–9.

78 Spencer SS, Gates JR, Reeves AT, *et al.* Corpus callosum section. In: Engel, J, ed. *Surgical treatment of the epilepsies.* New York: Raven Press, 1987:425–44.

79 Donabedian A. Evaluating the quality of medical care. *Milbank Memorial Fund Quarterly,* 1966;**44**(suppl):166–206.

80 Kessner DM, Kalk CE, Singer J. Assessing health quality: the case for tracers. *N Engl J Med* 1977;**189**:194.

81 Department of Health and Social Security. *Report of the working group on services for people with epilepsy.* London: HMSO, 1986.

82 Fitzpatrick R. Measurement of patient satisfaction. In: Hopkins A, Costain D, eds. *Measuring the outcome of medical care.* London: Royal College of Physicians, 1990.

4 Head injury

GRAHAM M TEASDALE

The problems posed by head injuries are vast, varied, and vexed. One million patients attend hospital in the United Kingdom every year; they present a wide range of types and severities of injury and sequelae; and there is much controversy, particularly between different specialties, about the appropriate procedures for management from acute to late stages. Head injuries are a major health problem because of their peak occurrence in young men; they account for many years of potential loss of life in people aged up to 65 years and (for many people) for lifelong disability. There are estimated to be as many people neurologically disabled due to head injury as due to stroke. No single approach to management can cater for the needs of all patients and their families, but a reasonable, rational approach follows from a consideration of the nature of head injuries and their consequences, of the scale of the problem, of the methods of treatment, and of the personnel and facilities available.

Definition

A practical operational definition, used in surveys in Scotland, incorporates a definite history of a blow to the head, a laceration of the scalp or head, or altered consciousness no matter how brief.[1] Unfortunately the International Classification of Diseases gives no single code for head injury, which is covered by up to 10 rubrics that are not mutually exclusive and that are related to pathological rather than clinical features. This has greatly limited the collection of reliable statistics, except as part of special surveys, but the 10th edition does include an assessment of the duration of unconsciousness.

88

Epidemiology

The best guide to the incidence of head injury is the number of patients presenting to the hospital after injury, in Scotland 1976 per 100 000 a year,[2] in the United Kingdom a total of nearly one million a year.[3] Almost half of these are children under 15, and males outnumber females by more than two to one. Most injuries (41%) are due to a fall and many (20%) to an assault. The importance of road traffic accidents increases with the severity of injury; they cause only 13% in those attending hospital, but account for a third of patients transferred to neurosurgery and 58% of deaths. Less than one adult in five and less than one child in 10 is admitted to hospital, an overall rate in Scotland of 313 per 100 000 a year.[1] For all ages, the death rate from head injury in the United Kingdom is nine per 100 000 a year; this accounts for 1% of all deaths but for 15–20% in people aged between 5 and 35. Death rates from head injury are already declining in road users as a reflection of existing preventive measures, and further reductions should follow the increasing use of air bags.

Traumatic brain damage

Brain damage after head injury can be classified by pattern and by time course. The patterns of damage recognised by pathologists and, increasingly by imaging in life, are essentially separated into focal and diffuse varieties (box 4.1). It must be accepted that in many patients the most accurate description may be of a multifocal distribution—for example, multiple cortical contusions or multiple ischaemic lesions. In the time course, the differentiation is between primary damage—developing at the moment of impact—and secondary damage due to the subsequent complications, which may be intracranial or extracranial insults (box 4.2). Classification can also be based on mechanisms of injury—for example, missile v non-missile—and on whether or not there is a compound fracture, and an open or closed injury.

Diffuse axonal injury is the single most important lesion in traumatic brain damage.[4] It is thought to be responsible for the extent of the impairment of consciousness in the acute stage and to account for much of the disability experienced by survivors in the later stages after all types of injury.[5] It consists of scattered damage and division of axons throughout the white matter of

89

Box 4.1 Lesions causing focal or diffuse patterns of damage after head injury

Lesions causing focal patterns	*Lesions causing diffuse patterns*
Contusion	Axonal injury
Haematoma	Hypoxia or ischaemia
Extradural	Diffuse vascular
Subdural	Fat embolism
Intracerebral	Subarachnoid haemorrhage
Swelling	Meningitis
Infarct	
Pressure necrosis	
Abscess	

Box 4.2 Complications after head injury that cause secondary insults to the damaged brain

Intracranial complications	*Systemic complications*
Haematoma	Hypoxia
Swelling	Hypercarbia
Raised intracranial pressure	Hypotension
Vasospasm	Severe hypocarbia
Infection	Fever
Epilepsy	Anaemia
Hydrocephalus	Hyponatraemia

---

the brain. Injury to individual axons can be recognised only by microscopy on fatal cases—silver stains show "retraction balls" which represent swollen blobs of axoplasm. These lesions are distributed centripetally and, with increasing injury, extend from the subcortical white matter into the centrum semiovale, internal capsule, and brain stem. In more severe cases, they are accompanied by haemorrhage from small macroscopic tissue tears. These are located typically in the parasagittal subcortical white matter—previously called a gliding contusion—the corpus callosum, the superior cerebellar peduncle, and the dorsolateral aspect of the brain stem. These lesions can be recognised on the cut surface of the brain in fatal cases, and are now being detected in many patients in life by computed tomography or magnetic resonance imaging.[6 7]

Ischaemic brain damage is by far the most common secondary insult[8] and is still found in more than 80% of fatal cases, despite modern intensive management.[9] The frequency of ischaemic damage is contributed to by impairment, as a consequence of injury, of the normal regulating mechanisms by which cerebral vascular responses maintain an adequate supply of oxygen.[10 11] The frequency of secondary ischaemic insults, particularly in patients with other injuries, has been highlighted by recent findings made by analysing continuous monitoring.[12–14] In a series of patients with varying severity of head injury, 92% were found to have one or more insults lasting for at least five minutes, despite being in a well equipped and staffed intensive care unit.

Primary and secondary traumatic brain damage are becoming less easy to differentiate. Thus it is recognised that axonal injury, once thought to occur at the moment of impact and be irreversible, may in fact evolve from a partial injury, in continuity, to complete disruption over some hours.[15] The sequence includes unfolding of the axolemma, loss of membrane properties, damage to the cytoskeleton, and interruption of axoplasmic flow leading to local swelling and then disruption. Also, secondary damage from insults such as hypoxia may occur within minutes, before even paramedical roadside attention, and merge with the damage resulting from the biomechanical forces acting at the moment of injury. Nevertheless, the distinction is still a useful clinical concept and underlines the importance of focusing management on the avoidance or reversal of secondary events.

Clinically the processes of primary and secondary damage are reflected in three principle patterns of change, each with implications for management. (1) Patients lose consciousness or develop other neurological features at the time of injury, but their condition improves as time passes; this correlates with damage that is principally primary from which natural recovery is taking place. (2) Patients do not lose consciousness at the moment of injury but their condition then deteriorates or (having lost consciousness initially) then begins to worsen; each of these signals the development of secondary damage and demands immediate action. (3) Features of brain damage develop at the moment of or soon after injury and persist without change; such patients may go on to show natural recovery but are also at increased risk of secondary complications.

Many of the issues in early treatment of head injuries concern the appropriate approach to investigation and management of these cases. The issues facing the clinician, therefore, are how severely injured the patient already is, and what the risks are of future deterioration and increased damage.

Classification: severity

Much of the confusion—scientific, clinical, and medico-legal—that clouds discussion and fuels controversy about head injuries can be traced to variations and discrepancies between different approaches to classification of severity of injuries. It is therefore important to discuss the purposes of classification and the approaches that are used; clarification of the confusion and the adoption generally of a coherent, consistent approach should lead to more fruitful discussion and agreement.

The first purpose of classification of severity is to help manage the acute stage: the critical factors are the patient's condition on arrival at hospital, how this is changing, and what complications can be expected. The second purpose is to assess the potential for recovery, after initial assessment and acute management have been completed—when the continuing assessment of the depth and duration of neurological impairment is of primary interest. The third concerns the interrelation between the injury and late sequelae. Here the total quantum of injury is important, both initial and due to subsequent complications, and early severity is often assessed retrospectively—for example, by duration of amnesia. This is particularly relevant to medicolegal issues. The difference in perceptions between those who have seen the patient at the acute stage (accident and emergency consultants, general and orthopaedic surgeons, and neurosurgeons) and those who usually become involved only later in the assessment of sequelae (neurologists, psychologists, and psychiatrists) reflect these varying standpoints.

Coma, concussion, amnesia

Changes in consciousness provide the basis of most approaches to the classification of severity;[16] this reflects the importance of

Box 4.3 Glasgow coma scale, coma score, and modifications for children under 5

In adults (score in normal adults is 15):

Eye opening response:

Spontaneously	4
To speech	3
To pain	2
None	1

Best motor response (of arms):

Obeys commands	6
Localisation to painful stimuli	5
Normal flexion to painful stimuli	4
Spastic flexion to painful stimuli	3
Extension to painful stimuli	2
None	1

Best verbal response:

Oriented	5
Confused	4
Inappropriate words	3
Incomprehensible sounds	2
None	1

Modifications of normal responses in children under 5

	Best motor response	Best verbal response
<6 months	Flexion	Smiles and cries
6–12 months	Localisation	Smiles and cries
1–2 years	Localisation	Sounds and words
2–5 years	Obeys commands	Words and phrases

diffuse axonal injury in the initial events and in causing later sequelae. The Glasgow coma scale (box 4.3) separately assesses eye, verbal, and motor performance.[17] This separation, which is appropriate conceptually (because each may change independently) and very convenient in practice, may have contributed to the wide acceptance of the Glasgow approach. The temptation, however, to summate the scores of the different components into an overall coma score ranging from 3–15 could not be resisted[18 19] and the total "coma score" now provides the most widely used basis for classification (table 4.1).[20] Nevertheless, its use needs critical review

Table 4.1 Classification of head injuries by the Glasgow coma score (GCS) into severe, moderate, mild, and minor

		% of patients		% with multiple injury	Risk of ICH in		Dead (%)
	GCS on arrival	Attended	Admitted		All patients	Fracture patients	
Minor	15	95	42 ⎱	32	1:10 000	1:100	<1
Mild	13/14 ⎱	4	38 ⎰	37	1:380	1:15	3–5
Moderate	9–12 ⎰	1	13	63	1:50	1:8	9
Severe	3–8		7				35–40

ICH = intracerebral haematoma.

and some redefinition may be necessary, particularly in less severe injuries,[21] even if this is at the price of some initial controversy.

The most widely definition for severe head injury is now a patient with a Glasgow coma score of 3–8. Originally, the definition used in the international studies coordinated from Glasgow,[22 23] was that the patient was in a coma for six hours, coma being defined as no eye opening, no comprehensible verbal response, and not obeying commands.[24] In some 80% of cases the notation for coma translates into a coma score of 8 or less, hence the adoption of the score. The six hour duration has become difficult to apply because people with severe head injuries are now almost uniformly sedated, intubated, and ventilated and are hence unassessable for many hours, and initial severity is usually assessed by the findings on admission.

Moderate head injury was defined as a patient with a coma score of 9–12.[25] This group until recently did not receive as much attention as either the severe or lesser injuries. The group may be difficult to identify consistently and the definition needs scrutiny before much further work is carried out.[26]

The most unsatisfactory definition is of mild or even minor head injury as a patient with a Glasgow coma score of 13–15.[27] The problem is that patients with a coma score of 15 make up by far the overwhelming majority of patients classified in this group.[27 28] In practice, a patient with a coma score of 15, compared with those with scores of 13 or 14, has a much lower risk of complications at the acute stage[29 30] and fewer and less persistent subsequent sequelae. The inclusion within the same category of all patients with a coma score of 13–15 underestimates the true severity of the injury in patients with scores of 13 or 14. It also gives an impression of undue seriousness to those with a coma score of 15. It is more appropriate to separate out patients with a coma score of 15 and refer to these as having had a minor injury.

Description of severity in later stages is based on the duration of alteration in consciousness—either of observed coma or of amnesia.[31] The duration of amnesia after the injury—post-traumatic amnesia—is a widely accepted index. It may be difficult to estimate precisely and is best regarded as a logarithmic scale: very mild, less than five minutes; mild, five to 60 minutes; moderate, one of 24 hours; severe, one to seven days; very severe—one to four weeks; extremely severe, more than four weeks.[16 32]

The classification of severity based solely on changes of consciousness may sometimes overlook the importance of focal injury. Computed tomography and magnetic resonance imaging show that cortical contusions can occur in the absence of prolonged unconsciousness but lead to prolonged confusion and sequelae, such as memory impairment and epilepsy.[33]

Prevention

Prevention is possible at three stages: forestalling the accident; minimising the degree of injury occurring on impact; and reducing the risk of secondary complications—the focus of medical management in the acute stage. Accident prevention requires modification of behaviour by the public and is effective usually only when enforced by legislation. The introduction of speed limits, the use of safety belts by vehicle occupants, and the wearing of helmets by motor cyclists have all proved effective. More stringent limits on the alcohol level allowed in drivers and the universal use of air bags, with rigorous enforcement, could further contribute to a reduction in injuries due to road accidents. This would leave alcohol still a major contributor to injuries from assaults and falls and in pedestrian victims of road accidents. There is increasing evidence that the wearing of helmets by cyclists prevents injuries, but this remains to be backed up by legislation. The dangers of brain damage from boxing are well recognised.[34] What doctors should do is to emphasise the inadequacy of current prefight medical examinations in minimising the risk and to point to the long term dangers, highlighted by the increasing evidence of a biological connection between head injury and dementia.[35]

Diagnosis

Two questions need to be answered in every suspected head injury: is it a head injury, and is it only a head injury? There is little doubt about the occurrence of a head injury when a clear history is available from either the victim or an onlooker. Difficulties arise in the person presenting with impaired consciousness of unknown onset and duration, especially when there is evidence of alcohol intake. There is compelling evidence that when in doubt it is safer to regard the victim as having a head injury than to attribute impaired consciousness to alcohol ingestion or, in the old person with focal signs, to the effects of a stroke.[36] Confirmation of an injury to the head may come from careful clinical examination or from the result of a skull radiograph. Conversely, when a patient with head injury has impaired consciousness, there is a temptation to focus too much attention to the head and to overlook important injuries elsewhere.[37] The initial clinical examination should note carefully any abnormal neurological symptoms or signs as a reference point for comparison with subsequent examinations and interviews. The niceties of the comprehensive neurological examination are, however, of considerably less relevance than regular reliable assessments of consciousness.

Management of head injury

The essence of management of head injury is the provision of optimum circumstances for recovery from damage already sustained—principally primary damage—and the avoidance of the development or exacerbation of damage due to complications—principally secondary damage. In the acute stage natural recovery can be expected in most patients with minor, mild, or moderate injury. The focus in these patients is therefore on identifying patients at risk of secondary complications, principally a traumatic haematoma. The patient with a severe head injury who is in a coma has both evidence of already having sustained a substantial amount of brain damage and also a much greater risk of both intracranial and extracranial complications.

Assessment, diagnosis, investigation, observation, monitoring, treatment, and rehabilitation each have a crucial part in the management of head injury. The diversity of injuries and variations in resources available mean that there is not a single approach that is optimum for all victims. On the other hand, attempts to tailor management to each individual patient, based on a process of deduction and deliberation, does not provide effective care for head injuries. Instead, as with all trauma, an approach based on a series of recommendations, criteria, or guidelines is both more efficient and effective. These permit an approach that is consistent between cases and between centres, they reduce confusion, enhance communication, and improve outcome.[38 39] Widely accepted approaches to head injury management have been reviewed recently.[40-43]

Assessment

The approach to assessment varies with the perceived severity of injury. When the patient has impaired consciousness, assessment and resuscitation must follow the principles of life support, as it is taught in the advanced trauma life support (ATLS) system.[44] The identification and correction of an obstructed airway, inadequate ventilation, or shock must take priority over the detailed assessment of the patient's neurological state.[43]

Assessment can begin at the roadside, and ambulance staff can now evaluate patients on the Glasgow coma scale and report the level of blood pressure and heart rate. Unfortunately, many patients still arrive at specialised units either from the scene of an accident or from another hospital with hypoxia, shock, or other factors that worsen prognosis.[45] On arrival at hospital, assessment and resuscitation must be completed before the patient is moved for further investigation or treatment. The temptation to focus on the head and carry out premature computed tomography or other investigations must be resisted in favour of a proper, thorough, general survey and management.[46]

Assessment of the patient's neurological state is quickly and effectively carried out with the Glasgow coma scale for overall consciousness, noting any side to side differences in limb movement to detect hemiparesis or other focal neurological deficit, and examining the pupil size and response to light.[18] The eye opening, verbal, and motor responses of the Glasgow coma scale are well known and can be modified for application to children under 5 years old.[47] Neurological assessment should be repeated and documented often (at least every 10 minutes) during the first hour and then afterwards according to progress. The findings are a valid guide to the extent of brain damage only when the patient is adequately oxygenated and has a normal blood pressure. Any deterioration is a signal to seek complications such as hypoxia, hypotension, or intracranial haematoma.

Investigation: radiology

Computed tomography proved its clinical value rapidly in the diagnosis of intracranial complications after head injury.[48] Despite its advantages in diagnosis, however, improvement in the outcome of head injury occurred only when the availability of computed tomography was allied to policies aimed at ensuring investigation at an earlier stage, preferably before the occurrence of neurological deterioration.[38] Magnetic resonance imaging is more sensitive to parenchymal abnormalities,[7 49] but the greater availability and practicability of computed tomography make it still the mainstay of acute investigation of head injury, and still where its value in improving outcome is most clear.

The issue that computed tomography brought into clear focus, and that continues to be controversial, is the triage of patients; what is the optimum match between the number of computed tomograms that it is feasible to carry out and the likelihood that the investigation will contribute to management?

Guidelines for selection of patients for computed tomography were first promulgated a decade ago, when scanners were largely restricted to neurosurgical units.[50 51] More recently the increasing availability of scanners in general hospitals has led to a reappraisal and a widening of the criteria for scanning (box 4.4).[30] Unfortunately, the opportunity provided by the availability of computed tomography[52] in many hospitals is often not turned to the advantage of patients with head injury because access to the scanner is limited to the normal working day, whereas most injuries occur at nights and at weekends. When this is the case, neurologists and neurosurgeons should press for the establishment of an "out of hours service" with, if necessary, image transfer for consultation with the neurosurgical unit. Without an emergency service, the restricted availability of the scanner in a general hospital can lead to inappropriate delay before the patient is investigated—and a delay in the diagnosis of remediable intracranial complications.[53]

It is neither feasible nor desirable that all patients with head injuries should undergo computed tomography. Instead, there is now evidence from several studies that the factors that identify the likelihood of a patient having either an abnormal scan or a remediable intracranial lesion can be deduced from clinical features.[30 31 54] The key factors are the depth and duration of alteration of consciousness, the result of a skull radiograph (fig 4.1) and, in a few cases, the presence of focal neurological signs. In the past, when scanning required neurosurgical transfer, this could be advocated only in patients with both impaired consciousness and a skull fracture—in whom the risk of haematoma was as high as one in four.[51] It is now more reasonable that all patients with persisting impairment of consciousness after arrival

---

Box 4.4   Indications for computed tomography and referral of recently head injured patients (from Teasdale et al[30])

Indications for referral to neurosurgical unit

Without preliminary computed tomography
- Coma persisting after resuscitation
- Deteriorating consciousness or progressive focal neurological deficits
- Open injury: depressed fracture of vault or basal skull fracture
- Patient fulfils criteria for computed tomography in a general hospital when this cannot be performed within a reasonable time—for example, three to four hours

After computed tomography in general hospital
- Abnormal tomogram (after neurosurgical opinion on images transferred electronically)
- Tomogram considered to be normal but patient's progress is unsatisfactory

Indications for computed tomography in general hospitals

- Full consciousness but with a skull fracture
- Confusion persisting after initial assessment and resuscitation
- Unstable systemic state precluding transfer to neurosurgery
- Diagnosis uncertain

---

at hospital are considered for computed tomography (fig 4.2).[30] In the patient in a coma, scanning should follow transfer to the regional neurosurgical unit; in the patient with a coma score between 9 and 14 whose condition does not return to normal within one or two hours of injury, scanning should be carried out locally.

Skull radiographs can be omitted from initial assessment if computed tomography is to be carried out. A skull radiograph, however, retains an important place in the investigation of patients who are fully conscious, in whom the finding of a skull fracture raises the risk of intracranial complications by more than 200-fold. Computed tomography should be performed if a skull fracture is present. The use of scanning in all cases is unjustified, because of the greater radiation exposure (some twofold) and the greater cost (twofold to fourfold) than with a skull radiograph.

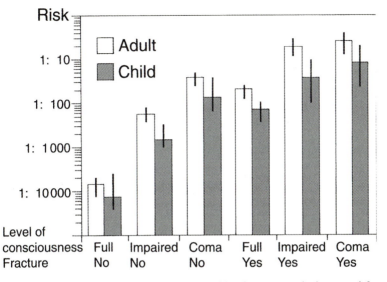

Figure 4.1 *The effect on increasing the risk of a traumatic intracranial haematoma of age, a skull fracture, and impaired consciousness and coma. (Based on data from Teasdale, Murray, Anderson, et al[30]).*

Skull radiographs still have value in detecting fluid levels in the sphenoid sinus, intracranial air, or depressed skull fracture—each of which signals an open injury and the risk of intracranial infection. Indications for skull radiographs include high or medium velocity impact with a broad hard surface[55] and association with other features, such as post-traumatic amnesia, leakage of CSF, or bleeding from the nose or ears, a large scalp haematoma, or laceration. In the unconscious patient, radiographs should also include films of the cervical spine, chest, and any areas suspected of having associated fractures.

Clinical observation

The twin purposes of observation and monitoring are to assess the pattern of change is a patient's neurological state and to detect complications. The intensity of observation and monitoring is therefore determined by the extent of any existing brain damage and the perceived risk of deterioration.

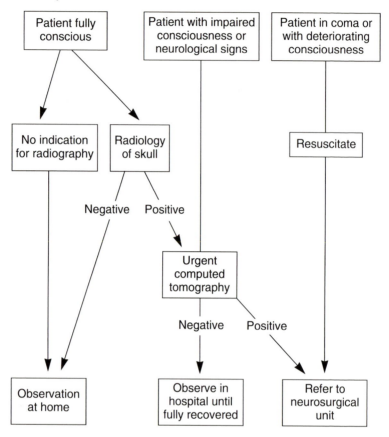

Figure 4.2   *Flow chart for managing patients with head injuries according to level of consciousness and skull radiograph and computed tomogram findings in district general hospitals and regional neurosurgical units (from Teasdale, Murray, Anderson, et al[30]).*

For the patient who is conscious and who does not have a skull fracture, the decision is whether or not to admit to hospital for observation. At least four out of five patients are discharged for observation at home, and the proportion of patients admitted can be reduced further without adverse effects.[36][57] Every accident and emergency department dealing with head injuries should have an established policy, clearly displayed and widely known. Box 4.5 shows accepted indications for admission. Patients who are conscious and have no skull fracture can be discharged for

102

Box 4.5   Indications for admission for observation of head injuries

The following list of indications for admission of patients with head injuries should be displayed in accident and emergency departments:

- Confusion or any other depression of consciousness at the time of the examination
- Skull fracture
- Neurological symptoms or signs, or both
- Difficulty in assessing the patient—for example, because of ingestion of alcohol, epilepsy, or other medical conditions that cloud consciousness; children are also difficult to assess
- Lack of a responsible adult to supervise the patient at home or other social problems
- Brief amnesia after trauma with full recovery is not necessarily an indication for admission
- If the patient is to be observed outside hospital he or she should be discharged with a head injury "warning card" into the care of a responsible person

---

observation under the care of a relative or responsible adult, who should be given a list of instructions in the form of a "warning card" about what to observe and what to do. In such low risk cases, admission to hospital confers no advantage when a haematoma does develop.[58]

In the patient who has impaired consciousness but is still talking, assessments of consciousness should be repeated every one to two hours. Cardiovascular, respiratory, and other "vital functions" can be assessed by customary clinical methods, with recordings made intermittently. The more severe the impairment of consciousness, however, the more likely it is that these traditional methods will fail to disclose important deviations from values that ensure satisfactory cerebral perfusion and oxygenation and the greater the indication for continuous and invasive methods.

Monitoring

Detailed continuous monitoring is needed in all patients who are not obeying commands, or who have a head injury and other

---

Box 4.6 Monitoring techniques used in severely head injured patients (*from Della Corte*[59])

Routine techniques	*Selective techniques*
Glasgow coma score	Intracranial pressure
Pupils	Cerebral perfusion pressure
Temperature	Central venous or pulmonary artery pressure
Arterial oxygen saturation	Electroencephalogram
End tidal carbon dioxide	Jugular bulb oxygen saturation
Arterial blood pressure	Transcranial doppler
Electrolytes and haematology	Computed tomography to be used on admission to hospital and postoperatively (24 hrs and 72 hrs) if intracranial pressure is raised or there is clinical deterioration

---

serious injuries (box 4.6). Arterial pressure should be monitored, using an indwelling arterial cannula to provide a continuous record. This will provide access for intermittent measurements of blood gases, as indicated by the results of continuous monitoring of arterial oxygen saturation using pulse oximetry. An electrocardiogram should be monitored continuously, and monitoring central venous or pulmonary artery blood pressure may be indicated when shock has occurred or is suspected. In a ventilated patient, the measurement of end tidal carbon dioxide with a capnograph is a useful check on the adequacy of ventilation, supplemented by the controls built into modern ventilator systems.

The role of monitoring intracranial pressure in head injuries is still controversial. Although it is not used in all units dealing with severe head injuries, it has at least two clear benefits.[42] The first is in providing an indication of severity of space-occupying effects from a focal intracranial lesion. The second, when coupled with arterial pressure measurements, is in calculating cerebral perfusion pressure, the critical determinant of overall cerebral blood flow. All techniques are to a degree invasive, however, and have a risk of intracranial infection of 2–8% and of causing intracranial haemorrhage (<1%) and epilepsy (1%).

The value of monitoring intracranial pressure in the management of a patient with an intracranial clot became established when it became apparent that computed tomography was showing many more focal lesions than could be expected to require evacuation.[60] Deciding as soon as possible whether to evacuate a clot in a stable patient minimises the risk of neurological deterioration and improves outcome. Certain scan features show strong correlation with a rise in intracranial pressure and by themselves are indications for evacuation.[40 41] Such features are: pronounced midline shift (1 cm), loss of visualisation of the third ventricle and peri-mesencephalic cisterns, and dilatation of the ventricle contralateral to the lesion, particularly the temporal horn. When scan features leave doubt about the need for operation, continuous monitoring of intracranial pressure should be instituted and the lesion evacuated if pressure is sustained above 20–25 mmHg. If the pressure remains below this level for 24 hours, then the likelihood of deterioration is very small. Intracranial pressure should be monitored after evacuation of an intracranial clot to provide an early warning of the development of a recurrent or new haematoma and because brain swelling and raised pressure are common after evacuation of a subdural or intracerebral clot.

Intracranial pressure can be monitored by inserting a fluid-filled catheter into the ventricle or, increasingly, by insertion of a solid state fibreoptic system into the CSF pathways or direct into brain parenchyma. The first usually requires a burr hole to be made in the operating theatre, whereas the second can be carried out with a twist drill in the intensive care unit. Although the techniques for monitoring intracranial pressure are not necessarily restricted to neurosurgical intensive care, just as an overconcern about the head injury in a comatose patient with multiple injuries can be dangerous, so too can an over-narrow focus on observing and treating intracranial pressure. Unless monitoring is accompanied by the knowledge and experience necessary to appreciate the importance of first considering the cause of raised pressure before any treatment, and of the need for easy access to and use of repeat computed tomography and other investigations needed to interpret intracranial pressure findings, benefits from monitoring may be outweighed by adverse effects. Thus it is inappropriate and harmful to attempt to lower intracranial pressure by medical measures when its primary cause is an expanding intracranial lesion requiring evacuation. It is also crucial to be aware that an apparently satisfactory reduction of intracranial pressure—for instance, by hyperventilation or barbiturate treatment—may be at the price of inducing cerebral ischaemia as a result of vasoconstriction,[13 61] or net lowering of cerebral perfusion pressure with concomitant hypotension[62] and result in a worse outcome.[63]

Continuous monitoring of jugular venous oxygen saturation can provide valuable information when treating raised intracranial pressure.[64] A decrease in venous blood oxygenation indicates increased extraction either due to reduction in blood flow or due to an increase in metabolism. Conversely, very high levels of venous oxygenation indicate cerebral hyperaemia. Jugular oxygen saturation can be measured continuously with indwelling fibreoptic catheters but, at the present stage of development, readings have to be interpreted with considerable caution because abnormal values can result from technical factors. The catheter should be recalibrated at least every 12 hours against the findings of a co-oximeter on withdrawn blood samples, and samples should be repeated to check any apparently abnormal values. In the presence of arterial hypoxaemia and anaemia, it is probably preferable to measure the absolute content of blood and hence the cerebral oxygen extraction rather than rely on saturation values. The precise values of venous saturation that are optimum are still being debated, values below 50–60% indicate excessive extraction and potential for ischaemia, at least regional, and values of 85% indicate hyperaemia.

Cerebral blood flow can be assessed intermittently from a variety of techniques, but none of these has as yet found a place in routine management. An index of cerebral blood flow is provided by the velocity of blood flow in the intracranial arteries, and this can be measured intermittently or continuously, typically in the middle cerebral artery, using transcranial Doppler sonography.[65] This non-invasive technique also finds application in the care of patients with subarachnoid haemorrhage and is becoming increasingly available in neurosurgical units. Changes in mean velocity or in indices of pulsatility—the difference between systolic and diastolic flow velocities—aid the interpretation of information from intracranial pressure measurements and cerebral oxygen extraction values. Velocity falls and pulsatility increases with reducing cerebral perfusion pressure and blood flow. A high velocity can be caused by hyperaemia or narrowing of the vessels due to traumatic cerebral vasospasm.

Studies of cerebral electrical activity can provide information about brain function in patients who are unconscious, either due to the head injury or because of pharmacological treatment. The potentials evoked by somatosensory stimulation provide a useful index of integrity and are prognostically useful but have not established a value in practical care. When neuromuscular paralysis is employed to permit ventilatory treatment, however, there are advantages in continuous monitoring of cerebral activity using a simplified device such as a cerebral function monitor.

Monitoring with which staff are not familiar or which produces technically capricious results is useless and even dangerous. The increasing complexity of monitoring used in the management of patients with serious head injury is a strong argument for concentrating such cases, and hence experience, in specialised regional centres where the expertise to carry out the measurements and interpret and act on their findings can be developed and sustained.

Management of traumatic brain damage

The early scepticism, if not pessimism, about the prospects for recovery of a patient who remained in a coma, despite effective early resuscitation, has been dispelled by the evidence from many sources that half or more of such victims can regain consciousness and make an independent recovery. The prospects for improving the outcome of such injuries have been considerably heightened by evidence from modern methods of monitoring the occurrence of secondary insults, which are likely to exacerbate brain damage, that were not detected by methods available a decade or more ago.[12] Such insults worsen outcome,[13] which opens the way to improving outcome by preventing secondary insults or minimising their consequences. Also, the greater understanding of the pathophysiology of injury that has come from animal experiments and clinical observation in the past decade has allowed the development of more rational policies for management and more appropriate targeted treatment in individual cases.[66] This is encompassed within the concept of neurointensive care, distinguished in its concepts and techniques from general intensive care. No longer is it satisfactory for patients with head injury to be sedated, paralysed, and ventilated in the absence of appropriate neurological monitoring and investigation facilities.

Non-surgical management of severe head injury

Conservative management covers a range of techniques employed to prevent and treat complications considered to be liable to produce secondary damage. Many of these complications are systemic—for example, hypotension, hypoxia, hypercapnia, hypothermia, or electrolyte imbalance—rather than intracranial. The need for meticulous standards of management of severely injured or ill patients, and the methods involved, apply just as much to a serious head injury. As a general principle, such systemic disturbances are both more common and more serious in their effects than intracranial disturbances,[67] even after the initial resuscitation and emergency measures have been carried out.[14] By contrast with the unanimity about the importance of these factors, there is still considerable variation of opinion about employing methods primarily aimed at treating raised intracranial pressure and brain swelling after head injury. This is partly because such methods have not been shown by a randomised controlled trial to substantially improve outcome, and it is difficult to conceive of the feasibility of carrying out such a trial. Also, it reflects the fact that brain swelling and raised intracranial pressure may be a consequence of brain damage, rather than a primary factor in producing damage. There is, nevertheless, an acceptance that the supervention of raised intracranial pressure and reduction in cerebral perfusion pressure and ischaemia on an already damaged brain that has heightened vulnerability as a result of injury[68] cannot be other than undesirable.[69]

Ventilation of unconscious patients is used widely (box 4.7). The aim should be to keep arterial oxygen saturation as close as possible to 100%, using increases in inspired oxygen and positive end expired pressure when necessary. Ventilation should be adjusted to maintain arterial CO_2 tension normal or slightly abnormal. The practice of equating ventilation of head injury with hyperventilation must be abandoned in view of the evidence of the cerebral hypoxia and impaired outcome that result.[13 63] Hyperventilation should be used only briefly, not least because its effects are only temporary. Hypotension, whether as a consequence of hypervolaemia due to inadequate fluid replacement, or the use of sedative depressant drugs, must be avoided.

When raised intracranial pressure occurs, and simple causes such as neck position, airway obstruction, abnormal breathing patterns,

---

Box 4.7   Indications for intubation and ventilation of recently head injured patients (from Gentleman et al[43])

Immediately:
- Coma (not obeying, not speaking, not eye opening)—that is, Glasgow coma score 8 or less
- Loss of protective laryngeal reflexes
- Ventilatory insufficiency (as judged by blood gases):
  —hypoxaemia (PaO_2<9 kPa breathing air or <13 Pa breathing oxygen)
  —hypercarbia ($PaCO_2$>6 kPa)
- Spontaneous hyperventilation causing $PaCO_2$<3·5 kPa
- Respiratory arrhythmia

Before intrahospital or interhospital transport:
- Appreciably deteriorating conscious level, even if not in a coma
- Bilaterally fractured mandible
- Copious bleeding into mouth (for example, from skull base fracture)
- Seizures

An intubated patient must also be ventilated

Aim for PaO_2>15 kPa and $PaCO_2$ 4·0–4·5 kPa.

PaO_2 = arterial oxygen tension.
$PaCO_2$ = arterial carbon dioxide tension.

---

fever, and seizures have been excluded and surgically remediable space-occupying intracranial lesion has been ruled out, two principal approaches to treatment are employed. The first is the use of osmotic diuretics such as mannitol with a view to withdrawing fluid from either the normal brain or areas of brain oedema. The usual starting dose is 0·5 g/kg body weight with adjustment as determined by the effects on intracranial pressure and cerebral perfusion pressure. Additional measures include giving frusemide to sustain the osmotic gradient, infusing colloid to maintain circulating volume, and avoiding hyperosmolarity (serum osmolarity more than 320 mmol/l). The alternative is to use sedative or hypnotic drugs, such as propofol or thiopentone, to reduce cerebral metabolism and hence induce a fall in blood flow and blood volume.

Mannitol is considered to be most effective in raised pressure due to focal space-occupying lesions, whereas sedatives are more appropriate in patients with raised intracranial pressure due to vascular dilatation — typically children with preserved cerebrovascular carbon dioxide activity and cerebral electrical activity.[65] In all circumstances, care must be taken to avoid hypotension and it is sometimes more appropriate to maintain cerebral perfusion pressure by raising blood pressure pharmacologically than to strive to reduce intracranial pressure.

Drug treatment of head injury

Neuroprotection

Various agents have been used or are being considered that aim to interfere with the molecular, biochemical, cellular, and microvascular processes affected in traumatic brain injury.[70] None has yet been shown clearly to be of benefit. This is particularly true of steroids. After many years of debate, several trials at various doses have failed to show beneficial effects, and even adverse consequences have been noted.[71] This contrasts with the benefit of steroids in brain swelling due to tumour, and highlights the mechanistic differences in the processes.

The increased understanding of traumatic and ischaemic brain damage that has come from intense research in recent years has pointed to the importance of mechanisms such as increased intracellular calcium, excitotoxicity from excessive glutamate and other excitatory amino acids, and lipid peroxidation.[72] Experimental studies give promising indications of benefit from a range of neuroprotective drugs—calcium ion channel antagonists, glutamate receptor blocking agents, and antioxidants—and also hypothermia. Clinical studies are under way or planned.

Most neuroprotective agents have side effects on cardiovascular and CNS function, and achieving an acceptable efficacy and safety margin is likely to depend on the patient receiving effective neurocritical care. This will certainly be necessary in the trials needed to determine efficacy, and the concentration of severely injured patients in appropriate facilities should be encouraged.

Anticonvulsants

The frequency of seizures (5%), both in the acute and late phase after head injury,[73] has prompted the use of anticonvulsant drugs

110

as a prophylactic measure rather than as a response to a declared epileptic event. It was hoped that prophylactic treatment, and the suppression of seizure events, would lead to a reduced occurrence of late continuing seizures. Trials have shown that this is not the case for such late epilepsy,[74 75] but one study has shown a clear reduction in seizures in the first week after injury.[76] The precise level of risk of seizures that merits treatment remains debated. Like most British neurosurgeons, I prefer to withhold treatment until such time that a seizure occurs.

Antibiotics

There is also controversy about the use of antibiotics in the prophylaxis against infection in patients with an open injury, particularly due to a fracture at the base of the skull causing CSF rhinorrhoea or otorrhoea or intracranial air. One school of thought argues that the use of broad spectrum antibiotics does not reduce infection and simply promotes the occurrence of antibiotic resistant bacteria. On the other hand, I believe that there is reasonable recent evidence to support the value of prophylaxis, with penicillin or allied agents, against pneumococcus,[77] which is the most common organism and which can cause explosive and irreversible deterioration.

Operations after head injury

Most intracranial haematomas after a head injury are intradural—subdural, intracerebral, or both. Effective surgical management of these lesions demands more access than can be achieved by a burr hole and requires neurosurgical and neuroanaesthetic expertise and facilities. With early referral for computed tomography, there now should be very few, if any, occasions that a non-neurosurgeon needs to contemplate intracranial surgery—even for the simpler but much more rare solitary extradural haematoma. When a haematoma is detected or strongly suspected, a large bolus of mannitol—for example, 1g/kg—can "buy time" for transfer to the neurosurgical operating theatre.

Intracerebral contusions and smaller haematomas can pose difficult decisions. Some surgeons favour a conservative approach: intracranial pressure is monitored and, if raised (especially if cerebral perfusion pressure is reduced) medical methods are used;

operation is performed only if these fail. Although a conservative approach may be reasonable initially, if intracranial pressure is raised and the computed tomogram shows a focal space-occupying mass effect then operation should be preferred. Evacuation does not risk injury to surrounding recoverable brain tissue—a scan showing areas of low density adjacent to a contusion identifies cytotoxic oedema in irreversibly damaged brain. Evacuation of a mass lesion will always be a more secure method of improving relationships of intracranial pressure to volume, and fatal herniation can occur from local shift while intracranial pressure is being "controlled" medically.

Open injuries are less urgent indications for operation. Debridement and repair of a compound depressed skull fracture within 12–24 hours of injury avoids or minimises infection. Repair of a basal skull fracture is usually postponed until any associated leakage of CSF has persisted for several days, at which time the frontal lobe swelling, due to the contusions customary in such cases, has subsided. There is a trend for early (<12 hours) operation in craniofacial injury, the optimum time for correcting deformity, but this should be avoided if an associated head injury is of any more than minor or mild severity.

Where should head injuries be treated?

Provision of care for head injuries needs to incorporate the assessment and arrangement for home observation of the minor injuries that make up 80% of hospital attenders; arrangements for admission and observation of mild and moderate injuries; computed tomography, either before or after neurosurgical referral and transfer; and, for the resuscitation, continuing care and definitive management of patients with a severe head injury combined with serious injuries elsewhere.[78]

Facilities needed for initial assessment include staff trained and able to assess consciousness, to apply guidelines for skull radiography, to interpret its findings, and to apply guidelines for discharge or hospital admission. These must be available at all times within a district general hospital that deals with trauma cases. The arrangements for cases needing admission to hospital will depend on whether the hospital also contains a neurosurgical unit. If it does not, people with head injuries admitted for observation should preferably be grouped together in a specific short stay or observation unit where expertise and experience in assessment, and when necessary referral onwards, can be maintained. It is less satisfactory for patients to be admitted for observation on acute surgical wards, whether general surgical or orthopaedic.

Transfer of a patient both within a hospital and from a district hospital to a neurosurgical unit is fraught with hazard.[12 79] The distance travelled is less important than the risk of changes in homeostasis developing insidiously, unnoticed, and untreated because of inadequate monitoring equipment or inexperienced escort.[45 80–82] Dedicated transfer teams, travelling from major centres to collect severely ill patients, have been shown to be of value[83] but most often the responsibility will lie with the staff of the referring hospital. Before transfer, the patient must be rendered stable; life threatening extracranial injuries demand priority.[84] Intubation and ventilation should be established if there is any concern about airway or oxygenation. The staff accompanying the patient should be experienced in the care of unconscious injured patients. The minimum is a doctor, preferably an anaesthetist or a doctor with anaesthetic training and experience, and a trained nurse or paramedic. They must be familiar with the patient's condition before the journey, with what can go wrong during transport, and with the procedures and equipment needed. During transport there must be reliable intravenous access and the electrocardiogram should be monitored continuously, as should the blood pressure and arterial oxygen saturation by pulse oximetry. The monitoring equipment should preferably have the ability to display trends, to store data, and to print hard copy for later analysis. Facilities must be available to reposition or replace an endotracheal tube to continue ventilation if the oxygen supply fails, to continue or replace intravenous treatment, and to deal with cardiac arrest. With an appropriately equipped ambulance and adequately experienced staff, road transport will be appropriate for most transfers, air transfer being needed only for inaccessible locations or for very long distances.[85]

The preferred location for the definitive and continued management of the severely injured patient is the regional neurosurgical centre, and neurosurgical intervention is highly cost effective.[86] Although district general hospitals can increasingly undertake computed tomography and provide general intensive care, the temptation to retain severely injured patients whose scans seem not to show a surgical complication should be resisted. The expertise needed to interpret scans, to decide on the need for repeat scanning, to carry out and interpret comprehensive "neuromonitoring", and to apply its results requires building up and continuing expertise; and experience depends on a case load of sufficient numbers that is likely to be found only in a regional centre. Acting against this are the factors, professional prestige and market forces, that lead to pressures not to transfer such patients for neurosurgical care but to manage them in general intensive care units in a general hospital. This limits the employment of comprehensive neurocritical care and also divorces the victims' families from the informed advice, counselling, support, and follow up that should be available in a specialised unit.

The merits of "trauma centres" are currently under debate and investigation. Proponents emphasise the benefits of early multidisciplinary intervention in patients with serious multiple injuries. Others point to the very small proportion of accident victims requiring such intervention and the difficulties in selecting out such patients, in arranging for their transport to a dedicated single centre, and in the centre being adequately staffed at all times when appropriate cases may be sporadic and unpredictable. Whatever the cause of multiple injuries, an injury to the head has the greatest influence on outcome.[87]

When a trauma centre exists or is being developed in a hospital in which there is also a neurosurgical unit, neurosurgical advice and intervention should be readily available but should not take priority over the diagnosis and management of serious systemic injuries, hypotension in particular being an adverse factor to the recently injured brain. In practice, injuries requiring the intervention of another surgical speciality occur in only a few patients with head injury, even those with a severe injury. Miller (personal communication) found that of 440 patients admitted with head injuries, only 14 needed an orthopaedic operation, four a maxillofacial operation, and three a general surgical operation—but 80 needed a neurosurgical procedure. It is therefore more appropriate for a patient with head injury to be transferred after initial resuscitation, with appropriate safeguards, for neurosurgical assessment and management in a fully equipped unit with round the clock neurosurgical cover. The Society of British Neurological Surgeons has strongly recommended that trauma centres should be developed in only hospitals with a neurosurgical service. It is doubtful that without this any centre can regard itself as offering comprehensive trauma care.

Outcome, prognosis, and prediction

The outcome that can be expected after a head injury is of much concern to a victim's relatives and carers.[88] The traditional approach of doctors has been to stress the uncertainty of the situation—borrowing the Hippocratic aphorism "no head injury is too trivial to ignore nor too serious to despair of", coupled with an emphasis on pessimism ("hanging crepe"), to prepare the relatives for death for death or disability and to protect staff from criticism if this ensues. Reasonably reliable predictions of expected outcome can, however, be made on the basis of the wealth of data described over the past two decades.[16 89 90] When considering prognosis, certain safeguards must be applied; an estimate made too soon after injury is fallible if the patient's condition is partly a reflection of high alcohol or low oxygen levels (correction of which may lead to rapid recovery) or if delayed complications supervene and lead to subsequent deterioration. A balance needs to be struck between the greater accuracy of later predictions and their lesser usefulness in practice.

In the individual patient one of the most important prognostic factors is age, outcome worsening progressively with increasing age. By incorporating the additional information about the severity and type of brain damage gained from clinical observations (consciousness, motor patterns, pupil reactions, and eye movements)[91] and investigations such as computed tomography,[92] an increasingly clear and reliable estimate of the probable outcome can be given for individual patients. Murray et al[89 90] used a simple computer programme to calculate outcome probabilities for a large series of patients with head injury and studied the effect of providing clinicians with predictions at the time that a patient was under acute management. Although this did not alter management overall, intensive methods were used less among patients with a very poor prognosis and were redirected towards patients with an intermediate, uncertain prognosis, for whom outcome was presumably less predetermined and who had more potential to respond.

Outcome after head injury depends predominantly upon the degree of mental sequelae, in particular changes in personality and information processing and, in only a few patients, on the degree of any persisting physical limitations.[93] For this reason, scales developed for patients with stroke or other types of neurological damage are inappropriate in the head injury population. The Glasgow outcome scale described by Jennett and Bond[94] distinguished three classes of conscious survival, described in terms of consequent handicap: the severely disabled patient who is unable to live independently and unable to shop or travel on public transport; the moderately disabled patient who is independent but does not resume previous employment or social lifestyle; and the patient who makes a good recovery but is not necessarily free from neurological or neuropsychological limitations.

After severe head injury, 10–20% of patients remain severely disabled for six months or longer. At this stage only 1–3% are categorised as being vegetative; hardly any of these subsequently improve to be even severely disabled and none makes an independent recovery. On either side of these outcomes, the distributions of deaths and independent recovery have an inverse relation, depending on the population considered. For severe injuries, defined as not obeying commands, the proportion of deaths is 30%,[95] when in addition the patient is in a coma, with no eye opening and no comprehensible verbal response, mortality is 35–40%[96] and when this state has been present for six hours or more, mortality approaches 50%.[1]

After moderate, and in particular mild, head injury most patients are at worst only moderately disabled, and the original Glasgow coma scale[94] has been criticised as being too crude for such populations.[97] The device of defining upper and lower levels in each category of conscious survival only partially removes this difficulty.[93] A wide range of neuropsychological tests[98] and inventories of emotional, behavioural, and social status have been described but no single one has yet been widely adopted. In assessing outcome, it is crucial that information is not obtained only from the patient or even from the family practitioner.[99] A true picture of the patient's state, and in particular of its impact upon the family as a whole, can be obtained only when psychologists are involved in the assessment and when the family and carers are interviewed. This is particularly important if a patient is being assessed for the purposes of a claim for damages, when an underestimate of the consequences of injury may have adverse effects upon the settlement for the patient and perhaps expose the assessor to subsequent criticism.

Postacute care

After discharge from acute care, a range of problems arise. On one hand, patients with persisting limitations need effective rehabilitation, support, and reintegration to minimise handicap. On the other, there is the problem of the management of patients without obvious physical or mental sequelae but with persisting symptoms and restrictions in activity.

Although there has been considerable controversy about the benefits of rehabilitation for head injury, there is evidence that it is beneficial particularly when begun soon after injury and provided intensively by specialists in neurological problems.[100 101] Unfortunately, many patients fail to receive the "seamless" continuity of management that is optimum.[102] This deficiency reflects (a) the shortage in the United Kingdom of appropriately trained and experienced specialist services and (b) the chasm that often lies between acute medical services and community services. Moreover, most rehabilitation services and therapists are directed towards specific physical limitations and their consequent disability, whereas mental limitations after head injury are much more important in causing disability and handicap and limiting return to previous social and working lifestyles.

Macauley's aphorism "The business of everybody is the business of nobody"[103] can be applied to head injuries. A wide range of professional disciplines, support services, and charitable and voluntary organisations can contribute to the recovery of a victim of head injury. They need to be coordinated effectively, and specific interventions should be used appropriately and selectively. Unfortunately, all too often coordination and communication is lacking and, given the range of problems after head injury, it can be tempting to regard the patient as "somebody else's problem". In some parts of Britain no effective organisation exists, in others the organisation is appropriate but facilities needed for benefit are inadequate; in a few centres, comprehensive progressive rehabilitation and community reintegration are available. All concerned should press for the institution in every region of an integrated policy for postacute care of head injury. Someone should be given the responsibility of establishing the service and for arranging for its implementation; in effect this person's job should be to make sure that everyone else does their job![104]

At the time of discharge from hospital the patient and the family should be counselled about the nature of the head injury, its likely sequelae in the short term, and the likelihood of progressive recovery. Sufficient information should also be conveyed to the general practitioner about the nature and severity of the head injury and the initial approach to subsequent care. In the patient with a minor or mild injury all that may be needed is reassurance, relief of symptoms—for example, headache—and arrangements for review and return to activities after an interval that is determined by the severity of injury and subsequent symptoms. In the uncomplicated mild or minor injury, review by the general practitioner after a week may show a satisfactory progress, enabling return to work. This should be discouraged, however, if symptoms that were present at discharge—for example, headache, dizziness, or mental limitations—persist or become exacerbated. At around a month after injury, patients who continue to have an appreciable problem should be referred or recalled for assessment and for planning of rehabilitation and reintegration socially, professionally, etc. This service would be facilitated if a regional register of head injuries was established, with close liaison with neurosurgical unit staff. Subsequently, further remedial services may be required for a year or longer, depending on the patient's progress and the findings of subsequent assessments.

Quality of care: audit

Analysis of the management of and the outcome from head injuries has already resulted in changes in practice that have been rewarded by better results. In the early 1970s some studies showed that avoidable mortality in patients with head injury occurred often because recognition of the presence of an intracranial haematoma had been delayed.[36 105 106] The recognition that computed tomography could detect haematomas before they caused deterioration, together with the identification of clinical features correlating with the likelihood of a haematoma, led to the production of guidelines aimed at early referral to neurosurgery. These were first used informally within the neurosurgical unit in Glasgow,[49] and were then published and widely adopted

---

Box 4.8 Introduction of guidelines for management of head injuries and associated improvements in outcome of patients with a traumatic intracranial haematoma

	No (%) dead
1974–7—Referred to neurosurgery when clinically deteriorating	305 (38)
1978–84—Local criteria for earlier acceptance	659 (30)
1985–8—Published national guidelines for earlier referral	222 (23)

---

nationally.[51] Continuing audit of outcome has shown that these changes in procedure were accompanied by reductions in mortality in patients operated on (box 4.8).[49 89]

Insults during transfer from district hospital to neurosurgery were identified as another source of brain damage, death, or disability, which might be avoided by a better standard of care during transfer.[45] In 11 years dissemination of this knowledge led to a rise from 11% to 82% in the use of endotracheal intubation and ventilation during transfer. This was associated with a fall in hypoxaemia on arrival from 22% to 8% and reductions in numbers of unidentified or undertreated major extracranial injuries from 31% to 11% and in hypotension from 11% to 6%. Mortality fell from 45% to 32% and independent recovery rose from 40% to 58%.[79]

It will be important in the future to ensure that the gains resulting from the foregoing neurosurgically-led and neuroanaesthetically-led improvements in practice are maintained against the background of alterations in the organisation of medical care (for example, trust hospitals, internal markets, and the dissemination of previously centralised facilities such as computed tomography scanners). Each health purchasing authority should identify standards of practice, based on the guidelines for the process of care. Contracts with providers should contain these specific recommendations and should require that audit is carried out to ensure that they are being used properly.

Questions to be asked include what proportion of people presenting with head injury undergo skull radiography, hospital admission, and neurosurgical transfer—and with what outcome? Samples should be surveyed in detail to discover if practice in regard to individual patients conforms with the agreed standards. The quality of interpretation of investigations should be checked. When skull radiographs are interpreted by accident and emergency staff, all radiographs should be reviewed by a senior radiologist. Likewise, computed tomograms made outside the neurosurgical department should be reviewed—either at the time, through image transfer and consultation with an experienced clinician in the neurosurgical centre, or as a matter of routine periodical quality assessment.

Every death of a patient who arrives at hospital with a head injury, or at the very least all cases in which the patient was known to have talked after injury, should be subject to detailed review at regional level. Without overview at this level, the dispersal of patients with head injuries to different hospitals and even different departments means that audit at unit level will not be satisfactory.

Improved outcomes for head injuries have been achieved by the standards in management that have developed in the past decade. It is essential to safeguard these standards as the foundation for building systems for even better care in future.

Management of head injury

- Patients with impaired consciousness should be resuscitated (by correcting impaired airway, inadequate ventilation, or shock)
- The Glasgow coma scale should be used to assess the severity of the injury and degree of consciousness
- Patients who have no skull fracture and have not lost consciousness can be discharged, with a warning card, in the care of an adult
- Radiography is indicated if skull fracture is suspected but consciousness is not impaired
- Computed tomography is indicated if impairment of consciousness continues after transfer to hospital
- To detect possible complications, severely head injured patients need intensive monitoring of: arterial pressure, blood gases, electrocardiogram, end tidal carbon dioxide (in ventilated patients), and possibly: intracranial pressure, jugular venous oxygen saturation, cerebral blood flow velocity, and cerebral electrical activity
- To prevent and treat brain damage patients with severe head injury should be treated by:
  —ventilation to ensure oxygenation and carbon dioxide elimination
  —reduction of raised intracranial pressure or raising of blood pressure, or both, to ensure adequate cerebral perfusion pressure
  —operation to evacuate intracranial haematoma and damaged tissue and to repair compound fractures
  —administration selectively of anticonvulsants, antibiotics, and neuroprotective drugs
- Continued treatment of severely injured patients should be in regional neurosurgical centres
- Patients being discharged from hospital, and their families, need counselling about their prognosis
- Patients with persisting disabilities need specialist rehabilitation, support, and reintegration to minimise handicap

1 Jennett WB, Murray A, MacMillan R, *et al.* Head injuries in Scottish hospitals. Scottish head injury management study. *Lancet* 1977;2:696–8.
2 Strang I, MacMillan R, Jennett B. Head injuries in accident and emergency departments at Scottish Hospitals. *Injury* 1987;10:154–9.
3 Jennett WB, MacMillan R. Epidemiology of head injury. *BMJ* 1981;282:101–7.
4 Adams JH, Doyle D, Ford I, *et al.* Diffuse axonal injury in head injury: definition, diagnosis and grading. *Histopathology* 1989;15:49–59.
5 McLellan DR, Adams JH, Graham DI, Kerr AR, Teasdale GM. The structural law of the vegetative state and prolonged coma after non-missile head injury. In: Papo I, Cohadon F, Massarotti I, eds. *Le coma traumatique.* Padova: Liviana Editrice, 1986;165–85.

6 Zimmerman RA, Bilaniuk LT, Harkney DB, *et al.* Head injury: early results of comparing CT and high field MR. *Am J Radiol* 1986;**147**:1215–22.

7 Jenkins A, Teasdale GM, Hadley D, *et al.* Brain lesions detected by magnetic resonance imaging in mild and severe head injury. *Lancet* 1986;ii:445–6.

8 Graham DI, Adams JH, Doyle D. Ischaemic brain damage in fatal non-missile head injuries. *J Neurol Sci* 1978;**39**:213–34.

9 Graham DI, Ford I, Adams JH, *et al.* Ischaemic brain damage is still common in fatal non-missile head injury. *J Neurol Neurosurg Psychiatry* 1989;**52**:346–50.

10 Lewelt W, Jenkins LW, Miller JD. Autoregulation of cerebral blood flow after experimental fluid percussion injury of the brain. *J Neurosurg* 1980;**53**:500–11.

11 Lewelt W, Jenkins LW, Miller JD. Effects of experimental fluid percussion injury of the brain on cerebrovascular reactivity to hypoxia and hypercapnia. *J Neurosurg* 1982;**56**:332–8.

12 Andrews PJD, Piper IR, Dearden NM, Miller JD. Secondary insults during intrahospital transport of head injured patients. *Lancet* 1990;**335**:327–30.

13 Gopinath SP, Robertson CS, Contant CF, *et al.* Jugular venous desaturation and outcome after head injury. *J Neurol Neurosurg Psychiatry* 1994;**57**:717–23.

14 Jones PA, Andrews PJD, Midgley S, *et al.* Measuring the burden of secondary insults in head injured patients during intensive care. *J Neurosurg Anesthesiol* 1994;**6**:4–14.

15 Povlishock JT. Traumatically induced axonal injury: pathogenesis and pathobiological implications. *Brain Pathology* 1992;**2**:1–12.

16 Jennett WB, Teasdale GM, Braakman R, *et al.* Predicting outcome in individual patients after severe head injury. *Lancet* 1976;ii:1031–4.

17 Teasdale GM, Jennett B. Assessment of coma and impaired consciousness. *Lancet* 1974; ii:81–4.

18 Teasdale GM, Jennett WB. Assessment and prognosis of coma after severe head injury. *Acta Neurochir* 1976;**34**:45–55.

19 Teasdale GM, Murray G, Parker L, Jennett WB. Adding up the Glasgow coma score. *Acta Neurochir* (Paris) 1979;**1**(suppl 28):13–6.

20 Williams DH, Levine HS, Eisenberg HM. Mild head injury classification. *Neurosurgery* 1990;**27**:663–4.

21 Gómez PA, Lobato RD, Ortega SM, *et al.* Mild head injury: differences in prognosis among patients with a Glasgow coma score of 13–15 and analysis of factors with an abnormal CT scan. *Neurosurgery* 1994 (in press).

22 Jennett WB, Teasdale GM, Galbraith S, *et al.* Severe head injuries in three countries. *J Neurol Neurosurg Psychiatry* 1977;**40**:291–8.

23 Jennett WB, Teasdale G, Braakman R, *et al.* Prognosis of patients with severe head injury. *Neurosurgery* 1979;**4**:283–9.

24 Teasdale GM. Assessment of head injuries. *Br J Anaesth* 1976;**48**:761–6.

25 Rimmell RW, Giordani B, Barth JT, Jane JA. Moderate head injury: completing the clinical spectrum of brain trauma. *Neurosurgery* 1982;**11**:344–51.

26 Johnstone AJ, Lohlun JC, Miller JD, *et al.* A comparison of the Glasgow coma scale and the Swedish reaction level scale. *Brain Injury* 1993;**7**:501–6.

27 Rimmell RW, Giordani B, Barth JT, *et al.* Disability caused by minor head injury. *Neurosurgery* 1981;**9**:221–8.

28 Swann IJ, MacMillan R, Strang I. Head injuries at an inner city accident and emergency department. *Injury* 1981;**12**:274–8.

29 Mendelow AD, Teasdale GM, Jennett B, *et al.* Risks of intracranial haematoma in head injured adults. *BMJ* 1983;**287**:1173–6.

30 Teasdale GM, Murray G, Anderson E, *et al.* Risks of traumatic intracranial haematoma in children and adults: implications for managing head injuries. *BMJ* 1990;**300**:363–7.

31 Russell WR. *The traumatic amnesias.* Oxford: Oxford University Press, 1961.

32 Teasdale GM, Brooks N. Traumatic amnesia. In: Fredericks JAM, ed. *Handbook of clinical neurology.* Vol 1. Clinical neuropsychology. Amsterdam: Elsevier, 1985:185–91.

33 Wilson JTL, Teasdale GM, Hadley DM, *et al.* Post-traumatic amnesia: still a valuable yardstick. *J Neurol Neurosurg Psychiatry* 1993;**56**:198–201.

34 Roberts AJ. *Brain damage in boxers.* London: Pitman Medical, 1969.

35 Roberts GW, Gentleman SM, Lynch A, *et al.* β-Amyloid protein disposition in the brain after severe head injury: implications for the pathogenesis of Alzheimer's disease. *J Neurol Neurosurg Psychiatry* 1994;**57**:419–25.

36 Galbraith S. Misdiagnosis and delayed diagnosis in traumatic intracranial haematoma. *BMJ* 1976;**1**:1438–9.

37 McLaren C, Robertson C, Little K. Missed orthopaedic injuries in the resuscitation room. *J R Coll Surg Edinb* 1983;**28**:399–401.

38 Teasdale GM, Galbraith S, Murray L, *et al.* Management of traumatic intracranial haematoma. *BMJ* 1982;**285**:1695–7.

39 Miller JD. Neurological emergency. Head injury. *J Neurol Neurosurg Psychiatry* 1993;**56**: 440–7.

40 Bullock R, Teasdale GM. Head injuries—surgical management: traumatic intracranial haematomas. In: Braakman R, ed. *Vinken and Bruyn's handbook of clinical neurology: Head Injury.* Amsterdam: Elsevier Science Publishers, 1990;**24**:249–98.

41 Bullock R, Teasdale GM. Head Injuries I and II. In: D Skinner, P Driscoll, R Earlam, eds. *ABC of major trauma. BMJ* 1990;**300**:1576–9.

42 Miller JD, Dearden NM. Measurements, analysis and the management of raised intracranial pressure. In: Teasdale GM, Miller JD, eds. *Current Neurosurgery.* Edinburgh: Churchill Livingstone, 1992:119–56.

43 Gentleman D, Dearden NM, Midgley S, Maclean D. Guidelines for resuscitation and transfer of patients with serious head injury. *BMJ* 1993;**307**:547–52.

44 American College of Surgeons Committee on Trauma. *ATLS course manual.* Chicago: American College of Surgeons, 1993.

45 Gentleman D, Jennett B. Hazards of inter-hospital transfer of comatose head injured patients. *Lancet* 1981;ii:853–5.

46 Henderson A, Coyne T, Wall D, Miller B. A survey of interhospital transfer of head injured patients with inadequately treated life-threatening extracranial injuries. *Aust NZ J Surg* 1992;**62**:759–62.

47 Reilly PL, Simpson DA, Sprod I, Thomas L. Assessing the conscious level in infants and young children. A paediatric version of the Glasgow coma scale. *Child's Nervous System* 1988;**4**:30–3.

48 Ambrose J, Gooding M, Uttley D. EMI scan in the management of head injuries. *Lancet* 1976;i:847–8.

49 Teasdale GM. Management of head injuries. *The Practitioner* 1982;**226**:1667–73.

50 Teasdale GM, Teasdale E, Hadley D. Computed tomography and magnetic resonance imaging classification of head injury. *J Neurotrauma* 1992;**9**:S249–57.

51 Briggs M, Clarke P, Crockard A, *et al.* Guidelines for initial management after head injury. Suggestions from a group of neurosurgeons. *BMJ* 1984;**288**:983–5.

52 Jennett WB, Macpherson P. Implications of scanning recently head injured patients in general hospitals. *Clin Radiol* 1990;**42**:88–90.

53 Marsh H, Maurice-Williams RS, Hatfield R. Closed head injuries: where does the delay occur in the process of transfer to neurosurgical care. *Br J Neurosurg* 1989;**3**:3–13.

54 Servadei F, Piazza G, Seracchioli A, *et al.* Extradural haematomas: an analysis of the changing characteristics of patients admitted from 1980 to 1986. Diagnostic and therapeutic implications in 158 cases. *Brain Injury* 1988;**2**:87–100.

55 Nee PA, Hadfield JM, Yates DW. Biomechanical factors in patient selection for radiography after head injury. *Injury* 1993;**24**:471–5.

56 Miller JD, Jones PA. The work of a regional head injury service. *Lancet* 1985;i:1141–4.

57 Miller JD, Jones PA, Dearden NM, Tocher JL. Progress in the management of head injury. *Br J Surg* 1992;**79**:60–4.

58 Miller JD, Murray LS, Teasdale GM. Development of a traumatic intracranial haematoma after a "minor" head injury. *Neurosurgery* 1990;**27**:669–73.

59 Della Corte F. Guidelines for monitoring during the first 72 hours in severe brain injury. *Second international symposium on severe head injury.* Parma, 1994. Paper 55.

60 Galbraith S, Teasdale GM. Predicting the need for operation in the patient with an occult traumatic intracranial heamatoma. *J Neurosurg* 1981;**55**:75–81.

61 Cruz J. Combined continuous monitoring of systemic and cerebral oxygenation in acute brain injury: preliminary observations. *Crit Care Med* 1993;**21**:1225–32.

62 Schwartz ML, Tator CH, Rowed DW, *et al.* The University of Toronto injury treatment study: a prospective randomised comparison of pentobarbital and mannitol. *Can J Neurol Sci* 1984;**11**:434–40.

63 Muizelaar JP, Marmarou A, Ward JD, *et al.* Adverse effects of prolonged hyperventilation in patients with severe head injury: a randomised clinical trial. *J Neurosurg* 1991;**75**:731–9.

64 Dearden NM. Jugular bulb venous oxygen saturation in the management of severe head injury. *Current Opinion in Anaesthesiology* 1991;**4**:279–86.

65 Chan KH, Dearden NM, Miller JD, *et al.* Multimodality monitoring as a guide to treatment of intracranial hypertension after severe brain injury. *Neurosurgery* 1993;**356**:547–53.

66 Bannan P, Teasdale G. Neuroprotection in head injury. In: Reilly P, Bullock R, eds. *Head injuries.* 1994 (in press).

67 Piek J, Chesnut RM, Marshall LF, *et al.* Extracranial complications of severe head injury. *J Neurosurg* 1992;**77**:901.

68 Jenkins LW, Moszynski K, Lyeth BG, *et al.* Increased vulnerability of the mildly traumatised rat brain to cerebral ischaemia: the use of controlled secondary ischaemia as a research tool to identify common or different mechanisms contributing to mechanical and ischaemic brain injury. *Brain Research* 1989;**477**:211–24.

69 Marmarou A, Anderson RL, Ward JD, *et al.* Impact of ICP instability and hypotension in outcome in patients with severe head trauma. *J Neurosurg* 1991;**75**:S59–66.

70 Faden AI, Salzman. Pharmacological strategies in CNS trauma. *Trends in Pharmacological Sciences* 1992;**13**:29–35.

71 Todd N, Teasdale GM. Steroids in human head injury: clinical studies. In: R Capildeo, ed. *Steroids in diseases of the central nervous system.* Chichester: Wiley, 1989:151–61.

72 McIntosh TK. Novel pharmacological therapies in the treatment of experimental traumatic brain injury: a review. *J Neurotrauma* 1993;**10**:215–61.

73 Jennett WB. *Epilepsy after non-missile head injuries.* London: Heinemann, 1975.

74 Young B, Rapp RP, Norton JA, *et al.* Failure of prophylactically administered phenytoin to prevent late post traumatic seizures. *J Neurosurg* 1983;**58**:236–241.

75 Penry JK, *et al.* A controlled prospective study of the pharmacological prophylaxis of post traumatic epilepsy. *Neurology* 1979;**29**:600–1.

76 Temkin NR, Kilmea SS, Wilensky AJ, *et al.* A randomised, double blind study of phenytoin for the prevention of post-traumatic seizures. *N Engl J Med* 1990;**323**:497–502.

77 El Jamal MS. Antibiotic prophylaxis in unrepaired CSF fistulae. *Br J Neurosurg* 1993;**7**:501–6.

78 Bryden JS, Jennett WB. Neurosurgical resources and transfer policies for head injuries. *BMJ* 1983;**286**:1791–3.

79 Gentleman D. Causes and effects of systemic complications among severely head injured patients transferred to a neurosurgical unit. *Int Surg* 1992;**77**:297–302.

80 Miller JD, Sweet RC, Narayan R, Becker DP. Early insults to the injured brain. *JAMA* 1978;**240**:4319–442.

81 Kohi YM, Mendelow AD, Teasdale GM, *et al.* Extracranial insults and outcome in patients with acute head injury—relationship to the Glasgow outcome scale. *Injury* 1984;**16**:25–9.

82 Gentleman D, Jennett B. Audit of transfer of unconscious head injured patients to a neurosurgical unit. *Lancet* 1990;**335**:330–4.

83 Bion JF, Wilson IH, Taylor PA. Transporting crucially ill patients by ambulance: audit by sickness scoring. *BMJ* 1988;**296**:170.

84 Munro HM, Laycock JRD. Interhospital transfer standards for ventilated neurosurgical emergencies. *British Journal of Intensive Care* 1993;**3**:210–4.

85 Stanforth P. Head injuries—to be transferred or not [Editorial]. *Injury* 1994;**25**:491–2.

86 Pickard JD, Bailey S, Sanderson H, *et al.* Steps towards cost benefit, analysis of regional neurosurgical care. *BMJ* 1990;**301**:629–35.

87 Gennarelli TA, Champion HR, Sacco WJ, *et al.* Mortality of patients with head injury and extracranial injury treated in trauma centers. *J Trauma* 1989;**29**:1193.

88 Barlow P, Teasdale G. Prediction of outcome and the management of severe head injuries: The attitudes of neurosurgeons. *Neurosurgery* 1986;**19**:989–91.

89 Murray LS, Teasdale GM, Murray GD, *et al.* Does prediction of outcome alter patient management? *Lancet* 1993;**341**:1487–91.

90 Murray LS, Teasdale GM, Murray GD, Jennett WB. Guidelines for decision making improves outcome after head injury. *J Neurotrauma* 1993;**10**:S101.

91 Jennett WB. Assessment of the severity of head injury. *J Neurol Neurosurg Psychiatry* 1976;**39**:647–55.

92 Marshall LF, Marshall SB, Klauber MR, *et al.* A new classification of head injury based on computerised tomography. *J Neurosurg* 1991;**75**:S14–20.

93 Jennett WB, Snoek J, Bond MR, *et al.* Disability after severe head injury: observations on the use of the Glasgow outcome scale. *J Neurol Neurosurg Psychiatry* 1981;**44**:285–93.

94 Jennett WB, Bond MR. Assessment of outcome after severe brain damage. *Lancet* 1975;i:480–4.

95 Bailey I, Bell A, Gray J, *et al.* A trial of the effect of nimodipine on outcome after head injury. *Acta Neurochirurgica* 1991;**110**:97–105.

96 Choi SC, Barnes TY, Bullock R, *et al.* Temporal profiles of outcome in severe head injury. *J Neurosurg* 1994;**81**:169–73.

97 Hall K, Cope DN, Rappaport M. Glasgow outcome scale: comparative usefulness in following recovery in traumatic head injury. *Archives of Physical Medicine and Rehabilitation* 1985;**66**:35–7.

98 Clifton GL, Kreutzer JS, Choi SC, *et al.* Relationship between Glasgow outcome scale and neuropsychological measures after brain injury. *Neurosurgery* 1993;**33**:34–8.

99 Anderson SI, Housley AM, Jones PA, *et al.* Glasgow outcome scale: an inter-rater variability study. *Brain Injury* 1993;**7**:309–17.

100 Malec JF, Smigielski JS, De Popolo RW, *et al.* Outcome evaluation and prediction in a comprehensive integrated post-acute operative brain injury rehabilitation programme. *Brain Injury* 1993;**7**:1529.

101 Spivack G, Spettel CM, Ellis D, *et al.* Effects of the intensity of treatment and length of stay in rehabilitation outcome. *Brain Injury* 1992;**6**:419–434.

102 Hetherington H, Earlam RJ. Rehabilitation after injury and the need for co-ordination. *Injury* 1994;**25**:527–31.

103 Macauley TB. Historical essays contributed to the *Edinburgh Review. Hallam's constitutional history*. 1828.

104 Teasdale GM. Who cares about head injuries. *Br J Hosp Med* 1985;**33**:67.

105 Rose J, Valtonen S, Jennett B. Avoidable factors contributing to death after head injury. *BMJ* 1977;**2**:615–8.

106 Jeffreys RV, Jones JJ. Avoidable factors contributing to the death of head injury patients in general hospitals in Mersey region. *Lancet* 1981;**2**:459–61.

5 Stroke and transient ischaemic attacks

PETER HUMPHREY

Definitions

The management of stroke is expensive and accounts for about 5% of NHS hospital costs. Stroke is the commonest cause of severe physical disability. About 100 000 people suffer a first stroke each year in England and Wales. It is important to emphasise that around 20–25% of all strokes affect people under 65 years of age. The annual incidence of stroke is two per 1000.[1] About 10% of all patients suffer a recurrent stroke within one year. The prevalence of stroke shows that there are 250 000 in England and Wales. Each year about 60 000 people are reported to die of stroke; this represents about 12% of all deaths. Only ischaemic heart disease and cancer account for more deaths. This means that in an "average" district health authority of 250 000 people, there will be 500 patients with first strokes, with a prevalence of about 1500.

Transient ischaemic attacks (TIAs) are defined as acute, focal neurological symptoms, resulting from vascular disease, which resolve in less than 24 hours; most settle in less than 30 minutes. The incidence of TIAs is a quarter of that of stroke.

Over the past 20 years, mortality from stroke has fallen in both the United Kingdom and the United States by about a quarter. There has also been a fall in the incidence of stroke.[2] This is probably real but may be partly accounted for by the reclassification of stroke. The more successful treatment of hypertension is also likely to be relevant, but is unlikely to be a complete explanation as this improvement had also been seen during 1950–60, before the treatment of hypertension was widely practised.

Stroke is not a diagnosis. It is merely a description of a symptom complex thought to have a vascular aetiology. It is important to classify stroke according to the anatomy of the lesion, its timing, aetiology, and pathogenesis. This will help to decide the most appropriate management.

Classification of stroke

Many neurologists have described vascular syndromes in erudite terms. Most of these are of little practical use. A broadbased anatomical knowledge is important, however, as this has significance in pathogenesis and management.

Anatomical classification

Carotid v vertebrobasilar arterial territory

Carotid—Classifying whether a stroke is in the territory of the carotid or vertebrobasilar arteries is important, especially if the patient makes a good recovery. Carotid endarterectomy is of proved value in those with carotid symptoms. Carotid stroke usually produces hemiparesis, hemisensory loss, or dysphasia. Apraxia and visuospatial problems may also occur. If there is a severe deficit, there may also be a homonymous hemianopia and gaze palsy. Episodes of amaurosis fugax or central retinal artery occlusion are also carotid events.

Horner's syndrome can occur because of damage to the sympathetic fibres in the carotid sheath. This especially follows carotid dissection.

After an internal carotid occlusion, there may be exaggerated pulsation in the branches of the external carotid artery (especially the superficial temporal artery). Increased collateral blood flow through this artery shunts blood via the orbital vessels into the ophthalmic artery and then into the circle of Willis in an attempt to compensate for the internal carotid occlusion, patients thus performing their own extracranial–intracranial anastomosis. This is an almost universal finding on ultrasonography in internal carotid artery occlusion. Sometimes the collateral flow is so pronounced that an orbital bruit is heard and the superificial temporal artery on the side of the occlusion becomes tender and painful. This can mimic temporal arteritis. It is particularly important that biopsy of

127

the temporal artery is not performed or a major collateral source of blood supply will be obliterated.

Vertebrobasilar—The terminal branches of this system are formed by the posterior cerebral artery. Ischaemia of its territory usually produces unilateral field defects. Bilateral symptoms are not uncommon, with complete blindness or bilateral visual hallucinations, such as an impression of frosted glass or water running across the whole field of vision.

Sometimes amnesic symptoms may be seen. In most patients, however, transient global amnesia is no longer thought to be caused by a TIA.[3]

The posterior cerebral artery also supplies part of the thalamus: infarction here produces sensory impairment over the contralateral side of the body. This may be accompanied by a very unpleasant pain which may be spontaneous or induced by light touch (thalamic pain) and often only reaches its peak some months after the stroke.

The brain stem signs after vertebrobasilar ischaemia depend on the level of the lesion.[4] Midbrain ischaemia may result in pupillary changes with impaired vertical gaze or oculomotor nerve dysfunction. Damage to the pons produces horizontal gaze palsy with facial weakness or sensory loss. In either case a tetraparesis or hemiparesis may occur.

A wide range of other syndromes is reported to follow ischaemia of localised areas of the brain. The basic pattern is one of ipsilateral cranial nerve palsies and cerebellar disturbance combined with contralateral paresis or sensory loss which may affect the face, arm, leg, or arm and leg, depending on the level in the brain stem at which this occurs. Horner's syndrome may be seen.

In the "locked in" syndrome, patients appear to be unconscious but are actually fully conscious. They can only move their eyes vertically; sometimes they can move their eyelids. It is good practice to introduce oneself to patients who appear to be unconscious, and immediately ask them to move their eyes before accepting that they are truly unconscious.

One word of caution—carotid artery dissection often presents with ipsilateral Horner's syndrome and contralateral hemiparesis. It has also been described with ipsilateral cranial nerve palsies (especially affecting nerves IX–XII) because the expanded carotid artery damages these nerves in the neck. Classical teaching would have mistakenly put this vascular syndrome in the vertebrobasilar territory.

Box 5.1   Common lacunar infarcts

Clinical type | Site of lesion

Pure motor hemiplegia — Internal capsule, pons, cerebral peduncle

Pure hemi-anaesthesia — Thalamus

Ataxic hemiparesis — Pons, internal capsule

Sensorimotor stroke — Thalamus

Lacunar infarcts

These small, deep microinfarcts described by Fisher are commonly seen in hypertensive and diabetic patients.[5] They rarely occur in patients with carotid artery stenosis. It is important to recognise these lacunar syndromes because of their good prognosis and different pathogenesis. Lacunar infarcts commonly present as pure motor stroke, pure sensory stroke, sensorimotor stroke, or ataxic hemiparesis (box 5.1). Acute focal movement disorders may also be lacunar. Patients have either complete face, arm, and leg or major face and arm or leg involvement. Those with more restricted deficits—for example, weak hands only—are not included but are considered to have partial anterior circulation infarcts in the cortex.

Sometimes multiple lacunar infarcts occur. In such patients there is often, but by no means always, a history of preceding minor stroke. The resulting syndrome is of a pseudobulbar palsy with dementia, dysarthria, small stepping gait (*marche à petits pas*) unsteadiness, and incontinence.

Clinical classification

Bamford and colleagues[6] have used the Oxford community stroke data to classify strokes clinically into—(*a*) lacunar infarcts; (*b*) total anterior circulation infarcts; (*c*) partial anterior circulation infarcts; and (*d*) posterior circulation infarcts (vertebrobasilar)—(*b*) and (*c*) are classified as carotid artery territory stroke.

Total anterior circulation infarct presents with a combination of higher cerebral dysfunction deficit (dysphasia, dyscalculia, and

129

visuospatial disorder); homonymous visual field defect; and motor or sensory deficit, or both, of at least two areas of the face, arm, and leg. Partial anterior circulation infarcts present with only two of the three components of the total anterior circulation infarct syndrome—with higher cerebral function alone or with a motor or sensory deficit more restricted than those classified as lacunar infarcts (for example, confined to one limb, or to face and hand but not to the whole arm).

Patients with posterior circulation infarct present with any of the symptoms described in the section on vertebrobasilar disease.

Using these simple clinical criteria, it proved possible to classify most strokes into one of these four different categories. This may be important because the prognosis, aetiology, and risk of recurrent strokes varies in the different groups. The total anterior circulation infarct group had a very poor prognosis, with high mortality but a low recurrence rate, presumably as most of the carotid territory had been destroyed by the infarct. The partial anterior circulation infarct group had a good prognosis but a high early recurrence rate, as this type of stroke is frequently embolic, probably from internal carotid artery atheroma. These patients have much to lose if a second stroke occurs. The lacunar group had an intermediate prognosis but a low risk of recurrence. This type of stroke is rarely due to embolic disease but follows microvascular thrombosis or haemorrhage, often as a result of hypertension with or without diabetes.

The posterior circulation infarct group had a good prognosis but high early recurrence rate. This Oxford community study dispels the notion that brain stem strokes in general have a poor prognosis in the acute phase: it also emphasises the appreciable risk of recurrence and the need to give advice about risk factors, and offer early medical treatment, to those with posterior circulation infarcts.

Subclavian steal syndrome

This syndrome is largely an irrelevance. Subclavian stenosis is common in asymptomatic patients. The classic syndrome of brain stem ischaemia on exercising the arm is rarely present. It has a very low risk of stroke (under 2% annually).[7] It can usually be diagnosed by measuring the blood pressure in both arms. It is not necessary to consider any form of surgical intervention unless there are intractable vertebrobasilar TIAs. Angioplasty is a less invasive option.

Border zone infarcts

Sometimes infarction follows a generalised reduction in cerebral blood flow. This is most commonly seen after a cardiac arrest or hypoxic damage during cardiac surgery. Ischaemia is then especially pronounced in the border zone between the territory of individual arteries because here perfusion is least. The parieto–occipital zone is the area most often affected, where border zone infarcts produce visual field defects (often partial and easily missed on routine examination), reading difficulties, visual disorientation, and constructional apraxia.[8] In the frontal border zone, slowing up, pathological grasp reflexes, gait disturbances, and incontinence may occur.

The clinical description is therefore helpful in formulating an opinion about the anatomical site, aetiology, prognosis, and risk of recurrence. This may well have management consequences.

Timing and pathogenesis of strokes and TIAs

The timing of events is important in our understanding of pathogenesis. Most TIAs are embolic and usually arise from the internal carotid artery or from the heart. A small percentage are haemodynamic—these usually occur when there is severe, widespread occlusive disease.

Sometimes it is possible to identify patients with haemodynamic TIAs clinically. Embolic TIAs usually occur for no apparent cause. Haemodynamic TIAs, however, may have a trigger; for instance, standing, exercising, lowering blood pressure, eating, and straining have all been described as precipitating events. Haemodynamic amaurosis fugax may be triggered by a bright light or sunlight. Unlike patients with embolic amaurosis fugax who usually describe a shutter or black shadow descending across the visual field, those with haemodynamic attacks often initially describe increased contrast between black and white, and then whiteness of vision, before their vision goes. Haemodynamic amaurosis fugax is often more gradual than embolic amaurosis. Sometimes haemodynamic TIAs may be preceded by symptoms of presyncope such as dizziness and faintness. Finally, they may occur many times a day over a considerable period of time: this is unusual in embolic TIAs.

Although haemodynamic TIAs are rare compared with embolic TIAs, it is important to identify them, because antiplatelet therapy

---

Box 5.2   Causes of cerebral haemorrhage

- Hypertension
- Berry aneurysm
- Perimesencephalic haemorrhage
- Arteriovenous malformation
- Anticoagulants
- Bleeding into tumour
- Mycotic aneurysm
- Coagulation disorders
- Arteritis
- Amyloid angiopathy
- Drug abuse—cocaine
- Venous thrombosis

---

is unlikely to help these symptoms. Reconstructive vascular surgery is more likely to be appropriate.[9]

Stroke is usually secondary to thromboembolic disease. About 15% of all strokes are haemorrhagic. Five per cent of these are secondary to subarachnoid haemorrhage and 10% to intracerebral haemorrhage (box 5.2).

Thromboembolic stroke accounts for 85% of all stroke.[10] It is usually possible on clinical grounds to differentiate it from subarachnoid haemorrhage. The management of subarachnoid haemorrhage[11] is not discussed in further detail here.

The clinical differentiation of thromboembolic disease from intracerebral haemorrhage is difficult. Various authors have attempted to develop a clinical score.[12] Early loss of consciousness, early vomiting, bilateral extensor plantars, and pronounced rise in blood pressure all suggest haemorrhage. TIAs and the presence of peripheral vascular disease suggest thromboembolic disease.

No clinical score is sufficiently accurate, however, to permit reliable differentiation. Computed tomography, provided that it is performed within two weeks of the first symptom, is the only reliable method. It should be used in patients with stroke because the proper assessment and treatment of thromboembolism and haemorrhage differ.

What percentage of strokes are thrombotic and embolic is even more difficult to ascertain. It is estimated that about half of all

---

Box 5.3   Cardiac sources of emboli

Left atrium:
    Thrombus (usually secondary to atrial fibrillation)
    Myxoma
    Paradoxical embolism
    Atrial septal aneurism

Mitral valve:
    Rheumatic endocarditis
    Infective endocarditis
    Marantic endocarditis
    Prosthetic valve
    Mitral valve prolapse
    Mitral annulus calcification

Left ventricle:
    Thrombus—myocardial infarction, cardiomyopathy

Aortic valve:
    Rheumatic endocarditis
    Infective endocarditis
    Marantic endocarditis
    Bicuspid valve
    Aortic sclerosis and calcification
    Prosthetic valve
    Syphilitic aortitis

Congenital cardiac disorders

Cardiac surgery:
    Air embolism
    Platelet/fibrin embolism

---

thromboembolic strokes are embolic (box 5.3) and half thrombotic. The percentage of all strokes caused by other factors such as primary hypoperfusion (see above, border zone infarcts), vasospasm, and arteritis is small.

Accuracy of diagnosis

The differential diagnosis of TIA and stroke includes epilepsy, migraine, tumour, demyelination, syncope, subdural haematoma, malignant hypertension, hyperventilation, hypoglycaemia, and giant intracerebral aneurysm.[13]

133

Focal motor seizures may be mistaken for TIAs, especially in patients with a very severe carotid stenosis, in whom the jerking of the limbs occurs as part of the TIA. Focal sensory seizures are even more difficult to distinguish, although the march of the sensory symptoms in a focal seizure may be helpful.

Migraine occasionally presents diagnostic difficulties. The slow build up of a migrainous aura, which often lasts 20 to 30 minutes, would be unusual in a TIA. Visual migraine often consists of positive visual symptoms, such as scintillating scotomas, unlike the blackness of amaurosis fugax. A typical migrainous headache is unlikely in a TIA. Headache occurs in 16% of patients with TIAs.[14]

The United Kingdom TIA Study Group has recently presented their data on tumours mimicking TIAs. Patients who present with sensory or jerking TIAs, loss of consciousness, or speech arrest should all be suspected of having a tumour until proved otherwise.[15]

Demyelination is usually suspected because of the age of the patient, history of previous attacks, and a more gradual onset of hemiparesis compared with that seen in a vascular hemiparesis.

Subdural haematomas rarely present with vascular-like symptoms. They do, however, present a particular diagnostic difficulty. The diagnosis of a carotid TIA is usually reasonably consistent,[16 17] but vertebrobasilar TIAs are more variable. It is important to be wary of labelling the following as TIAs: loss of consciousness; dizziness; mental confusion; incontinence of faeces or urine; or bilateral loss of vision with reduced level of consciousness. These are all often secondary to hypoperfusion, after primary cardiac disease.

Single symptoms such as vertigo, diplopia, dysphagia, dysarthria, loss of balance, tinnitus, sensory symptoms confined to one part of one limb or face, amnesia, drop attacks, and scintillating scotomas, should always be interpreted cautiously when they occur in isolation. They may, however, be consistent with TIAs, especially if they occur together or with other more definite symptoms of TIAs. The reliability of the diagnosis can be improved if clear cut criteria in plain language are used in the assessment of TIAs.[17]

In the diagnosis of stroke, the false positive rate with no investigations is between 1% and 5%, if a careful history is taken of the event.[10] It is important to emphasise that computed tomography is no more accurate than clinical opinion[13]; this is probably because some events that are clinically strokes are mistakenly diagnosed on computed tomography as tumours, a diagnosis that is not substantiated with time.

Risk factors

Age is the most important risk factor for stroke. Hypertension is the most important treatable risk factor.[18] The risk of stroke after a TIA is 30% in five years, the highest risk being in the first year.[19] Other proved risk factors include cardiac disease, diabetes mellitus, smoking,[20] and hypercholesterolaemia.[21] High cholesterol levels are also a major risk factor for heart disease which will be the cause of death in most patients with cerebrovascular disease.

Alcohol, taken in excess, is probably a risk factor for cerebrovascular disease, especially haemorrhage. Raised homocysteine and fibrinogen levels may be independent risk factors for vascular disease.[22 23]

It is not known whether obesity, stress, or physical activity have any part to play in the aetiology of stroke—if so, it is likely to be small.

Investigations

Few basic investigations are necessary for most patients with TIAs. Measurements should include a full blood count, erythrocyte sedimentation rate, urea and electrolyte levels, glucose and cholesterol levels. Many physicians request a chest radiograph and electrocardiogram, although it is debatable whether these are necessary if there are no symptoms of cardiac disease.

Patients with carotid TIAs or stroke with recovery should also be assessed with Doppler/duplex ultrasonography to detect carotid stenosis—this is highly accurate but very dependent on the operator's skills[24-26]; our own experience has shown that most radiology departments setting up Doppler/duplex ultrasound services produce some highly inaccurate results, and all such units should have their results substantiated either by angiography or a proved ultrasound service.

Box 5.4 lists other tests that should be considered.

Treatment

Medical

Vascular risk factors

Hypertension is the most important risk factor for stroke. The risk of stroke rises exponentially as diastolic blood pressure increases

135

in the range 70–100 mmHg. A 7·5 mmHg rise in diastolic pressure within the range 70–110 mmHg is associated with a doubling in the risk of stroke.

This underlines the importance of blood pressure control. There is a risk of precipitating hypotension in a small number of patients, especially the elderly; this is often overstated as a reason for not

---

Box 5.4   Additional investigations in patients with TIAs

Thyroid function tests (especially when cholesterol is raised or the patient is in atrial fibrillation)

Computed tomography if there is:
   doubt about the diagnosis especially if the stroke onset was gradual or the history unclear
   a need to exclude cerebral haemorrhage (ideally all strokes)
   cerebellar stroke with a deteriorating level of consciousness

Cerebral angiography
   Digital subtraction/magnetic resonance may be indicated if the patient is a candidate for carotid endarterectomy
   To look for evidence of arteritis
   In cerebral haemorrhage

Echocardiography if:
   abnormal cardiac findings are present, suggestive of valvular heart disease or evidence of recent myocardial infarction, or left ventricular aneurysm either clinically or on chest radiograph or electrocardiogram
   all young patients with stroke (<50 yrs) if no clear cut cause is found
   multiple territory stroke for no clear cause
   antiphospholipid syndrome or systemic lupus erythematosus? Libman-Sacks endocarditis
   positive blood cultures

Blood cultures if the patient is febrile, to detect subacute bacterial endocarditis

Temporal artery biopsy to detect giant cell arteritis

24-Hour electrocardiography in case of arrhythmia (very rarely necessary: grossly overused)

Work up for young patients with stroke (see box 5.6)

---

being more aggressive in the treatment of high blood pressure, especially isolated systolic hypertension.

In the population at large, a modest fall of 5 mmHg in mean diastolic pressure, achievable by reducing the mean daily salt intake by 50 mmol/l, might reduce overall stroke mortality by 22%.[27] This would have a greater effect on the total number of strokes than just treating high blood pressure in people with diastolic pressures of over 100 mmHg.

Treating all hypertensive patients would reduce the mortality of stroke by 15%. This compares with aspirin, which reduces the overall incidence of stroke by 1–2%, and carotid endarterectomy, which reduces the overall incidence by 0·5%.[28] Recent data suggest that inadequate monitoring and treatment of high blood pressure is common and is the most important, and avoidable, risk factor.[29] These figures emphasise that treating high blood pressure will do more for stroke prevention than any other treatment, either surgical or medical.

Advice about tobacco smoking is clearly important. Good control of diabetic symptoms is also to be encouraged, although there are no data proving that good control reduces the risk of stroke.

There is no consensus about the value of cholesterol lowering drugs. There is, however, no doubt that the lower the cholesterol, the lower the chance of a heart attack. Prescription costs for lipid lowering drugs are increasing by 20% per year. Drug trials are beginning to show some benefit from lipid lowering drugs; the United Kingdom heart protection study is about to start, in which 20 000 subjects are expected to be recruited to receive either placebo or simuastatin.

A small number of patients, who have a packed cell volume of over 50%, need assessment for polycythaemia followed by appropriate treatment.

Acute stroke

High blood pressure after acute stroke is common, often settles spontaneously, and does not need to be treated in most people. Treatment should be started only if hypertensive encephalopathy is considered to be likely (systolic more than 230 mmHg: diastolic over 130 mmHg) or the patient has had a proved cerebral haemorrhage and the blood pressure is very high. It is also important to check the blood pressure in all patients with stroke one or two months after discharge from hospital, as an appreciable number will show a persistent rise in blood pressure that is severe enough to require treatment, even though their blood pressure was satisfactory when they were discharged.

In recent years there has been much debate over the value of stroke units. A recent overview leaves little doubt that patients treated in stroke units do better than those treated in general medical wards.[30] There is no specific reason for this: it may just be an organisational matter rather than due to any one specific treatment.

More difficult is the question of whether patients do better at home or in hospital. The recent papers from Gladman *et al*,[31] and Young and Forster,[32] have suggested that home treatment may be better. More work needs to be done on this. If patients are kept at home, it is clearly important that they should still be investigated in the most appropriate manner. Trials comparing home treatment with stroke units are needed. We should not assume that hospital is better. Motivation and "do it yourself" physiotherapy are probably greatly enhanced by staying at home, provided that adequate support from social services, paramedical teams, and the family is available.

There is no proved medical treatment for acute stroke. Dextran has been shown not to be beneficial. The trials of calcium antagonistics, steroids, and glycerol are inconclusive,[33] and this is an area of active research.

The international stroke trial (IST) is comparing heparin, aspirin, and placebo. The multicentre acute stroke trial (MAST) is assessing thrombolysis. These trials have recently been reviewed.[34] Despite the lack of any proved treatment, it is one of the most exciting frontiers in the field of acute neurology. There is no doubt that successful treatment will be found: the increase in, and interest created by, large multicentre trials is rightly unstoppable. Stroke units make these trials much easier to perform. We have only to see how the international studies of infarct survival (ISIS) have transformed the care of myocardial infarction to know that we must encourage stroke units to investigate treatments for this most debilitating disease.

TIAs and stroke with recovery

There is no doubt that aspirin reduces the risk of stroke and death in patients with TIAs by approximately 25%.[35] The exact dose is unclear. The evidence is best for doses of around 300 mg.

Some believe smaller doses (of 37·5 or 75 mg) may be adequate, but it is possible that the relevant trials may be too small and that a difference between 37·5 mg and larger doses may have been missed because of a type II statistical error.

Ticlopidine is also an effective antiplatelet agent, perhaps more effective than aspirin.[36] It is available in the United States but is not on general release in the United Kingdom. Unfortunately it sometimes causes rash, diarrhoea, and reversible neutropenia—patients, therefore, need more careful monitoring. A related drug, clopidogrel, is now undergoing trials comparing it with aspirin.

Warfarin is indicated for definite cardiac emboli. Lone atrial fibrillation has now been added to this list. The European atrial fibrillation study shows that warfarin reduces the risk of subsequent stroke by 60–70% compared with placebo in patients who have had an episode of cerebral ischaemia. The annual risk of serious bleeding was only 3% with 0·2% intracranial bleeds.[37]

I also use warfarin if a patient has had several TIAs that were not controlled by aspirin. I give warfarin for six to 12 months and then switch back to aspirin, provided that no further ischaemic events occur. There are no good data to support this as yet but trials are being performed in the United States, Italy, and the Netherlands comparing aspirin with warfarin.

A very common question is when to start warfarin after a definite stroke. The risk of recurrent emboli is high after the first event but there is the danger of secondary haemorrhage into an infarct if warfarin/heparin is started too early. The Cardiac Embolism Study Group has shown that the risk of secondary haemorrhage is very low 11 days after the initial event. The risk is also very low in the first 11 days if the infarct is small or the deficit mild. I therefore start anticoagulants immediately if the deficit is mild but delay for 11 days if the deficit is severe (for example, severe hemiparesis, sensory loss, and dysphasia with a large infarct visible on computed tomogram. Clearly on the first day, computed tomography may be negative and the decision then has to be made on the severity of the clinical deficit only).[38]

Surgical treatment

In 1954 the first carotid endarterectomy was performed. The annual risk of stroke in patients with a carotid stenosis who have had a TIA is about 10%. The surgical risk of carotid endarterectomy varies from 1% to 25%. It is not surprising therefore that, for 37 years, it was not known if this operation was worthwhile. It was only with the publication of the European carotid surgery trial (ECST) and the North American trial (NASCET) in 1991 that the true value of this operation became known.[39]

The incidence of serious complications in Europe was 3·7% and in North America 2·1%. Patients were randomised to surgery and medical treatment or best medical treatment. In the group with 70–99% stenosis, there was a highly significant benefit from surgery—there were 75% fewer strokes in those treated with carotid endarterectomy. Clearly the lower the surgical complication rate, the sooner the patient benefits from surgery. In the European trial, the crossover was at approximately five months and in the North American trial three months. All fit patients with a tight symptomatic stenosis should therefore be offered surgery. They should be told the risk of stroke—that is, 10% annually—and the local operative risk, and advised that operation reduces the risk of stroke to 2–3% annually. Patients can then make up their own minds. If the surgical risk is over 10%, then the benefit is lost: all units should aim for less than 5%.

There are a possible 5000 candidates for carotid endarterectomy in England and Wales: operation in this group would prevent 500 strokes in the first year. It is not a cheap form of treatment but, for a person with a carotid TIA and a tight stenosis, surgery reduces the risk of a stroke by 75%.

The average district general hospital in the United Kingdom serving a population of 250 000 would expect to have about 20 patients who are fit, symptomatic, and have a carotid stenosis of more than 70%. The value of this operation is dependent on low operative mortality and morbidity. I believe that there should be a small number of designated surgeons in each region who do this operation. Each should do at least 50 operations a year and the results should be independently audited.

It is important to appreciate that this operation is only for patients with recent carotid symptoms, such as amaurosis fugax, hemiparesis, hemisensory loss, and dysphasia. Just how much this operation has been overused is emphasised by the report in 1988 (before the results of the European and North American trials) which showed that only 35% of patients had this operation for appropriate reasons in a sample of 1302 patients in the United States.[40]

Ultrasonography and angiography

None of these surgical trials included the angiographic risk. Although the risk of stroke after carotid angiography is generally quoted as 1%,[41] it is almost certainly higher in patients with carotid stenosis, leaving about 2% with a permanent disability.[42] Doppler/duplex ultrasonography is undoubtedly the best screening test but it is very dependent on the skill of the operator. Some units operate on the results of ultrasonography alone; unfortunately, obtaining information on the intracranial circulation is difficult with ultrasound. Combined with magnetic resonance angiography (MRA), ultrasound gives highly accurate information about the carotid artery in the neck, as well as an angiographic picture of the whole intracerebral circulation.

Our policy is to operate on the basis of an entirely non-invasive work up with ultrasound and magnetic resonance angiography if both tests agree. We have found that, in patients with 70–99% stenosis, the tests agree in 96%: we only pursue digital subtraction angiography in the other 4%. If magnetic resonance angiography proves to be less dependent on the operator and becomes widely available, it may replace the need for ultrasonography; however, this would require an enormous expansion in magnetic resonance angiography to all district general hospitals.

In expert hands, a bruit is the best clinical guide to detect an underlying internal carotid stenosis.[44 45] The bruit is lost, however, in very tight stenoses (false negative).

A false positive bruit is not infrequent in the presence of a contralateral occlusion, external carotid stenosis, or just internal carotid atheroma. Furthermore, if the presence of a bruit is to be of value, it needs to be useful to those who are making the initial assessment. The presence or absence of a bruit mentioned in the referral letter to a cerebrovascular clinic showed a specificity of 70% and sensitivity of 57% for patients with 70–99% stenosis (Davies and Humphrey[45a]). On this basis, many patients with a carotid stenosis would be denied surgery if only those with a bruit were referred.

All patients with carotid TIA or who have recovered from stroke should have carotid ultrasonography in a department with a proved

141

track record. I no longer listen for a bruit; if I wish to detect a carotid stenosis I use ultrasonography.

My own personal work up for carotid endarterectomy is therefore a careful history, simple examination of the cardiovascular system (occasionally I examine the neurological system!), routine blood tests, chest radiography, and electrocardiography. This, combined with Doppler/duplex ultrasonography, is all done at the first clinic visit. If the patient is found to have a carotid stenosis and is prepared to take the risk of surgery, then an urgent magnetic resonance angiography is booked in the outpatient department.

Computed tomography and magnetic resonance imaging

I do not routinely perform computed tomography or magnetic resonance imaging on patients with stroke or a TIA. The value of computed tomography was evaluated in a prospective study of 469 patients being considered for carotid endarterectomy—the cost was considerable and the results did not alter management.[46] In this increasingly cost conscious health service, we need to look for value for money.

Tumour "TIAs"[15] are rare and can often be suspected on clinical grounds—patients with speech arrest, pure sensory TIA, blackouts, and jerking during their attacks should all raise the suspicion of alternative pathology. Computed tomography need only be performed in this group.

Assessment for surgery

I remain convinced that a neurologist or physician with a major interest in vascular disease should perform the initial assessment. Patients with stroke or a TIA should not be referred primarily to the vascular surgeons. In our cerebrovascular clinics, of the 25 new patients we see each week, only two or three on average meet all the criteria for carotid endarterectomy. The differential diagnoses recently seen in our clinic include migraine, epilepsy, hyperventilation, tumours, Parkinson's disease, and motor neuron disease, to name but a few. In a population of a million people, there are about 50 to 100 who are candidates for carotid endarterectomy each year: this compares with around 15 000 with asymptomatic carotid stenosis. The scope for inappropriate surgery is substantial. It is unreasonable to expect a vascular surgeon to differentiate stroke or TIAs from these other conditions.

There is little doubt that the risk of a stroke is highest in the first six months after the initial event and, if the time from first symptom to assessment, investigation, and surgery takes several months, then we are failing to meet the needs of many patients. In the United Kingdom we need to assess these patients within a few days of their symptoms and prepare them for surgery, if appropriate, within two weeks after TIAs and six to eight weeks after recovery from stroke. This will require changes in organisation, more neurologists with an interest in vascular disease, and perhaps more vascular surgeons.

Hydrocephalus

Hydrocephalus is a complication of cerebellar strokes (both haemorrhage and infarction) which may be amenable to surgical treatment.

Asymptomatic bruits

These are common in the elderly population (about 7% over the age of 65). The annual risk of ipsilateral stroke is about 2%. Surgery is of no proved value, although trials are in progress.

Other aspects

Emotional

Psychiatric factors are very important; few doctors have sufficient time to address these fully. Depression and anxiety are common: with reassurance, especially about the risk of recurrence and advice about treatment to prevent further events, this will often improve. Counselling the spouse and close family is also important.[47]

Emotionalism is also common: it is present in both bilateral and unilateral strokes. It is usually sufficient to explain to the patient that this is a physical symptom which will improve with time. Small doses of amitriptyline (10–25 mg) may be beneficial.[48]

Epilepsy

Early epilepsy occurs in about 10% of all patients with stroke. It should be energetically treated with, for example, intravenous phenytoin, as the cerebral metabolic rate doubles during a fit. Late epilepsy after a stroke is a common cause of epilepsy in the elderly population. It is rare in the individual patient, however, and

143

indicates that the validity of the diagnosis of cerebrovascular disease should be reassessed.

Dysphagia

This is common, even after unilateral strokes. It usually improves but predisposes to aspiration, chest infection, dehydration, and death. As it can be assessed by simply asking the patient to drink 50 ml of water, this test should be mandatory in all patients with stroke.[49]

Thalamic pain

This is more common than is generally appreciated; it frequently starts weeks after the patient is discharged from hospital. It is a cause of great distress and may be helped by a variety of strategies.[50]

Other common problems

After acute stroke, deep venous thrombosis occurs in more than 50% of paretic legs, although a relatively small number develop symptomatic pulmonary embolism. It can usually be managed with elasticated stockings. Pressure sores, septicaemia (often secondary to urinary tract or chest infection), and hyperglycaemia may arise. Frozen shoulder is a common problem and can noticeably slow recovery.

Prognosis

The risk of a stroke after TIA is about 30% in five years. It is highest in the first year: in patients with carotid stenosis it is about 10–12%. The figures for stroke are similar. It is therefore important to reassure all patients that a second stroke is not imminent. Even patients with bilateral internal carotid occlusions only have a recurrent stroke risk of 13% a year.

Death in most patients with TIAs and stroke is caused by ischaemic heart disease.[5]

After an acute stroke, 20–30% of patients die. A poor prognosis is associated with reduced consciousness, conjugate gaze palsy, signs of severe brain stem dysfunction, pupillary changes, and incontinence persisting beyond the first few days. Strokes resulting in cognitive impairment, such as apraxia and neglect, and visuospatial dysfunction also carry a poor prognosis for recovery.

One year after a stroke, 33% of patients will be dead, 22% dependent, and 45% independent. Most recovery occurs in the first few weeks; less occurs in months three to six and even less (but still useful recovery) occurs in months six to 12. It is known that some symptoms, such as hemiplegic leg, can improve over a long period of time, but others often do not improve unless there is early recovery—for example, retinal infarction, homonymous hemianopia, and isolated spinothalamic sensory loss. In the hemiplegic hand, if there is no active hand grip after three weeks, there is unlikely to be much improvement. It is crucial to take the history of disability into account when planning rehabilitation.

Six months after a stroke, almost half the patients will be physically independent, 15% will have speech problems, 11% will be incontinent of urine and 7% incontinent of faeces, and 33% will still need assistance with feeding.

Stroke in the young

Stroke in youth is often not caused by premature atheroma (box 5.5). It should be investigated by a neurologist. The most common causes are emboli from the heart, carotid or vertebral dissection, antiphospholipid syndrome, arteritis, cerebral venous thrombosis, and premature atherosclerotic or hypertensive vascular disease. These require active assessment and treatment (box 5.6).[52] Cerebral venous thrombosis should possibly be treated by anticoagulation.[53]

Care of patients with TIA and stroke

In England and Wales there are about 100 000 patients with first stroke each year and 25 000 with initial TIAs.

TIA

Most TIAs will be managed by general practitioners. All reasonably fit patients with carotid events aged under 80 years should be referred to a neurologist or physician with an interest in vascular disease, to investigate the possibility of carotid stenosis, provided that the patient is prepared to take the risk of operation. All patients should be told the local surgical risk. The results should be independently audited to ensure a low complication rate.

145

Box 5.5   Causes of stroke in the young

Common:
  Premature atherosclerosis
  Cardiac embolism
  Dissection—carotid or vertebral
  Antiphospholipid syndrome including Sneddon's syndrome
  Migraine
  Arteritis (including postinfective e.g. ophthalmic zoster)
  Venous thrombosis
  Pregnancy

Uncommon:
  Fibromuscular dysplasia
  Drug abuse especially cocaine, heroin, amphetamine
  Late effect of radiotherapy
  Moya moya syndrome
  Takayasu's syndrome, Behçet's syndrome
  Amyloid angiopathy
  Homocystinuria
  Fabry's disease
  Pseudoxanthoma elasticum, Marfan's syndrome, Ehlers-Danlos
    syndrome
  Haematological causes
  Mitochondrial cytopathy
  Syphilis
  AIDS
  Neoplastic angioendotheliosis

I believe that patients under 50 years of age with TIAs should receive specialist opinion. I spend much time reassuring patients and refuting the diagnosis of vascular disease, usually with enormous relief to the patient. Patients with TIAs not controlled by aspirin or causing diagnostic difficulty should also be seen for specialist opinion.

Stroke

This is more difficult—the first question is whether the patient should be admitted to hospital. This is partly dependent on the severity of the deficit and age but, more often, on social factors such as the presence of carers and support services. Whatever

---

Box 5.6   Additional tests in young patients with stroke

- Magnetic resonance imaging or angiography*
- Echocardiography*
- Serology for syphilis*
- Serology for lupus anticoagulant, antinuclear factor*
- Serology for anticardiolipin antibody*
- Conventional angiography
- Haemoglobin electrophoresis
- Haematological opinion including pro-antithrombin III
- 24-Hour electrocardiography
- Screening tests for homocysteinuria
- Lumbar puncture
- Brain biopsy/meningeal biopsy
- White blood cell α-galactosidase
- Muscle biopsy
- HIV screen

* Should be performed in all young patients with stroke.

---

policy is followed, patients should be investigated appropriately and, ideally, all should have computed tomography.

I have no doubt that there will be treatment for acute stroke soon (as in myocardial infarction), and that acute stroke units will be needed to administer this. Acute investigations will all be performed at the same time. After a short period in such a unit (perhaps 24–72 hours), there are likely to be three options. Patients who have a mild deficit and will do well in any case can go home, needing only a small amount of domiciliary services. Severely disabled patients who will not do well whatever is done may be managed at home or in nursing homes or other long stay institutions. It is a waste of time and resources putting these people through a long and arduous rehabilitation programme that will do nothing except lead to frustration and disappointment for staff, patient, and family alike. Realistic goals must be set at all times and the patient and carers must understand what these are.

The rehabilitation of patients with intermediate disability is discussed in a separate chapter in this book.

Clinical criteria to identify these groups are slowly being formulated. Where doubt exists, the patient should be assumed to be able to benefit from rehabilitation. New data are beginning to identify patients at an early stage who will not benefit from rehabilitation.

A decision is needed about whether rehabilitation is best delivered at home or in hospital. It is also necessary to ascertain what aspects of disability respond to physiotherapy, speech therapy, and occupational therapy. Could one type of generalised therapist deliver most of this care and advice, only calling on a more specialised service if necessary? This would certainly simplify much domiciliary care.

Rehabilitation research needs to answer questions such as this to provide a useful, long term answer about the role of these therapists. Multicentre trials with simple protocols are just as relevant to rehabilitation as drug trials.

I suspect that rehabilitation is best managed at home: one hour daily (at best) of inpatient physiotherapy will be trivial compared with the amount of "physiotherapy" motivated patients will do in their own home. The two most important factors affecting length of stay in hospital are stroke severity and the absence of a carer at home.[54] Routine follow up every three to six months may help to reverse or slow down the late decline in mobility seen after stroke.[55] An integrated stroke service must be coordinated by a team leader. In hospital, this will be the consultant in charge of the stroke unit. In the community, the integrated stroke service liaising with the general practitioner will organise the necessary service. We do not want two completely separate services, one led by the hospital and one by the general practitioner. Large, randomised trials with detailed costings are needed to find out what is the most effective method of delivering optimum care. In addition, all therapists must be aware of their role as counsellors.[56]

It is essential that we use the charities fully. In the United Kingdom, the Stroke Association is becoming more and more active, and a host of support clubs are springing up. Booklets about many aspects of stroke, from TIA to wheelchairs and from epilepsy after stroke to stroke in the young, are available.

Delivering stroke care is expensive; it uses a large percentage of the NHS budget and we need to deliver care in the most efficient and cost effective manner. No view, however steeped in tradition, should be exempt from proper clinical assessment with large, properly conducted trials. The progress made in the past 10 years tells us that this must be the way forward; it is exciting to answer questions that everyone involved in the care of patients with stroke will face daily. The ultimate beneficiary is the patient.

Management of stroke and transient ischaemic attacks

- The initial assessment should try to show which anatomical territory has been affected—cortical, lacunar, vertebrobasilar, or carotid
- Risk factors should be assessed and vascular screening performed on all patients
- Blood pressure is the most important risk factor
- All patients with strokes should have computed tomography to differentiate haemorrhage from infarction
- Aspirin 300 mg should be given to all patients with ischaemic strokes, if possible, unless there is an indication for anticoagulation
- Carotid endarterectomy should be considered in patients who have recovered from a carotid event, are medically fit, and have a stenosis larger that 70%
- Young stroke is often not atheromatous

1 Oxfordshire Community Stroke Project. Incidence of stroke in Oxfordshire. First year's experience of a community stroke register. *BMJ* 1983;**287** 713–6.
2 Whisnant JP. The decline of stroke. *Stroke* 1984;**15**:160–8.
3 Hodges JR, Warlow CP. The aetiology of transient global amnesia. *Brain* 1990;**113**:639–57.
4 Caplan LR. Vertebrobasilar disease. *Stroke* 1981;**12**:111–4.
5 Fisher CM. Lacunar strokes and infarcts: a review. *Neurology* 1982;**32**:871–6.
6 Bamford J, Sandercock P, Dennis M, Burn J, Warlow C. Classification and natural history of clinically identifiable subtypes of cerebral infarction. *Lancet* 1991;**337**:1521–6.
7 Hennerici M, Klemm C, Rautenberg W. The subclavian steal phenomenon: a common vascular disorder with rare neurologic deficits. *Neurology* 1988;**36**:669–73.
8 Ross Russell RW, Bharucha N. The recognition and prevention of border zone cerebral ischaemia during cardiac surgery. *Q J Med* 1978;**47**:303–23.
9 Ross Russell RW, Page NGR. Critical perfusion of brain and retina. *Brain* 1983;**106**: 419–34.
10 Sandercock P, Molyneux A, Warlow CP. Value of computed tomography in patients with stroke: Oxfordshire Community Stroke Project. *BMJ* 1985;**290**:193–7.
11 Van Gijn J. Subarachnoid haemorrhage. *Lancet* 1992;**339**:653–5.
12 Allen CMC. Clinical diagnosis of acute stroke syndrome. *Q J Med* 1983;**52**:515–23.
13 Norris JW, Hachinski VC. Misdiagnosis of stroke. *Lancet* 1982;i:328–31.
14 Koudstaal PJ, Van Gijn J, Kappelle LJ. Headache in transient or permanent cerebral ischaemia. *Stroke* 1991;**22**:754–9.
15 Coleman RJ, Bamford JM, Warlow CP. For the UK TIA Study Group. Intracranial tumours that mimic transient cerebral ischaemia: lessons from a large multicentre trial. *J Neurol Neurosurg Psychiatry* 1993;**56**:563–6.

16 Kraaijeveld CL, Van Gijn J, Schouten HJA, Staal A. Interobserver agreement for the diagnosis of transient ischaemic attacks. *Stroke* 1984;**15**:723–5.

17 Landi G, Candelise L, Cella E, Pinardi G. Interobserver reliability of the diagnosis of lacunar transient ischaemic attack. *Cerebrovasc Dis* 1992;**2**:297–300.

18 Kannel WB, Wolf PA. Epidemiology of cerebrovascular disease. In: Ross Russell RW, ed. *Vascular disease of the central nervous system*. Edinburgh: Churchill Livingstone, 1983:1–24.

19 Dennis M, Bamford J, Sandercock P, Warlow C. Prognosis of transient ischaemic attacks in the Oxfordshire Community Stroke Project. *Stroke* 1990;**21**:848–53.

20 Donnan GA, McNeil JJ, Adena MA, Doyle AE, O'Malley HM, Neill GC. Smoking as a risk factor for cerebral ischaemia. *Lancet* 1989;ii:643–7.

21 Qizilbash N, Duffy SW, Warlow CP, Mann J. Lipids are risk factors for ischaemic stroke, overview and review. *Cerebrovasc Dis* 1992;**2**:127–36.

22 Clarke R, Daly L, Robinson K, *et al*. Hyperhomocysteinaemia: an independent risk factor for vascular disease. *N Engl J Med* 1991;**324**:1149–55.

23 Qizilbash N, Jones L, Warlow CP, Mann J. Fibrinogen and lipid concentrations as risk factors for transient ischaemic attacks and minor ischaemic strokes. *BMJ* 1991;**303**:605–9.

24 Humphrey P, Sandercock P, Slattery J. A simple method to improve the accuracy of non-invasive ultrasound in selecting TIA patients for cerebral angiography. *J Neurol Neurosurg Psychiatry* 1990;**53**:966–71.

25 Hankey GJ, Warlow CP. Symptomatic carotid ischaemic events: safest and most cost effective way of selecting patients for angiography, before carotid endarterectomy. *BMJ* 1990;**300**:1485–91.

26 Howard G, Cambless LE, Baker WH, *et al*. A multicentre validation study of Doppler ultrasound versus angiography. *J Stroke Cerebrovasc Dis* 1991;**1**:166–73.

27 Law M, Frost C, Wald N. By how much does dietary salt reduction lower blood pressure? II. Analysis of data from trials of salt reduction. *BMJ* 1991;**302**:819–24.

28 Dennis M, Warlow C. Strategy for stroke. *BMJ* 1991;**303**:636–8.

29 Payne JN, Milner PC, Saul C, Bowns IR, Hannay DR, Ramsay LE. Local confidential inquiry into avoidable factors in deaths from stroke and hypertensive disease. *BMJ* 1993; **307**:1027–30.

30 Langhorne P, Williams B, Gilchrist W, Howie K. Do stroke units save lives? *Lancet* 1993; **342**:395–8.

31 Gladman JRF, Lincoln NB, Barer DH. A randomised controlled trial of domiciliary and hospital based rehabilitation for stroke patients after discharge from hospital. *J Neurol Neurosurg Psychiatry* 1993;**56**:960–6.

32 Young JB, Forster A. The Bradford Community Stroke Trial, results at six months. *BMJ* 1992;**304**:1085–9.

33 Sandercock P, Willems H. Medical treatment of acute ischaemic stroke. *Lancet* 1992;**339**: 537–9.

34 Sandercock PAG, Van der Belt AG, Lindley RJ, Slattery J. Antithrombotic therapy in acute stroke: an overview of the completed randomized trials. *J Neurol Neurosurg Psychiatry* 1993; **56**:17–25.

35 Antiplatelet Trialists' collaboration. Secondary prevention of vascular disease by prolonged antiplatelet treatment. *BMJ* 1988;**296**:320–31.

36 Editorial. Ticlopidine. *Lancet* 1991;**459**–60.

37 European Atrial Fibrillation Study Group (EAFT). Secondary prevention in non rheumatic atrial fibrillation after transient ischaemic attack or minor stroke. *Lancet* 1993;**342**:1255–62.

38 Cerebral Embolism Study Group. Immediate anticoagulation of embolic stroke: brain hemorrhage and management options. *Stroke* 1984;**15**:779–89.

39 Brown MM, Humphrey PRD on behalf of the Association of British Neurologists. Carotid endarterectomy: recommendations for management of transient ischaemic attack and ischaemic stroke. *BMJ* 1992;**305**:1071–4.

40 Winslow CM, Solomon DH, Chassin MR, Kosecoff J, Merrick NJ, Brook RH. The appropriateness of carotid endarterectomy. *N Engl J Med* 1988;**318**:721–7.

41 Hankey GJ, Warlow CP, Sellar RJ. Cerebral angiographic risk in mild cerebrovascular disease. *Stroke* 1990;**21**:209–22.

42 Davies KN, Humphrey PRD. Complications of cerebral angiography in patients with symptomatic carotid territory ischaemia screened by carotid ultrasound. *J Neurol Neurosurg Psychiatry* 1993;**56**:967–72.

43 Young G, Humphrey PRD, Shaw MDM, Nixon TE, Smith ETS. A comparison of magnetic resonance angiography, Duplex ultrasound and digital subtraction angiography in the

assessment of extracranial internal carotid artery stenosis. *J Neurol Neurosurg Psychiatry* 1994;**57**:1466–78.

44 Harrison MJG, Marshall J. Indications for angiography and surgery in carotid artery disease. *BMJ* 1975;**1**:616–8.

45 Wilson LA, Ross Russell RW. Amaurosis fugax and carotid artery disease: indications for angiography. *BMJ* 1977;**ii**:435–7.

45a Davies KN, Humphrey PRD. Do carotid bruits predict disease of the internal carotid artery? *Postgrad Med J* 1994;**70**:433–5.

46 Martin JD, Valentime RJ, Myers SI, Rossi MB, Patterson CB, Clagett GP. Is routine CT scanning necessary in the preoperative evaluation of patients undergoing carotid endarterectomy? *J Vasc Surg* 1991;**14**:267–70.

47 House A. Depression after stroke. *BMJ* 1987;**294**:76–8.

48 House A, Dennis M, Molyneux A, Warlow CP, Hawton K. Emotionalism after stroke. *BMJ* 1989;**298**:991–4.

49 Gordon C, Langton Hewer R, Wade DT. Dysphagia in acute stroke. *BMJ* 1987;**295**:411–4.

50 Bowsher D. Pain syndromes and their treatment. *Curr Opin Neurol Neurosurg* 1993;**6**: 257–63.

51 Sacco RL, Wolf PA, Kannel WB, McNamara P. Survival and recurrence following stroke: the Framingham Study. *Stroke* 1982;**13**:290–5.

52 Caplan LR. Stroke in children and young adults. In: *Stroke: a clinical approach.* Oxford: Butterworth Heinemann, 1993;469–85.

53 Einhaupl KM, Villringer A, Meister W, *et al.* Heparin treatment in sinus venous thrombosis. *Lancet* 1991;**338**:597–600.

54 Wade DT, Langton Hewer R. Hospital admission for acute stroke. Who, for how long and to what effect? *J Epidemiol Commun Hlth* 1985;**39**:347–52.

55 Wade DT, Collen FM, Robb GF, Warlow CP. Physiotherapy intervention late after stroke and mobility. *BMJ* 1992;**304**:609–13.

56 Forster A, Young J. Stroke rehabilitation: can we do better? Emphasising physical recovery may be counter-productive. *BMJ* 1992;**305**:1446–7.

6 Meningitis

H P LAMBERT

Three organisms predominate in causing community-acquired bacterial meningitis, *Neisseria meningitidis*, *Haemophilus influenzae*, and *Streptococcus pneumoniae*. Meningococcal meningitis is most common in childhood but also affects adolescents and adults. In 1993 the Meningococcal Reference Unit examined 1297 isolates, 72% of which contained group B strains against which no vaccine is yet available. *H influenzae* meningitis chiefly affects children under 5 years old, although a few older patients are encountered. In 1992, 1089 blood or CSF isolates, or both, were recorded and a seven year study in the Oxford region has estimated the cumulative risk by the fifth birthday as 1:800.[1] Invasive haemophilus infections are already showing a gratifying reduction since the introduction of *H influenzae* type B (HIB) conjugate vaccines in October 1992.

The pattern of pneumococcal meningitis is more complex. It is seen at all ages but affects particularly the extremes of life and is also especially associated with immune defects such as asplenia, as in sickle cell disease, and with fractures of the skull or congenital defects allowing entry of bacteria to the CNS. This infection carries a high mortality, rarely recorded as less than 20%. The overall mortality from meningococcal and haemophilus meningitis is 5–6% in Britain, but the picture is often complicated by inclusion of acute meningococcal septicaemia, with a much higher death rate than that seen in meningitis alone. The overall mortality from childhood meningitis over a 10 year period in Nottingham[2] was 11·6% and at least one in 10 of the survivors suffered permanent sequelae; these consequences of meningitis are discussed later. In developing countries the incidence and mortality from meningitis are often much higher than in wealthier countries.

Meningitis caused by other bacteria is less common but important, as these infections often cause serious difficulties in diagnosis and management. The need to consider other agents has increased with the increasing number of patients with immune defects, especially HIV infection, and the associated resurgence of tuberculosis. To these bacterial causes must be added the problem of cryptococcal meningitis in association with HIV infection. In nosocomial meningitis, Gram negative organisms such as *Escherichia coli*, klebsiella, and pseudomonas have to be considered in the differential diagnosis, as also does *Listeria monocytogenes*. A similar distribution of organisms is seen in neonatal meningitis, a special problem not dealt with in this review.

Clinical diagnosis

In most patients the initial diagnosis of meningitis, or at least its possibility, is obvious from the combination of systemic and neurological features. Malaise, fever, severe headache, photophobia, and neck stiffness are common and sometimes consciousness is disturbed. The discussion will therefore mainly be concerned with difficulties in diagnosis and, as so often, these are greatest at the extremes of life. The problem of diagnosis in infancy is beyond the ambit of this review, but similar difficulties are sometimes encountered in the elderly. Consciousness may become rapidly depressed and soft neurological signs may lead diagnostic thoughts in the direction of a cerebrovascular accident. Fortunately meningism is a sign not easily masked and is usually, but not always, maintained even in comatose patients.

Meningococcal disease may present in several atypical and deceptive ways. At one extreme, fulminating meningococcal septicaemia, the illness may run its short course from onset to death with no element of meningitis. At the other end of the scale of severity patients, especially children, may experience a period of hours, or even days, of febrile illness with no meningeal features before the symptoms and signs of meningitis appear. This sequence has often led to medicolegal problems when a claim of delayed or missed diagnosis may rest on this point. One especially deceptive presentation of meningococcal meningitis, seen in adolescents and young adults, is as acute mania, directing the diagnosis towards acute psychosis, possibly drug-induced.[3] Neck stiffness may not yet have developed or may be impossible to test for.

153

The rash of meningococcal septicaemia, when present, is a valuable feature, as the combination of petechial-purpuric rash and meningitis is virtually diagnostic for this organism. The rash may vary from a few inconspicuous petechiae to extensive purpura with skin necrosis. Non-purpuric rashes—and occasionally petechial ones—are seen in some patients with enteroviral rashes, but this aetiology should never be assumed, as the early rash of meningococcal disease may be macular and unimpressive.

Focal neurological signs are relatively uncommon in pyogenic meningitis in previously healthy patients. Ocular palsies usually resolve within days or weeks. In sharp contrast, labyrinthine damage, which often develops early in the illness, is usually permanent. The frequency of convulsions varies greatly between different forms of meningitis, and is much higher in infancy than in older age groups. They are most frequent in pneumococcal meningitis, less common in haemophilus meningitis, and uncommon in meningococcal disease.[4] Fits are also distinctly uncommon in community-acquired meningitis in adult life in patients with no underlying neurological abnormality, When focal signs, convulsions, or disturbance of consciousness are prominent in the clinical picture, the possibility of encephalitis as the primary diagnosis should be considered.

In community-acquired meningitis in previously healthy patients there is often no specific aetiological clue such as rash, recent otitis media, or head injury. In such cases the patient's age may be the sole diagnostic pointer, as haemophilus meningitis is rare after the first few years of life, meningococcal meningitis is the most common form at school age and in young adults, whereas in the elderly S pneumoniae becomes more frequent. There are many exceptions to these generalisations, especially now that many reasonably well people in the community may have various forms of immune suppression, notably HIV infection or treatment with immunosuppressive drugs, and may present with uncommon forms of meningitis. Early and accurate laboratory diagnosis therefore remains important and should be achieved as often as possible.

Lumbar puncture

Until recently, suspicion of meningitis was accepted as an almost invariable indication for lumbar puncture, although it was always recognised that it should be avoided or deferred if there was suspicion of an alternative diagnosis that might mimic meningitis, such as brain abscess, cerebral haemorrhage, encephalitis, or posterior fossa tumour. In the past few years, however, concern about the possibility of coning has led to a more cautious approach to lumbar puncture in meningitis. The risk of coning is variously estimated. A recent retrospective survey, from an Australian paediatric referral centre receiving a preponderance of complicated or seriously ill children, noted cerebral herniation in 19 of 445 children (4·3%).[5] There was a strong suggestion that lumbar puncture led to this complication in some patients, although it can certainly occur in patients with meningitis when no lumbar puncture has been done. On the other hand, there are great advantages in making an accurate and early diagnosis, and a Gram-stained smear of the CSF deposit is still the most common way in which this can be achieved. Certainly "blind" treatment is often successful but if the responsible organism is unusual or antibiotic-resistant, or the patient's progress is unsatisfactory in any way, failure of identification creates an uncertain and unsatisfactory situation.

The dilemma can be resolved by defining genuine risk factors for coning while accepting that lumbar puncture is normally indicated in suspected meningitis. A common injunction is to avoid lumbar puncture if there is suspicion of raised intracranial pressure, a distinctly unhelpful precept as intracranial pressure is raised in nearly every patient with meningitis.[6] More realistic guidelines can be set using known clinical correlates of impending coning, namely coma or rapidly increasing depression of consciousness, focal neurological signs, and tonic or prolonged fits. Fits are common in childhood meningitis in some communities and are not an invariable contraindication to lumbar puncture although, as Mellor points out in a thoughtful review,[7] it is sensible to defer lumbar puncture for 30 minutes after a fit because of the transient cerebral oedema that accompanies it. Papilloedema is a contraindication but is very rare in meningitis and its presence should in any case indicate a wider diagnostic sweep.

Another indication for avoiding or delaying lumbar puncture is unrelated to the question of coning. This is the need for urgent treatment of patients with established or threatened bacterial shock (usually meningococcal septicaemia). The window of opportunity closes rapidly in these patients and treatment should on no account be delayed in order to do a lumbar puncture.

Computed tomograms or magnetic resonance scans are usually normal or mildly and non-specifically abnormal in meningitis and are not generally helpful in detecting coning.[7]

Tuberculous meningitis

In countries with a high prevalence of tuberculosis, tuberculous meningitis acts as one of the markers of the frequency of infection, and the diagnosis is in question in any patient, especially a child, with meningitis. Where tuberculosis has declined the diagnosis is hard to bear in mind, and the problem is compounded by the often deceptive ways in which this disease presents. Its importance is again increasing with the spread of HIV infection and the high prevalence in many countries of the poor social conditions and crowding that are associated with tuberculosis. The relation of success in treatment to the stage at presentation has rightly been stressed.

There is usually a prodromal illness of days or weeks, with low fever, malaise, and headache before meningeal features develop. The multiple pathology of tuberculous meningitis, with basal arachnoiditis, vasculitis, infarction, and obstructive hydrocephalus leads to an immense variety of possible focal features; most frequent are cranial nerve palsies and papilloedema. Spinal involvement may take a number of different forms, and rare presentations include a mainly encephalopathic picture. It is important, however, to remember that tuberculous meningitis may present as a meningeal illness with no specific features, so that the diagnosis must be entertained in any patient with non-purulent meningitis. Some persistent myths must be abandoned; the onset may be acute, the CSF glucose concentration is within the normal range in about 20% of cases, and the tuberculin test result is initially negative in a similar proportion. Because of these protean manifestations, laboratory diagnosis is particularly important (see below), but unfortunately tubercle bacilli are seen in the CSF in only a few cases, depending on the technical skills available, and cultures are not always positive. Indicative features in the clinical presentation include slow onset, contact or family history, ethnic origin, or immigrant status from an area of high prevalence, whereas a primary lung complex or any evidence of miliary tuberculosis will obviously virtually establish the diagnosis.

Cryptococcal meningitis

Cryptococcal meningitis also varies widely in its mode of onset. In immunocompromised patients the course tends to be more rapid than in immunocompetent people but in both groups onset may be insidious, with general malaise, low fever, and headache. This subtle form of presentation is common now that HIV infection is the most frequent type of immune abnormality preceding cryptococcal meningitis.[8] Indeed, features indicative of CNS involvement may be entirely absent and the indications for lumbar puncture must be more widely set in these patients than in immunocompetent people. Lumbar puncture in HIV-infected patients should be preceded by computed tomography because of the possibility of a silent mass lesion. A small proportion of patients with cryptococcal meningitis show focal neurological signs, including early visual loss.[9] In some patients the course of the illness is much more protracted, extending over many months before a diagnosis is reached, and sometimes greatly fluctuating in severity.

Listeria meningitis

Listeria meningitis is most frequently seen in neonates but also has a predilection for immunocompromised and elderly people. Presentation is usually as an acute purulent meningitis with no particular distinguishing features, but the subtle presentations mentioned in the context of cryptococcal meningitis are seen here also. Neurological signs and disturbance of consciousness are common with a mixed meningitic and encephalitic picture, which is more commonly seen with listeria than with other forms of bacterial meningitis. Listeria also causes a range of other CNS conditions, including single or multiple brain abscess, diffuse encephalitis and, rarely, brain stem encephalitis.

Laboratory diagnosis

This topic can be discussed only briefly, chiefly to stress its importance and the need for efficient and prompt acquisition of correct specimens by the clinician and for good liaison between ward and laboratory. Gram staining of the centrifuged CSF deposit remains the gold standard for early diagnosis, with occasional help from other specimens such as smears from skin lesions. Later, results of blood and CSF cultures provide the main diagnostic yield. Many methods of early diagnosis have been developed, the most useful of which are antigen detection methods, especially latex particle agglutination, which can be employed using CSF, serum, or urine. These techniques are not generally superior to traditional staining, but have definite value in reducing the diagnostic gap in patients who have been given antibiotics before admission.

Diagnosis of tuberculous meningitis still depends mainly on traditional staining methods on the CSF deposit, but new techniques are being developed, notably the polymerase chain reaction, which may greatly improve the low sensitivity of current diagnostic methods.[10]

Diagnosis of cryptococcal meningitis rests largely on cryptococcal antigen detection in CSF (but not blood), on India ink preparations of CSF to detect capsulated *Cryptococcus neoformans*, and on culture using large volumes of CSF.

Treatment (see table 6.1 for doses)

Treatment of the three common forms of pyogenic meningitis has been greatly complicated by increasing prevalence of several types of antibiotic drug resistance. Until these changes became widespread, antibiotic treatment of meningitis caused by these organisms could be accomplished using two safe, easily administered, and cheap agents benzylpenicillin (or ampicillin) and chloramphenicol. Benzylpenicillin is still appropriate for meningococcal and pneumococcal disease in most countries, but haemophilus meningitis, and meningitis of uncertain aetiology must now often be treated with extended spectrum cephalosporins, a particular tragedy in developing countries in which meningitis is common and in which the cost of these compounds is beyond the reach of publicly funded health budgets. It is therefore important

Table 6.1 Dosage of antibiotics commonly used in meningitis

| | Total dose per 24 hours | | | |
Agent	Adult (g)	Child (mg per kg)	Dose interval (hours)	Route
Benzylpenicillin	14·4	180–300	4	Intravenous
Ampicillin	12	200	4	Intravenous
Chloramphenicol*	3	50–100	6	Intravenous or oral
Cefotaxime	8	200	8	Intravenous
Ceftriaxone	4	80	24	Intravenous
Vamcomycin†	2	40	6	Intravenous

* Dosage unsuitable for neonates, † Control by blood levels required.

to remember that penicillin and chloramphenicol remain agents of first choice in many areas, and may indeed be the only agents available. Table 6.1 gives the dosages of antibiotics commonly used.

Meningococcal meningitis can be treated with equal efficacy by high dose penicillin or ampicillin given intravenously or by chloramphenicol, given by intravenous injection initially, and by mouth as soon as practicable. The role of cephalosporins was at first controversial, as the earlier compounds were relatively ineffective, but the newer compounds, although most widely used in *H influenzae* meningitis, are also of established efficacy in meningococcal infections. An important caveat is the emergence of penicillin resistance in meningococci, especially in Spain, but also increasingly recorded elsewhere. The level of risk of encountering a resistant strain that would necessitate a change from penicillin or ampicillin must be kept under review. One important difference between meningococcal and other forms of meningitis is the relative ease with which the organism can be eradicated. Although 10–14 day courses of treatment have traditionally been used in all forms of meningitis, shorter courses are fully adequate in meningococcal disease. Successful trials have included durations of seven, five, and even four days with penicillin.[11] Chloramphenicol is the best choice in patients allergic to penicillin. In field conditions in tropical Africa, several studies have been made of treatment in one or two doses using a long acting preparation of chloramphenicol in oil. For example, in a large, randomised trial involving 528 patients in Mali and Niger, the success of a two-dose scheme of this sort equalled that achieved by intravenous ampicillin given four times

159

daily for five days, and was clearly much more simple to administer. The mortality in all groups in these trials was much higher than that found in the West, again demonstrating the great impact of meningitis in these areas.[12]

Penicillin is also still the best agent for the treatment of pneumococcal meningitis, but pneumococci resistant to penicillin have become widespread and are now common enough in several countries, inluding Spain and Hungary, to preclude the use of penicillin in treatment. The treatment of penicillin-resistant pneumococcal meningitis presents a difficult and partly unsolved problem. The chief alternative, chloramphenicol, may be successful but has failed to eradicate infection in a number of cases. It has been shown, in work from South Africa, that many penicillin-resistant pneumococci, although susceptible to chloramphenicol on disc testing, require high minimum bactericidal concentrations of this agent, and that this form of partial resistance is associated with poor results of treatment.[13] Vancomycin, although a difficult drug to use, has had some success, but a number of treatment failures have led to the suggestion that it should be used in penicillin/chloramphenicol-resistant pneumococcal meningitis only if high dose cephalosporins have failed or if the patient has anaphylactic reactions to β lactam agents.[14]

H influenzae meningitis has its main impact in children under 4 years old, but is seen occasionally in older children and adults. Ampicillin, formerly widely used alone or together with chloramphenicol, has now lost its role because resistance to its action is now present in a large number of isolates, 15–25% in most countries. Chloramphenicol is still the best agent in many areas, but resistance is increasing, and many ampicillin-resistant strains are also resistant to chloramphenicol. For these reasons extended spectrum cephalosporins such as cefotaxime and ceftriaxone have become the chosen agents in haemophilus meningitis or meningitis of uncertain aetiology. Treatment may be modified when laboratory results are available. Although active against the three common pathogens,[15] cephalosporins have limited or no activity against some of the more unusual causes of meningitis, notably listeria and some of the less common Gram negative organisms. If the patient has an underlying disease that places him or her at risk for these unusual pathogens and treatment has to be started without microbiological information, the initial regimen should include ampicillin together with the cephalosporin.

Antibiotic treatment before admission diminishes the prospects of obtaining a positive finding by CSF microscopy or culture. Occasionally the CSF is altered more profoundly, with a lymphocytic picture. If partly treated pyogenic meningitis is in question (as well as other diagnoses such as brain abscess and tuberculous meningitis), it would be reasonable to begin provisional treatment with a cephalosporin in full dosage while other investigations are in train.

Tuberculous meningitis

Tuberculous meningitis stands apart from other forms of meningitis in many important ways. Diagnosis can be difficult, the course of the disease variable, and prognosis uncertain. These and other factors have led to a deficiency of the extensive controlled clinical trials that have established well validated regimens for the treatment of pulmonary and some forms or non-pulmonary tuberculosis. Treatment tends therefore to be based on limited trial data, the empirical opinion of physicians with experience of the disease, and on knowledge of the pharmacokinetics of antituberculous agents.[16] The broad relationship of prognosis to neurological deficit demands that treatment should be started as soon as possible, even when there is still uncertainty about the diagnosis. Fear that diagnosis will then be impossible to establish is largely unfounded, because it can often be made from post-treatment specimens of CSF, or from later results of culture of specimens taken before or after treatment. Alternatively, a different diagnosis may later be established—for example, by virological findings that allow the provisional treatment for tuberculosis to be discontinued.

The pharmacokinetics of antituberculous agents in the CSF are well established. Pyrazinamide shows excellent penetration into the CSF. The CSF/serum ratio in Chinese patients is about 75% two hours after the dose is given, and about 110% after five and eight hours. Isoniazid too penetrates well, with concentrations in CSF approaching those in serum. Rifampicin concentrations in CSF are 10–15% those in serum, representing the unbound moiety of the drug. Streptomycin achieves adequate concentration in the CSF after standard intramuscular dosage only when the meninges are inflamed, and this is true also of ethambutol, given orally. Ethionamide and prothionamide, by contrast, penetrate the CSF

161

well, whether or not the meninges are inflamed, although their value is limited by gastrointestinal and other unwanted effects. Initial treatment should employ at least a triple regimen of pyrazinamide, isoniazid, and rifampicin. It is still uncertain whether streptomycin is needed as an addition to this scheme. Workers in Hong Kong with great experience of the disease recommended its inclusion during the first two or three months of treatment, and it should certainly be used if rifampicin cannot be obtained because of its cost.[16] The three principal agents are all given by mouth in once daily dosage, or by gastric tube if the patient cannot swallow. The dose of pyrazinamide is 35 mg/kg for a child, 2 g for an adult, that of rifampicin 10 mg/kg. Isoniazid has customarily been given in higher dosages, 10 mg/kg, than are used in other forms of tuberculosis, but the conventional dose of 300 mg or 4–5 mg/kg is probably adequate. Pyridoxine 10 mg daily is given to prevent isoniazid neuropathy. Streptomycin is administered by intramuscular injection in a dose of 20 mg/kg to a maximum of 1 g daily but careful and continued attention should of course be paid to renal function. Intrathecal treatment can no longer be recommended, although there was evidence of its value in treatment regimens which preceded the use of rifampicin and pyrazinamide.

The optimum duration of treatment is unknown. Because the disease is so serious, it has been customary to use long courses of treatment. This is perhaps illogical because, despite the devastating pathology of the condition, the bacterial population concerned is small compared with that found, say, in cavitating pulmonary tuberculosis. Most authors continue treatment for one year, but shorter courses have been used, for example, a nine month regimen.

The role of steroids has been debated for decades, but rigorous analysis by controlled trial has never been achieved. A mixture of open studies, anecdotal evidence, and possibly shaky inference from the known effects of steroids on inflammatory processes has led to their use in the more neurologically advanced grades of the disease, in infants, in generally very ill patients, and in impending spinal block, which may nevertheless progress even during their administration. The situation with raised intracranial pressure in tuberculous meningitis is more clear cut. CSF block leading to hydrocephalus requires urgent control by shunting. Clinicians working in areas of high prevalence believe that early shunting is an important factor in improving prognosis. Rising intracranial pressure from enlarging tuberculoma can be controlled in most patients by high dose dexamethasone, and surgical decompression is rarely necessary.

Cryptococcal meningitis

Before the advent of HIV infection and AIDS, cryptococcal meningitis was rarely seen in Britain, and then mainly in association with defects of cellular immunity—for example, in patients with lymphoma, those receiving substantial doses of steroids, and in patients with sarcoid whether or not on steroids. In some other countries a substantial number of patients with cryptococcal meningitis had no overt predisposing factors. This picture changed dramatically with the spread of HIV infection and cryptococcal meningitis is now seen as one of the most common CNS infections associated with AIDS. Treatment is difficult and demanding. Failure and relapse are common even in patients without HIV infection; in the presence of HIV, as with other infections, eradication is especially difficult and for this reason much thought has been given to devising practical methods of long term prevention as well as to improving treatment of established infections.

Agents available for chemotherapy include amphotericin in various forms, flucytosine and some of the more recently developed triazole compounds, of which fluconazole has been most extensively studied. Trials completed before the onset of HIV established the value of amphotericin, despite its formidable toxicity, and showed how the unwanted effects could be partly mitigated by using the synergy, demonstable in vitro and in vivo, between this agent and flucytosine. A major multicentre study showed that a combination of amphotericin in a dose of 0·3 mg/kg daily together with flucytosine in a dose of 150 mg/kg daily given for six weeks gave results at least as good as with amphotericin alone at 0·4 mg/kg per day for 10 weeks. The patients given combination therapy showed superior results at a non-significant level by a number of criteria; eight of 34 patients in the combination group died compared with 15 of 32 given amphotericin alone.[17]

Since this trial the methods of using amphotericin have been to some extent refined, with a trend to give larger doses, 0·5–0·7 mg/kg daily, or 1·0–1·2 mg/kg on alternate days. Duration of treatment may also be varied. Four weeks may prove adequate for patients with no adverse prognostic factors. These factors include underlying immune defects (and therefore all those with cryptococcal meningitis superimposed on HIV infection), neurological deficit, a high cryptococcal antigen titre (>1:32) in the CSF and a low (<20 mm³) CSF leucocyte count. Treatment may, however, fail even in patients with no identifiable adverse features.

The onerous nature and limited success of these methods of treatment is even more notable in AIDS-associated cryptococcal meningitis, in which marrow suppression by disease or by other drugs used in therapy may limit or prevent the use of flucytosine. The potential of triazole compounds, with lower toxicity and the advantage of oral administration, is therefore especially interesting in this group of patients. After favourable early results, a formal comparison of fluconazole and amphotericin was made in a randomised, multicentre trial.[18] Fluconazole was given in a dose of 200 mg daily, amphotericin at 0·4–0·5 mg/kg daily. The gravity of this infection is clearly revealed, with successful treatment in only 40% of 63 patients in the amphotericin group and in 34% of 131 patients given fluconazole. There was no significant difference in overall mortality, but deaths were more frequent in the fluconazole group during the first two weeks of treatment and CSF culture reverted to negative more slowly than in the amphotericin group. Comments on this trial emphasised that dosage of both drugs might now be thought too low. Other schemes being evaluated use a higher (0·7 mg/kg) dose of amphotericin with or without flucytosine at 100 mg/kg, either as definitive treatment or for the first two weeks followed by fluconazole. Other studies involve higher doses: 400 mg or 800 mg of fluconazole. Favourable results are also being reported with itraconazole,[19] although this compound does not reach the CSF in detectable concentrations.

The prospects for preventing recurrence of cryptococcal meningitis after initial successful treatment are more promising. A comparison of fluconazole 200 mg daily, with amphotericin 100 mg weekly showed clearly superior results for fluconazole, with relapse in 2% compared with 18% in the amphotericin group.[20] The high relapse rate in patients with AIDS and other forms of immune suppression make it essential to use long term prophylaxis after initial treatment. What is still uncertain is whether, at least in areas where cryptococcal meningitis is a common feature of AIDS, primary prophylaxis should be attempted. A retrospective study reported only one patient with cryptococcal meningitis of 329 given daily fluconazole as against 16 in 329 historical "controls". This type of primary prevention may come to be vitiated by the development of fluconazole resistance, already emerging in *Candida albicans* infections.

Role of steroids

There is now abundant evidence that endogenously released factors play an important part in causing the inflammatory changes of meningitis, and increasing interest in the possibility that measures aimed at inhibiting this response might be beneficial.

Although much detail remains to be filled in, the relevant processes can be summarised briefly. In the case of meningococci and *H influenzae*, the initiating factor is endotoxin, a lipopolysaccharide component of the cell wall released in the form of vesicles from the bacteria. Similar processes are induced in pneumococcal infection by the release of other cell wall components, mainly teichoic acid and peptidoglycan. After a time lag of a few hours, pro-inflammatory cytokines are induced, including tumour necrosis factor, and interleukins 1, 6, and 8. These and other factors produced from macrophages and from platelets have been shown in experimental systems to induce the changes of acute inflammation in the CNS. An additional complicating factor is that neutrophils, although an important component of the defence systems against pyogenic infection, themselves contribute to the inflammatory process when, after adhesion and migration, they degranulate and produce pro-inflammatory factors including reactive oxygen species.[21]

The link between inflammatory mediators and the timing and intensity of CSF changes is well established in experimental work, and there is increasing evidence of their relevance to human meningitis. For example, the outcome of meningitis can be correlated with levels of endotoxin and pro-inflammatory cytokines in the CSF.[22 23] These processes are also clearly established in septicaemic meningococcal infection, in which there are close relations between plasma endotoxin levels and prognosis and between endotoxin levels and levels of tumour necrosis factor-α, interleukin-1, and interleukin-6.[24]

An especially taxing question is whether lytic antibiotics, given to cure the infection, might themselves have an adverse effect by causing rapid release of bacterial products and thus provoking an increased inflammatory burst. In experimental models of meningitis

165

it is clear that an increase of several mediators, and a consequent inflammatory burst, follows the administration of lytic antibiotics such as β lactams.[25] This increased inflammatory response can be significantly mitigated by dexamethasone if given at the same time as, but not one hour later than, the antibiotic.[26] Again, the evidence from human meningitis is necessarily more fragmentary. In one study, eight children with H influenzae meningitis had repeat lumbar puncture two to six hours after their initial dose of antibiotic, ceftriaxone. The second specimens showed increased concentration of endotoxin correlated with the decrease in viable bacteria, together with increase in lactate and decrease in glucose concentration in the CSF. In some cases tumour necrosis factor concentration in the CSF rose about four hours after starting treatment.[27] It is therefore possible that diminishing the endogenously mediated inflammatory processes might be beneficial.

It is against this background that the current renewed interest in a role for steroids in pyogenic meningitis has arisen, after a 20 year lapse since their first trial.[28 29] The first favourable evidence of a beneficial effect on outcome was gained from two trials involving 200 children, predominantly with haemophilus meningitis.[30] In one trial the antibiotic used was cefuroxime (not now considered entirely satisfactory as the cephalosporin of choice in meningitis), in the other ceftriaxone. In both, patients were randomly allocated to receive placebo or dexamethasone in a dose of 0·15 mg/kg six hourly for four days. The dexamethasone group showed a significant increase in the speed with which abnormal CSF findings resolved, and, at follow up, substantial hearing loss was found in 15 placebo and three dexamethasone recipients; hearing aids were needed in 12 and one respectively. A smaller trial of 60 patients gave similar, although non-significant results.[31] Notable reductions in the interlukein-1 β concentration were also demonstrated, together with improved prognosis, in dexamethasone-treated children. An open study in Egypt involved adults and children with meningitis, alternate patients being given dexamethasone. Seven of 52 patients with pneumococcal meningitis given dexamethasone died, compared with 22 of 44 controls. Sequelae were also less common in the dexamethasone group.[32]

Two more substantial controlled trials in childhood meningitis have taken account, in their design, of the importance of timing in experimental models. Children in Costa Rica[33] were given placebo or dexamethasone in the same dose as in the previous studies (0·15 mg/kg six hourly for four days) but beginning 15–20 minutes before the first dose of the antibiotic, cefotaxime. At 12 hours the dexamethasone-treated group showed improvement compared with the controls in CSF pressure and in inflammatory indices and cytokine concentrations in the CSF. At follow up seven of 51 dexamethasone-treated children (14%), and 18 of 48 controls (38%) had neurological or audiological sequelae (relative risk 3·8, 95% confidence interval (CI) 1·3 to 11·5). A Swiss trial[34] differed in the dose and duration of dexamethasone administration, 0·4 mg/kg 12 hourly for two days, starting 10 minutes before the first dose of antibiotic, ceftriaxone. Follow up at 3, 9, and 15 months showed sequelae in three of 60 dexamethasone recipients (5%) and nine of 55 placebo recipients (16%) (relative risk 3·27, 95% CI 0·93 to 11·47). Table 6.2 summarises the results of these important studies.

The trials also showed few adverse effects in the dexamethasone groups, mainly a higher incidence of gastrointestinal bleeding, usually detected only by investigation rather than by a significant clinical event. Moreover, cases of viral meningitis inadvertently treated with dexamethasone showed no adverse effects. It is reasonable to conclude that steroids, given in high dosage for a short time, and started early and preferably shortly before starting antibiotics, have a beneficial effect on outcome in childhood haemophilus meningitis, with lesser but suggestive evidence of benefit in other forms and at other ages. For example, a retrospective study of 97 children with pneumococcal meningitis indicated benefits both in the acute illness and in the neurological outcome for those who received steroids before, or concurrently with, the first dose of antibiotic.[34a]

Several other modes of damping the inflammatory response and its adverse pathophysiological consequences have been successful in experimental systems. They include non-steroidal anti-inflammatory agents, monoclonal antibodies against some of the cytokines involved, and antibody inhibiting leucocyte adhesion to endothelium. No method of modulating the inflammatory process, however, other than administration of steroids, is yet available for use in human meningitis.

Other aspects of management

Might any aspects of therapy other than antibiotics and steroids help to mitigate the continued high mortality and residual morbidity

Table 6.2 Neurological and audiological sequelae of meningitis. Trials of dexamethasone

Reference	No in study	No (%) with neurological sequelae		No (%) with moderate or severe deafness	
		Dexamethasone	Placebo	Dexamethasone	Placebo
30,31	260	4 (4)	9 (12)	11 (9)	21 (19)
33	101	5 (10)	15 (31)	3 (6)	7 (16)
34	115	3 (5)	5 (9)	3 (5)	7 (13)

associated with bacterial meningitis? Fits must, of course, be brought under control as promptly as possible, and mannitol infusions are of established value if signs of increasing intracranial pressure appear. Changes in the cerebral circulation in meningitis may be important, and certainly in experimental models the inflammatory process leads to a complex interaction of brain oedema and raised intracranial pressure, with changes in cerebral blood flow and perfusion. Especially notable is loss of autoregulation so that the cerebral blood flow becomes passively responsive to the systemic blood pressure.[35] Few measurements of the cerebral circulation have been made in human meningitis, and these largely in infants and children. Two important studies by non-invasive techniques are notable. Goh and Minns[36] made serial measurements of cerebral blood flow velocity using transcranial Doppler ultrasound. They found an increase in flow velocity as meningitis resolved with a decrease in the final resistance index, suggesting a decrease in cerebral perfusion during the acute phase of the illness. Mannitol infusion, by reducing intracranial pressure, increased cerebral perfusion pressure with a resultant decreased resistance index and increase in blood flow velocity. Another study, involving seriously ill children, employed stable xenon computed tomography.[37] This showed diminished blood flow in only a few patients (five as against 18 with normal cerebral blood flow) but did show pronounced regional variations in flow changes. Measurements in artificially ventilated patients at different arterial carbon dioxide tensions ($PaCO_2$) showed that hyperventilation to low $PaCO_2$ could reduce regional blood flow below ischaemic thresholds. In these and other studies cerebral autoregulation appeared to be generally preserved, and pressure passivity was seen only in some very ill children with grossly abnormal neurological signs.

Some tentative conclusions relevant to clinical management may be drawn from these studies. It would seem sensible, in patients seriously ill with meningitis, to aim at avoiding fluctuations of blood pressure in either direction which might lead to changes in cerebral blood flow. In particular, hyperventilation with the aim of reducing intracranial pressure may sometimes prove dis-advantageous and it is preferable to maintain the $PaCO_2$ within the normal range.

A common error in management is to limit fluid intake unduly with the aim of controlling inappropriate secretion of antidiuretic hormone and, it is supposed, thus reducing the likelihood of cerebral oedema. It has been shown in childhood meningitis, however, that the observed high levels of arginine vasopressin are an appropriate response to hypovolaemia and that levels return to normal when fluid replacement is achieved.[38] Fluid deficits in meningitis should be corrected with the appropriate replacement fluids and normal maintenance requirements provided.

Communication

The diagnosis of meningitis brings with it enormous fear and anxiety for many reasons. Will the patient die? Will the patient be brain damaged? Will other members of the family or other people "catch" meningitis? All these questions must be discussed as often as necessary. Especially difficult is the oft-expressed question, why did this particular person develop meningitis? A simple account of how these bacteria spread is often helpful to the family and needs including with discussion of the patient's progress. To this must be added the common anxiety of health service staff about the possibility of infection when treating patients with meningococcal meningitis or septicaemia. The consultant in communicable disease control must be informed as soon as possible so that preventive measures (see below) can be rapidly brought into operation. Close liaison with the laboratory is of course essential to ensure the best possible quality of specimens and thus the best chance of identifying the causal organism and its sensitivity to antibiotics.

Sequelae

Most previously healthy survivors of community-acquired meningitis recover completely but an important minority is left with residua ranging from mild neurological or audiological defects to profound and lifelong disability. Bacterial meningitis is the most common cause of acquired sensorineural deafness. Its frequency has been analysed in a thoughtful review by Fortnum[39] accepting only published series with well-defined criteria avoiding the many possible confounding factors in such studies (table 6.3). Deafness complicates meningitis in about 10% of patients, and will be bilaterally profound or total in 1–4%.

Pneumococcal meningitis is generally reported to carry a much higher risk of deafness than the other two common forms, although

Table 6.3 Permanent hearing loss after bacterial meningitis

Type of meningitis	No in study	No (%) with permanent sensorineural hearing loss of any degree
Unselected	1175	113 (9·6)
Haemophilus influenzae	876	99 (11·4)
Meningococcal	398	30 (7·5)
Pneumococcal	66	21 (31·8)

After Fortnum.[32]

the difference may not be as great as has been supposed. Certainly the risk of deafness exists in all forms of meningitis and at all ages, and no reliable predictors of this complication are available. Whether the trend towards steroid treatment will make an impact on the frequency of deafness remains to be seen.

The likelihood of other serious long term sequelae is hard to estimate but may occur at about the same frequency as severe deafness—for example, four of 48 children who survived haemophilus meningitis in Wales suffered long term neurological sequelae (8%).[40]

Relation between duration of illness and outcome

The relation between clinical features and the known pathophysiology of meningitis is important to our understanding of the disease. The question is also important in the medicolegal context as actions about neurological damage following meningitis often centre on a claim of missed or delayed diagnosis. Inflammatory changes in the CNS are related to bacterial load, which suggests a connection between prognosis and delayed diagnosis, but attempts to analyse the point reveal a more complex picture. One prospective analysis[41] showed that children with a history of less than 48 hours illness did significantly worse than those with longer histories. A recent exhaustive examination of 22 studies involving 4707 patients with meningitis attempted to analyse the question in more detail.[42] Many of the studies were unsuitable for formal meta-analysis, but the previous finding that children with a slow and insidious presentation had a better outlook than those with acute illness was confirmed. At the other extreme, in a small subgroup with fulminant meningitis, the influence of antibiotics seemed minimal. Between these lies the group with clinically overt meningitis but without septicaemic shock; data were insufficient to analyse these, the very patients in whom it would seem plausible that early treatment would be beneficial. These analyses reflect a familiar clinical observation, that there is often a substantial prodromal illness of hours to days before features of meningitis appear, especially in children. Although the entire illness is subsequently designated as meningitis, presumably the early phase corresponds with the bacteraemic illness preceding localisation to the meninges, or perhaps in some cases a preceding viral infection. In either case the host–parasite relation is more evenly balanced, and the illness less severe, than in fulminant meningococcal septicaemia.

A further point bearing on the complex relation between duration of illness and outcome is that deafness, the most common adverse event leading to long term disability, often develops very early in the course of meningitis.

Prevention

Vaccination

The persistently high mortality and residual morbidity from meningitis make it likely that substantial further progress can be made only by improvements in prevention. Recent years have seen encouraging advances in vaccination, with the promise of more to come.

Capsular antigen plays an important part in pathogenesis for all the common causes of bacterial meningitis, and antibody to capsular antigen is correspondingly important in protection. Unfortunately, children under 2 years old show poor and transient responses to these polysaccharide antigens.[43] This serious deficiency in the value of these antigens in immunisation programmes has been successfully addressed in the case of *H influenzae* by formulating conjugates of the capsular antigen with various protein moieties that render them fully immunogenic in infancy as well as in older age groups. The problem is complex as different conjugates so far devised vary in their immunological properties and in their potency as antigens in infancy. There are also variations in host response dependent on ethnic, nutritional, and demographic factors. Despite these intricacies, several conjugate vaccines have been developed

172

and widely used in many countries including Great Britain.[44] Their introduction has been followed by rapid reduction in the incidence of haemophilus meningitis and an additional, unexpected benefit, reduction of the nasopharyngeal carrier rate. In Finland, which has been in the forefront of immunisation against haemophilus meningitis, this form of meningitis has been almost eliminated.[45]

The great majority of invasive haemophilus infections are caused by one serotype, group b. The situation is more complex in meningococcal infection. Capsular polysaccharide vaccines have been developed against groups A and C strains, and are available for use in contacts and for outbreak control when one of these strains is responsible, for travellers to areas of high prevalence, and for individuals at special risk of meningococcal disease.[46] The development of vaccine against meningococci of group B, the predominant group in Britain, has proved difficult, but several approaches to this problem are now being pursued. One involves developing conjugate vaccines, another using outer membrane proteins (OMPs) rather than the polysaccharide capsular material as antigen. As these outer membrane proteins are strain specific, this approach necessitates the development of multivalent vaccines. Trials of outer membrane protein vaccines have been achieved in several countries, including Norway, Brazil, and Cuba, with overall efficacy rates varying between 50% and 90%, but with less efficacy in children.[47 48]

Pneumococcal vaccines[49] are relevant mainly in the prevention of respiratory disease and otitis media, but here too the successful development of conjugate vaccine against a high proportion of important serotypes might in future contribute to a general vaccine against the main types of bacterial meningitis. Alternatively, other anti-meningitis components may come to be added to combinations, already being developed, of diphtheria, pertussis, and tetanus with HIB vaccine.

Chemoprophylaxis

The risk of meningococcal and of haemophilus meningitis is significantly higher in certain contact groups than in control populations. For this reason chemoprophylaxis is used in these contacts to eradicate nasopharyngeal carriage of the causal organism and thus diminish the likelihood of disease.[50 51] Although the alarm that is engendered by the diagnosis of meningitis leads naturally to great emphasis on treatment of contacts, it has to be emphasised that chemoprophylaxis is a control measure of very limited value compared with preventive vaccination or early diagnosis and treatment of cases. There are several reasons for this, chiefly that in most patients with meningitis the source is unknown, and the patient could therefore not have received chemoprophylaxis. In addition, spread of both *H influenzae* and the meningococcus between carriers may be quite slow, and the risk to contacts extends long beyond any practicable period of chemoprophylaxis.[52] Moreover, sometimes the carrier state is not eradicated, and resistance may develop to the agent used.

Rifampicin is used for contacts of both these forms of meningitis, although there are important differences in dose and duration (10 mg/kg 12 hourly for two days for meningococcal contacts, 20 mg/kg daily for four days for haemophilus contacts, maximum 600 mg per dose). Two other authenticated forms of chemoprophylaxis are available, ciprofloxacin in a single oral dose, or ceftriaxone as a single injection. In general, close family, household, and nursery contacts are given chemoprophylaxis, and also the index case before leaving hospital, as, paradoxically, successful chemotherapy for meningitis does not eradicate the carrier state.

It is most important that contact between health professionals and families of patients with meningitis should include careful discussion of possible early features of meningitis, and the limitations of chemoprophylaxis.

Resource implications

Hospital management of meningitis requires well trained and well staffed medical and paediatric units with easy access to the relevant supporting services. Most essential is liaison with the laboratory on a 24 hour basis, and with the relevant clinical specialists, including especially neurological and infectious disease services. Access to a fully staffed intensive care unit may become essential for some very ill patients, with facilities for safe transfer if this is not available on site. Outside the hospital, communication with the relevant specialist in public health medicine should extend beyond the legal requirements of notification and should include detailed discussion of possible contacts and control measures.

Audit of services for meningitis might measure, in addition to mortality and morbidity, such factors as completeness of notification, duration of illness before admission, whether antibiotics were given before admission, time between admission and definitive treatment, and appropriateness of treatment regimens employed.

Management of meningitis

- Most common causes of pyogenic meningitis developing outside hospitals are *Neisseria meningitidis*, *Haemophilus influenzae* type B, and *Streptococcus pneumoniae*
- Less common causes include *Cryptococcus neoformans*, *Listeria monocytogenes*, and *Mycobacterium tuberculosis*
- CSF examination is central to diagnosis as some clinical presentations are deceptive
- Antibiotic treatment of children should be preceded or accompanied by high dose dexamethasone to prevent neurological sequelae, especially deafness
- Benzyl penicillin is first line treatment for meningococcal and pneumococcal meningitis in the UK
- Broad spectrum cephalosporins (cefotaxime or ceftriaxone) are used against *H influenzae* and where meningococci or pneumococci are resistant to penicillin, but are ineffective against several of the less common causal organisms
- Chloramphenicol is most important for pyogenic meningitis in many developing countries
- Cryptococcal meningitis—regimens of amphotericin, triazole compounds, and sometimes flucytosine are being developed; fluconazole is more effective than amphotericin to prevent recurrence in patients infected with HIV
- Tuberculous meningitis is treated by a regimen of at least isoniazid, pyrazinamide, and rifampicin; streptomycin is useful if resistance to one of these drugs is suspected; prompt treatment of rising intracranial pressure (caused by CSF block or by enlarging tuberculomata) is important
- Vaccines are outstandingly successful against *H influenzae*, effective (and available) against groups A and C meningococci, and being developed against group B meningococci and pneumococci
- Chemoprophylaxis is used for contact groups and index cases but has little impact on the burden of meningitis in a community

At a later stage, rehabilitation facilities will be needed for patients with residual disability. The needs of children with hearing problems have been well studied.[53] Early skilled assessment is required because, although some hearing loss in the acute illness and during recovery is conductive and may be transient, early identification of sensorineural loss is essential so that rehabilitation can begin promptly. It has been strongly argued that all children who have had meningitis should have auditory assessment, initially 4–6 weeks after discharge from hospital. This would involve 30–40 appointments annually for a health district with a population of 250 000. This requirement may well change with successful vaccination programmes, although there is evidence that at present not all patients who need assessment are referred.

1 Booy R, Hodgson SA, Slack MPE, Anderson EC, Mayon-White DT, Moxon ER. Invasive *Haemophilus influenzae* type b disease in the Oxford region (1985–1991). *Arch Dis Child* 1993;**69**:225–8.
2 Fortnum HM, Davis AC. Epidemiology of bacterial meningitis. *Arch Dis Child* 1993;**68**: 763–7.
3 Baldwin LN, Henderson A, Thomas P, Wright M, Acute bacterial meningitis in young adults mistaken for substance abuse. *BMJ* 1993;**306**:775–6.
4 Bohr V, Hansen B, Jessen O, *et al.* Eight hundred and seventy-five cases of bacterial meningitis. Part 1 of a three part series. *J Infect* 1983;**7**:21–30.
5 Rennick G, Shann F, de Campo J. Cerebral herniation during bacterial meningitis in children. *BMJ* 1993;**306**:953–5.
6 Minns RA, Engelman HM, Stirling H. Cerebrospinal fluid pressure in pyogenic meningitis. *Arch Dis Child* 1989;**64**:814–20.
7 Mellor DH. The place of computed tomography and lumbar puncture in suspected bacterial meningitis. *Arch Dis Child* 1992;**67**:1417–9.
8 Harrison MJG, McAllister RH. Neurologic complications of HIV infection. In: Lambert HP, ed. *Infections of the central nervous system.* London: Edward Arnold 1991:343–60.
9 Johnson SRD, Corbett EL, Foster O, Ash S, Cohen J. Raised intracranial pressure and visual complications in AIDS patients with cryptococcal meningitis. *J Infect* 1992;**24**:185–9.
10 Brisson-Noel A, Aznar C, Chureau C, *et al.* Diagnosis of tuberculosis by DNA amplification in clinical practice evaluation. *Lancet* 1991;**338**:364–6.
11 Viladrich PF, Pallares R, Ariza J, Rufi G, Gudiol F. Four days of penicillin therapy for meningococcal meningitis. *Arch Intern Med* 1986;**146**:2380–2.
12 Pecoul B, Varaine F, Keita M, *et al.* Long-acting chloramphenicol versus intravenous ampicillin for treatment of bacterial meningitis. *Lancet* 1991; **338**:862–6.
13 Friedland IR, Klugman KP. Failure of chloramphenicol therapy in penicillin-resistant pneumococcal meningitis. *Lancet* 1992;**339**:405–8.
14 Viladrich PF, Gudiol F, Linares J, *et al.* Evaluation of vancomycin for therapy of adult pneumococcal meningitis. *Antimicrob Agents Chemother* 1991;**35**:2467–72.
15 Peltola H, Anttila M, Renkonen O-U, and the Finnish Study Group. Randomised comparison of chloramphenicol, ampicillin, cefotaxime and ceftriaxone for childhood bacterial meningitis. *Lancet* 1989;**1**:1281–7.
16 Teoh R, Humphries M. Tuberculous meningitis. In: Lambert HP, ed. *Infections of the central nervous system.* London: Edward Arnold 1991:189–206.
17 Bennett LE, Dismukes WE, Duma RA, *et al.* A comparison of amphotericin B alone and combined with flucytosine in the treatment of cryptococcal meningitis. *N Engl J Med* 1979; **301**:126–31.

18 Saag MS, Powderly WG, Cloud GA, *et al.* Comparison of amphotericin B with fluconazole in the treatment of acute AIDS-associated cryptococcal meningitis. *N Engl J Med* 1992; **326**:83–9.

19 British Society for Antimicrobial Chemotherapy Working Party. Antifungal chemotherapy in patients with acquired immunodeficiency. *Lancet* 1992;**340**:648–51.

20 Powderly WG, Saag MS, Cloud GA, *et al.* A controlled trial of amphotericin B to prevent relapse of cryptococcal meningitis in patients with the acquired immunodeficiency syndrome. *N Engl J Med* 1992;**326**:793–8.

21 Quagliarello V, Sheld WM. Bacterial meningitis: pathogenesis, pathophysiology, and progress. *N Engl J Med* 1992;**327**:864–72.

22 Mustafa MM, Lebel MH, Ramilo O, *et al.* Correlation of interleukin 1β and cachectin concentrations in CSF and outcome from bacterial meningitis. *J Pediatr* 1989;**115**:208–13.

23 Arditi M, Manogue KR, Kaplan M, Yogev R. Cachetin/tumour necrosis factor and platelet-activating factor concentrations and severity of bacterial meningitis in children. *J Infect Dis* 1990;**162**:139–47.

24 Brandtzaeg P, Kierulf P, Gaustad P, *et al.* Plasma endotoxin as a predictor of multiple organ failure and death in systemic meningococcal disease. *J Infect Dis* 1989;**159**:195–204.

25 Tauber MG, Shibl AM, Hackbarth CG, Larrick JW, Sande MA. Antibiotic therapy, endotoxin concentration in CSF, and brain edema in experimental *E coli* meningitis in rabbits. *J Infect Dis* 1987;**156**:456–62.

26 Mustafa MM, Ramilo O, Mertsola J, *et al.* Modulation of inflammation and cachectin activity in relation to treatment of experimental *H influenzae* type b meningitis. *J Infect Dis* 1989;**160**:818–25.

27 Arditi M, Ables L, Yogev R. Cerebrospinal fluid endotoxin levels in children with *H influenzae* meningitis before and after administration of intravenous ceftriaxone. *J Infect Dis* 1989;**160**:1005–11.

28 de Lemos RA, Haggerty RJ. Corticosteroids as an adjunct to treatment in bacterial meningitis. A controlled clinical trial. *Pediatrics* 1969;**44**:30–4.

29 Belsey MA, Hoffpauir CW, Smith MHD. Dexamethasone in the treatment of bacterial meningitis: the effect of study design on interpretation of results. *Pediatrics* 1969;**44**:503–13.

30 Lebel MH, Freij BJ, Syrogiannopoulos GA. Dexamethasone therapy for bacterial meningitis. Results of two double-blind, placebo-controlled trials. *N Engl J Med* 1988;**319**:964–71.

31 Lebel MH, Hoyt MJ, Waagner DC, Rollins NK, Finitzo T, McCracken GH. Magnetic resonance imaging and dexamethasone therapy for bacterial meningitis. *Am J Dis Child* 1989;**143**:301–6.

32 Girgis NI, Farid Z, Mikhail IA, Farrag I, Sultan Y, Kilpatrick ME. Dexamethasone treatment for bacterial meningitis in children and adults. *Pediatr Infect Dis J* 1989;**8**:848–51.

33 Odio CM, Faingezicht I, Paris M, *et al.* The beneficial effects of early dexamethasone administration in infants and children with bacterial meningitis. *N Engl J Med* 1991;**324**:1526–31.

34 Schaad UB, Lips U, Gnehm HE, Blumberg A, Heinzer I, Wedgwood J. Dexamethasone therapy for bacterial meningitis in children. *Lancet* 1993;**342**:457–61.

34a Kennedy WA, Hoyt MJ, McCracken GH. The role of corticosteroid therapy in children with pneumococcal meningitis. *Am J Dis Child* 1991;**145**:1374–8.

35 Tureen JH, Dworkin RJ, Kennedy SL, Sachdeva M, Sande MA. Loss of cerebrovascular autoregulation in experimental meningitis in rabbits. *J Clin Invest* 1990;**85**:577–81.

36 Goh D, Minns RA. Cerebral blood flow velocity monitoring in pyogenic meningitis. *Arch Dis Child* 1993;**68**:111–9.

37 Ashwal S, Stringer W, Tomasi L, Schneider S, Thompson J, Perkin R. Cerebral blood flow and CO_2 reactivity in children with bacterial meningitis. *J Pediatr* 1990;**117**:523–30.

38 Powell KR, Sugarman LI, Eskenazi AE, *et al.* Normalisation of arginine vasopressin concentrations when children with meningitis are given maintenance plus replacement fluid therapy. *J Pediatr* 1990;**117**:515–22.

39 Fortnum HM. Hearing impairment after bacterial meningitis: a review. *Arch Dis Child* 1992;**67**:1128–33.

40 Howard AJ, Dunkin KT, Musser JM, Palmer SR. Epidemiology of *Haemophilus influenzae* type b invasive disease in Wales. *BMJ* 1991;**303**:441–5.

41 Kilpi T, Anttila M, Kallio MJT, Peltola H. Severity of childhood bacterial meningitis and duration of illness before diagnosis. *Lancet* 1991;**338**:406–9.

42 Radetsky M. Duration of symptoms and outcome in bacterial meningitis: an analysis of causation and the implications of a delay in diagnosis. *Pediatr Infect J* 1992;**11**:694–8.

43 Peltola H, Kayhty H, Virtanen M, Makela PH. Prevention of *Haemophilus influenzae* type b bacteremic infections with the capsular polysaccharide vaccine. *N Engl J Med* 1984;**310**: 1561–6.

44 Cartwright KAV. Vaccination against *Haemophilus influenzae* b disease. *BMJ* 1992;**305**: 485–6.

45 Peltola H, Kilpi T, Anttila M. Rapid disappearance of *Haemophilus influenzae* type b meningitis after routine childhood immunisation with conjugate vaccines. *Lancet* 1992;**340**: 592–4.

46 Frasch CE. Vaccines for prevention of meningococcal disease. *Clin Microbiol Rev* 1989; **2**(Suppl 1):S134–8.

47 Bjune G, Hiby EA, Grnnesby JK, Arnesen O. Effect of an outer membrane vesicle vaccine against group B meningococcal disease in Norway. *Lancet* 1991;**338**:1093–6.

48 Cassio de Moraes J, Perkins BA, Camargo MCC, *et al.* Protective efficacy of a serogroup B meningococcal vaccine in Sao Paulo, Brazil. *Lancet* 1992;**340**:1074–8.

49 Broome CV, Breiman RF. Pneumococcal vaccine—past, present and future. *N Engl J Med* 1991;**325**:1506–8.

50 Cartwright KAV, Begg NT, Hull D. Chemoprophylaxis for *Haemophilus influenzae* type b. *BMJ* 1991;**302**:546–7.

51 Jones DM. Control of meningococcal disease. *BMJ* 1989;**298**:542–3.

52 Cooke RPD, Riordan T, Jones DM, Painter MJ. Secondary cases of meningococcal infection among close family and household contacts in England and Wales, 1984–7. *BMJ* 1989; **298**:555–8.

53 Fortnum H, Davis A. Hearing impairment in children after bacterial meningitis: incidence and resource implications. *Br J Audiol* 1993;**27**:43–52.

7 Parkinson's disease

C D MARSDEN

Parkinsonism is a clinical syndrome dominated by a disorder of movement consisting of tremor, rigidity, elements of bradykinesia (slowness of movement), hypokinesia (reduced movement) and akinesia (loss of movement), and postural abnormalities. Parkinson's disease consists of the clinical syndrome of parkinsonism associated with a distinctive pathology consisting of degeneration of pigmented brain stem nuclei, including the dopaminergic substantia nigra pars compacta, with the presence of Lewy bodies in remaining nerve cells.

Parkinson's disease is a common and disabling illness affecting some 1 in 1000 of the population. Symptoms usually appear after the age of 50 years, but the young are not exempt. Prevalence in those over the age of 50 rises exponentially. A community-based survey in Aberdeen[1] showed age-specific prevalence rates per 100 000 of the population of 47 at the ages of 40–49 years, 78 at 50–59, 254 at 60–69, and 832 at 70–79. Men and women are affected, and the disease occurs worldwide, although perhaps less frequently in China and Africa than in Western countries.

The Office of Health Economics[2] calculated that there were probably between 60 000 and 80 000 people suffering from Parkinson's disease in the United Kingdom. Harris[3] estimated that there were 22 000 people disabled by Parkinson's disease living in the community, 22% of whom were severely handicapped, 48·3% were appreciably handicapped, and 29·7% of whom had a minor handicap. The Office of Health Economics[2] estimated that there were 15 000 patients with Parkinson's disease in hospital or residential care, 22 000 handicapped in the community, and more than 30 000 in the community but not handicapped.

The Association of British Neurologists[4] estimated that within a population of 250 000 people there would be 400 patients with

Parkinson's disease, of whom 342 would have significant disability (see Wade and Langton-Hewer, 1987).[5]

The cause of Parkinson's disease in unknown. There may be a genetic predisposition rendering individuals more vulnerable to toxic substances. Some surveys have hinted that exposure to a rural environment including well water or pesticides may be of significance, but no common environmental toxin has been identified.

The practical management of Parkinson's disease follows a series of steps in the individual's life history of their illness. For the purpose of this review, I will follow patients from the time of their initial symptoms, through diagnosis and early management, into the complications of long term treatment and the problems of increasing disability.

Early symptoms

The characteristic tremor of Parkinson's disease affects about 70% of patients. Many present with much vaguer symptoms. Sensations of numbness or pain without demonstrable sensory loss often are described. Muscles may be referred to as painful and tender and limbs may be said to be weak or stiff. Difficulty with handwriting, or inability to undertake repetitive sequential tasks such as cleaning the teeth, winding a watch, doing up buttons or manipulating spoons may be the sole complaint for many months. Fatigue is a common complaint, as is depression and a vague sensation that the patient has slowed down and life has become weary. Unexplained weight loss may be prominent.

Against this background, several alternative diagnoses are often entertained to begin with. Everything may be attributed to a depressive illness. Aches and pains may be interpreted as due to rheumatism. Fatigue and weight loss may suggest a more sinister cause. The initial tendency for the symptoms to begin on one side of the body may be misinterpreted as a hemiparesis.

Diagnosis

Eventually, the characteristic features of parkinsonism are recognised, and the question then becomes whether this is due to Parkinson's disease or some other condition. The diagnosis is clinical for there is no test specific for Parkinson's disease. Even the most experienced neurologist may have difficulty in making the diagnosis at this stage of the illness.

In two recent series of patients diagnosed as having Parkinson's disease in life who came to autopsy,[6 7] the pathological diagnosis was of some other condition in about a quarter of cases. The commonest alternative diagnoses were Steele-Richardson-Olszewski disease (progressive supranuclear palsy) and multiple system atrophy (Shy-Drager syndrome with autonomic failure, striatonigral degeneration, and olivopontocerebellar degeneration in various combinations). In the early stages of these conditions the eye movement disorder characteristic of progressive supranuclear palsy may not be apparent, and the symptoms and signs of autonomic failure and cerebellar deficit typical of multiple system atrophy may not be evident. Position emission tomography using ^{18}F-dopa and other ligands can discriminate typical Parkinson's disease from other parkinsonian syndromes in about 80% of cases, but is not specific or widely available.[8]

Hughes et al,[7] on the basis of the autopsy findings in 100 cases diagnosed as having Parkinson's disease in life, recommended the following clinical criteria to improve the success rate for diagnosing Parkinson's disease. There needs to be bradykinesia plus one of the following: a classic rest tremor, unilateral onset, progressive persistent asymmetry, an excellent response to levodopa (>70%), levodopa induced dyskinesias, and continued response to levodopa for at least five years. Parkinson's disease would be excluded if there were no response to levodopa, more than one affected relative, early dementia, early postural imbalance and falls, early autonomic findings, appreciable abnormality of eye movement, and cerebellar or pyramidal signs.

In a further series of 100 cases of pathologically proved Parkinson's disease[9] it was found that tremor was present at the onset in 69%, and in the course of the disease in 75% of cases. Only 77% of patients had a "good" or "excellent" initial levodopa response. Accordingly, failure to respond to an apomorphine or levodopa challenge test (using single injections of apomorphine or a single dose of Sinemet or Madopar) does not exclude the diagnosis of Parkinson's disease; nor does it completely exclude a subsequent positive response to longer term oral levodopa treatment. Conversely, some patients with Steele-Richardson-Olszewski disease or multiple system atrophy may show a response to levodopa initially.

181

Initial treatment

Having made the diagnosis of Parkinson's disease, important decisions have to be made about subsequent management. These depend on an open and frank discussion of prognosis, options for treatment and management, and the personal philosophy of patient and carer. These initial discussions will set the framework for a lifetime of living with Parkinson's disease.

Many patients seek as much information as they can find about their illness. The Parkinson's Disease Society provides a large range of excellent educational information. Patients need to know that Parkinson's disease cannot be cured, but that it can be effectively relieved by symptomatic treatment. Life expectancy is now near to normal, and the main issue is the maintenance of the best quality of life. Patients will also be reassured to know that there is only a small risk of passing the illness to their children. They need advice on diet, the need for exercise and sensible home exercise programmes,[10] and they will seek reassurance on the effect of lifestyle on their illness and their illness on lifestyle. Moderate alcohol intake does not affect Parkinson's disease adversely, and there are no major bars to recreational activities. Discussion of the effect of the illness on sexual activity may be reassuring, and specific problems associated with hygiene, childbirth, and hormone replacement therapy require discussion with women patients. The issue of driving should be raised and appropriate assessment undertaken. Most patients will not have major problems with speech, hand function, and walking at this stage, but those who do will benefit from contact with speech therapists, physiotherapists, and occupational therapists. Contact with social services may be required to sort out problems of housing, adaptation of the home, and financial difficulties.

As far as drug treatment is concerned, it should be pointed out that there are two categories of drug treatment to be considered; (a) treatment designed to slow the rate of progression of the disease (neuroprotection); and (b) symptomatic treatment.

Neuroprotection

Nothing is known to halt Parkinson's disease, but in recent years there have been suggestions that the administration of selegiline (Deprenyl), an irreversible monoamine oxidase B inhibitor, may have an effect on the natural course of the illness. The rationale for the use of selegiline in early Parkinson's disease was that inhibition of monoamine oxidase B might prevent damage caused by dopamine metabolism resulting in oxidative stress, and also that selegiline had been found to prevent the capacity for 1-methyl-4-phenyl-1,2,3,6-tetrahydropyridine (MPTP) to cause experimental parkinsonism in non-human primates. These concepts lay behind the major DATATOP study in North America which investigated the effects of selegiline and vitamin E treatment in de novo patients with Parkinson's disease.[11 12]

The major result of this study was that early selegiline treatment delayed the need for levodopa significantly (but vitamin E had no effect, either alone or in combination with selegiline). Selegiline itself was found to have a modest symptomatic antiparkinsonian action, so it proved impossible to decide definitely whether its effect in delaying the need for levodopa treatment was due to this symptomatic action or whether there was an additional true neuroprotective action.

Whether or not one should use selegiline at the time of diagnosis depends upon one's philosophy about levodopa treatment for Parkinson's disease. Levodopa and other antiparkinsonian drugs offer only symptomatic relief, so it is crucial here to distinguish between the *impairments* typical of Parkinson's disease (tremor, rigidity, akinesia, and postural deficits), the *disabilities* they cause, and the *handicaps* that result. Levodopa and other symptomatic antiparkinsonian drugs are employed to relieve disability and handicap.

If the strategy in an individual is to delay levodopa treatment for as long as possible (see below), then the early administration of selegiline at the time of diagnosis is a rational policy.

Symptomatic treatment

There has been controversy over which drugs to use and when to use them. Much of this debate has turned on the issue of whether levodopa should be given early or late in Parkinson's disease. In fact, although the published work on this topic may seem to be polarised, in practice there is much less discord.

Levodopa is the most reliable and effective symptomatic treatment for Parkinson's disease. Most patients with true idiopathic Lewy body Parkinson's disease will respond to levodopa

183

treatment. Indeed, failure to respond suggests (but does not prove) an alternative diagnosis.[7] In contrast, directly acting dopamine agonists such as bromocriptine and pergolide only benefit about a third to a half of patients when given alone.[13] The problem with levodopa is that many patients will develop complications of treatment after some years.[14] These complications represent a complex interaction between the long term effects of the drug and the progression of the disease itself. Fluctuations and dyskinesias are a major problem in those with disease of younger onset, whereas the emergence of cognitive and psychiatric problems along with imbalance and speech difficulty tend to occur in the more elderly patient. The objective of symptomatic drug treatment in Parkinson's disease is to keep the patient functioning independently for as long as possible. Life expectancy in Parkinson's disease is now near to normal.[15–17]

Taking all these facts together, the critical issue in the management of Parkinson's disease becomes the need to individualise treatment. Decisions will be based upon firstly, the patient's age. The younger patient with Parkinson's disease, facing a long life with the illness, may opt to delay levodopa treatment until it is absolutely necessary. The elderly patient, with a limited life span, may opt for early levodopa treatment to get its benefits as soon as possible. Secondly, the patient's disability and handicap must be considered. In the early stages of Parkinson's disease, although impairment is evident, there may be little disability or handicap. At this stage, symptomatic treatment may not be required at all. Thirdly, the patients' expectations in the light of their social and occupational demands will affect decisions. An elderly, retired person may tolerate a level of impairment that would be insufferable to a young, active patient.

All these factors have to be taken into account in a final decision about the use of symptomatic drug treatment at various stages of Parkinson's disease. The patient requires counselling on the options available, and the short and long term outlook faced. In the final analysis, patients will decide on the basis of their own individual philosophy, responsibilities, and requirements.

Symptomatic treatment when disability and handicap occur

There comes a time when Parkinson's disease progresses to the point that symptomatic treatment needs to be initiated. The most common problems that patients and clinicians consider important for the decision to begin symptomatic agents are threat to employment; threat to ability to handle domestic, financial, or social affairs; threat to the ability to handle activities of daily living; and worsening gait and balance.

At this stage, disability and handicaps still may be mild and some might opt to use an anticholinergic drug or amantadine to provide initial symptomatic relief. Both drugs can improve function by about 20%, which is much less than the benefit obtained with levodopa or a dopamine agonist. This may be sufficient, however, to maintain independence initially. Anticholinergics and amantadine tend to produce unacceptable adverse side effects, particularly in the elderly, where they may contribute to forgetfulness, memory difficulties, hallucinations, and even psychoses. Nevertheless, anticholinergics and amantadine may give valuable relief early in the illness, thereby avoiding the need for dopaminergic drugs. Anticholinergic drugs also may be helpful to suppress tremor resistant to other medications.

Eventually the time comes when stronger symptomatic treatment is required. The question then is whether to begin with levodopa or a directly acting dopamine agonist such as bromocriptine or pergolide. The aims now are to provide adequate symptomatic relief of disability and handicap, and to adopt a strategy least likely to lead to long term complications.

Strategies to delay or prevent long term complications

The dilemma in the choice between levodopa versus a dopamine agonist is due to the facts that (a) levodopa is more or less guaranteed to work but has a high incidence of long term complications and (b) bromocriptine and pergolide are less likely to be effective when given alone but, in those who can obtain adequate benefit, there is less risk of the long term development of fluctuations and dyskinesias.

Using dopamine agonists as monotherapy will provide adequate symptomatic relief in only a minority of patients (ranging from 30%[18] to around 50%[13 19 20]). In the study by the Parkinson's Disease Research Group in the United Kingdom,[21] of 263 patients entered into treatment with bromocriptine alone (mean dose 36 mg/day; range 7·5–120 mg/day) 181 withdrew, mainly due to lack of response (41 cases), deterioration despite treatment (30 cases), or adverse reactions (69 cases). The early use of dopamine agonist monotherapy, however, reduces the likelihood of developing complications such as fluctuations and dyskinesias in those who gain adequate relief.[19 20 22] Furthermore, delaying the initiation of levodopa delays the time when such complications occur.[23-26]

Again, the decision about whether to use a dopamine agonist or levodopa is often decided according to individual circumstances. The patient in whom disability and handicap has reached a stage that urgently threatens independence or employment may opt for immediate levodopa treatment as the best guarantee of relief. Those in whom the pressure is less may opt for a dopamine agonist first as the best insurance against long term problems. Younger patients may wish to delay levodopa for as long as possible. Elderly patients may opt for early levodopa treatment because long term side effects are of less concern and because the neuropsychiatric side effects of directly acting dopamine agonists are more of a hazard.

If the decision is for levodopa, the next problem is whether to use standard Sinemet or Madopar, or the delayed release forms of Sinemet CR or Madopar CR. There are theoretical reasons in favour of Sinemet CR or Madopar CR.[27 28] The large swings in levodopa plasma levels produced by standard Sinemet or Madopar may be deleterious and contribute to long term complications. Starting treatment with the more stable blood levels produced by Sinemet CR or Madopar CR may decrease long term complications, and this theory is under clinical trial at present.

A few patients experience nausea and vomiting when levodopa is introduced, even when taking the drug after food. Usually this can be prevented by prefacing each dose with domperidone 10–20 mg an hour beforehand.

One strategy that has been advocated as a compromise is to use a low dose of levodopa combined with a dopamine agonist. Rinne and colleagues[19 29 30] have advocated this as a means of reducing to some extent the long term complications of fluctuations and dyskinesias. Although an attractive option, the evidence that combined treatment does indeed reduce long term side effects has come under recent criticism.[31 32]

Strategies for treating complications of long term levodopa treatment

With long term treatment with levodopa (defined as greater than five years) only about 25% of patients continue to have a good, smooth response.[14][33] Most patients develop either troublesome fluctuations, troublesome dyskinesias, toxicity at therapeutic or sub-therapeutic dosages, or total or substantial loss of efficacy. There are three common patterns of late failure of chronic levodopa treatment; (a) the emergence of increasingly severe fluctuations and dyskinesias, which are particularly prevalent in younger patients; (b) the appearance of increasingly severe cognitive impairment and psychosis; often with (c) postural instability and falls, gait difficulties, and speech problems, which are particularly prevalent in the more elderly.

Fluctuations

The initial benefits of levodopa treatment are sustained. Most patients experience general improvement throughout the day with little response to each individual dose. With the passage of time, however, an increasing proportion of patients begin to experience fluctuations of their response.[34-36] Most patients will develop fluctuations within about five years after starting levodopa therapy. Initially these take the form of the "wearing-off effect" or "end-of-dose deterioration", which is defined as fluctuations in motor disability related to the timing of levodopa intake. With the passage of time and modification of treatment, such motor fluctuations become increasingly abrupt and random, culminating in the "on-off effect", which is defined as sudden unpredictable fluctuations in motor disability unrelated to the timing of levodopa intake.

The main risk factors for fluctuations appear to be the duration of treatment[25][26] and dosage.[37] As indicated above, using low doses of levodopa seems to delay the onset of this problem,[37] as does delaying the introduction of levodopa.[23] Fluctuations seem to be more common and occur sooner in patients who develop Parkinson's disease at a younger age.[38][39]

Fluctuations in motor disability are often accompanied by a variety of other disabling, variable symptoms.[40] The associated dyskinesias are discussed below. During "off" periods, many patients complain bitterly of pain and other sensory complaints,[41][42] akathisia,[43] respiratory distress,[44] depressive mood swings,[45-47] sweating and other autonomic symptoms,[48] hallucinations,[45] anxiety and panic attacks,[45][49] sometimes with screaming,[50] and slowing and impairment of thought processes.[51][52]

In the fully developed "on-off" state, the swings in motor function and other symptoms may become highly unpredictable and rapid ("sudden offs"). Some doses of levodopa may fail to have any effect at all ("dose failures"), or there may be a considerable delay before the patient switches on ("delayed-on"). Furthermore, many patients describe diurnal variation in their responsiveness to levodopa, getting most benefit in the morning particularly after the first dose of the day, but less and less response as the day goes on, with bad periods in the afternoon and evening.

Many mechanisms contribute to the emergence of fluctuations during long term levodopa treatment.[53-55] There seems to be no significant change in the peripheral pharmacokinetic handling of levodopa during long term treatment.[56] There is, however, a shortening of therapeutic benefit after each dose.[55] In addition, the character of the pharmacodynamic response to levodopa changes during long term treatment. When treatment is started the degree of improvement bears a more or less linear relation to dose and plasma levodopa level. In those who develop the "wearing-off" and particularly the "on-off" effect, however, this classic dose-response relation changes into a sigmoid curve. Patients switch "on" at a critical level of plasma levodopa, below which they are "off" and above which they are more or less fully "on".[57] Increasing the dose of levodopa at that stage does not improve the quality of the "on" period, but prolongs its duration. The absolute threshold for turning a patient with Parkinson's disease "on" with levodopa does not change during chronic treatment, but this critical threshold appears.

The emergence of a critical threshold has important implications for management. The natural response to the appearance of the "wearing-off" effect is to reduce individual levodopa doses and increase their frequency. This strategy, however, although initially effective, often fails quite quickly. The smaller doses may produce peak plasma levels below threshold, so that the patient does not turn fully "on", or remains just at threshold so that they oscillate between "on" and "off". In addition, the smaller dose and lower plasma levels mean a reduced duration of response, even if threshold is reached.

Now, with plasma (and brain) levodopa levels hovering around threshold, peripheral pharmacokinetic factors assume greater importance. Delayed gastric emptying,[58] or large protein meals competing for absorption or brain entry of levodopa,[53] may reduce brain levodopa levels to or below threshold, and reduce the duration of response even if it occurs.

In patients who have developed the "wearing-off" effect, and to a less predictable extent in those with the true "on-off" effect, maintaining a continuous supply of dopamine or a dopamine agonist to the brain, such as by intravenous[53 59 60] or intestinal[61 62] infusion of levodopa, can overcome such fluctuations. The same can be achieved by a constant subcutaneous infusion of the dopamine agonist apomorphine.[63]

Against this background, the following strategies are employed to try and overcome the emergence of fluctuations during chronic levodopa therapy.

Selegiline can be mildly effective in treating "wearing-off" problems.[64 65] The addition of slow release Sinemet CR or Madopar CR to maintain more constant blood levels of levodopa may also help, particularly in the early stages of the emergence of this problem.[66–72] Many patients will also require supplemental standard Sinemet or Madopar as well as Sinemet CR or Madopar CR to obtain an adequate response. It often takes over an hour for the delayed release medications to become effective, and patients frequently find that these formulations do not give a sufficient "kick-start" to switch them "on", especially with the first dose of the day. The addition of direct acting dopamine agonists, such as bromocriptine or pergolide,[73 74] which have a longer biological half life than levodopa, can also be used in combination with standard Sinemet or Madopar and Sinemet CR or Madopar CR. There is some evidence that pergolide is more effective and better tolerated than bromocriptine.[75]

Attention to gastric and dietary factors also becomes important. Dissolving levodopa in liquid before ingestion may help,[76] as may the use of the dispersible Madopar preparations, which act more quickly. Occasional patients may benefit from drugs enhancing gastric emptying or antacids.[77 78] Taking levodopa before rather than after meals also may produce a more reliable and rapid effect.[58] Reduction in dietary protein also may be of benefit.[79]

Despite these strategies, many patients evolve into the situation of sudden and unpredictable "off" periods. In these circumstances, subcutaneous apomorphine injections may be used to rescue patients from "off" periods, or apomorphine may be employed as a continuous subcutaneous infusion.[63 80]

189

Dyskinesias

As motor fluctuations begin to develop during long term levodopa treatment, various dyskinesias appear.[81][82] These are conventionally divided according to the time of their appearance after individual doses into: (a) those occurring at the peak of benefit—"peak dose dyskinesias"; (b) those occurring as mobility improves or wanes, or both—diphasic dyskinesias"; and (c) those occurring in "off periods" or in the early morning—"off period dyskinesias". Peak dose dyskinesias are commonly choreic, ballistic, or stereotyped; less commonly they are dystonic; they tend to be more unsightly than disabling. Diphasic dyskinesias are similar in type to peak dose dyskinesias, although dystonia is often more prominent and tends to be more severe and disabling. "Off period" dyskinesias tend to be dystonic, painful, and distressing. The pattern of dyskinesias, both in their character and timing, varies considerably from patient to patient, but is fairly consistent in each individual.

The mechanisms responsible for the appearance of dyskinesias are complex and not fully understood.[83][84] Whereas the threshold for motor benefit from levodopa does not appear to change during long term treatment, that for the production of dyskinesias decreases dramatically. Indeed, in those who have developed the typical "wearing-off" and "on-off" effect, the threshold for dyskinesias is similar to that required for motor benefit.[83] Diphasic dyskinesias[85] appear when the plasma level of levodopa is rising or falling but not during the peak. Thus, patients describe a flurry of dyskinesias as the initial evidence of a levodopa effect; such dyskinesias may settle during the period of maximum mobility, only to reappear as the patient turns "off". Off period dyskinesias, especially the painful cramps and dystonias, may be evident first thing in the morning as well as during "off" periods during the day. Although they occur when mobility is at its worst, they disappear if levodopa is entirely withdrawn for a time.

Management of dyskinesias is difficult. Reducing the dose of levodopa may often improve the dyskinesias, but at the expense of intolerable worsening of mobility. When peak dose dyskinesias are causing disability, however, reducing each individual dose may resolve the problem. Alternatively, substituting an increasing dose of a dopamine agonist such as bromocriptine or pergolide while lowering the dose of levodopa can help.

Diphasic dyskinesias are even more difficult to manage. As they occur with intermediate plasma levels of levodopa, it would seem

190

rational to increase levodopa intake.[86] Usually this eventually produces much more severe dyskinesias and other adverse effects. Lowering the dose is equally unsatisfactory because increasing parkinsonism ensues. The best strategy probably is to add increasing doses of an agonist such as pergolide while reducing levodopa intake.

"Off period" painful dystonia can be very disabling. The best way of preventing such dyskinesias is to try and overcome "off" periods by the strategies described above. Sometimes the addition of baclofen, an anticholinergic, or lithium is of benefit.

Freezing, postural imbalance, gait problems, and speech difficulties

Whereas long term levodopa treatment continues to help some problems of Parkinson's disease, albeit for shorter and shorter periods and increasingly unreliably, other disabilities begin to emerge that are less responsive.

As "wearing-off" emerges, freezing episodes often appear during "off" periods. These particularly affect gait. Patients begin to experience start hesitation, and freezing on the turn or when passing through enclosed spaces.[87] Accompanying such freezing episodes is increasing instability of gait. Postural reflexes become impaired. Patients become increasingly unsteady, and no longer correct when imbalanced. Not only do they fail to take appropriate action to prevent a fall, but they also lose rescue reactions and so cannot protect themselves if they fall. A common problem arises from sudden unexpected freezing when walking. The feet get glued to the ground, momentum carries the patient forward, they cannot correct this imbalance but fall and injure themselves. Unexpected falls with injury thus become a major problem, particularly in "off" periods.[88]

Speech also may be compromised, with increasing hypophonic dysfluency, hesitations, and even freezing during speech.[89][90] Swallowing too may be disturbed.[91]

Levodopa and dopamine agonists, during long term treatment, seem less capable of relieving these impairments of posture, gait, and speech.[88][92][93] Reasons for the emergence of these difficulties during long term levodopa treatment may relate to progressive pathology[23] and the effects of ageing.[93] In particular, neurons in

191

the nuclei in brain stem centres that control posture, locomotion, and speech may be degenerating.

Unfortunately, there is no effective way of managing these problems with medication, other than by attempting to control them with optimum levodopa and dopamine agonist replacement treatment. Once locomotor and speech problems begin to intrude, however, considerable help can be obtained from the physiotherapist, the speech therapist, and the occupational therapist.

Physiotherapy designed to improve gait patterns, and to educate the patient to minimise risks of falls, is of benefit. Teaching strategies to ease getting out of the bed or a chair, to initiate walking, and to manage turns is helpful. Walking aids are a problem to patients with Parkinson's disease. They tend to carry, rather than use, a stick or frame; a wheeled rollator is often of more benefit. Other valuable aids include elevating chairs, house lifts, automatic controlled beds, bed-hoists, strategically placed rails, toilet aids, bath seats and showers, and feeding utensils. Unfortunately, about a half of patients and their carers need aids and equipment to assist daily living.[94] Close and regular contact with the occupational therapist and physiotherapist is essential to assess the need for appropriate assistance, which often requires a visit to the patient's home, and to select the most useful aids for the individual patient.[95] Liaison between the occupational therapist, physiotherapist, and social services is crucial to ensure the provision of such assistance, and the designated social worker can provide invaluable advice and practical help in financial matters. The Parkinson's Disease Society also provides considerable help in all these areas. It is the responsibility of the specialist and general practitioner, in liaison, to ensure that patients are referred early rather than late, and repeatedly, to the appropriate professionals.

Speech and feeding problems also may be a major cause of disability and handicap at this stage,[91 94] and the advice of the speech therapist now may be invaluable.[96-98] Assessment of speech deficits, formal speech therapy and education, and the provision of appropriate communication aids may be required. Advice on dietary and swallowing strategies may be necessary and helpful.[99] Drooling of saliva, due to failure to swallow, is sometimes a major problem. An anticholinergic drug may help to dry the mouth.

It is also appropriate to consider the problems of the bladder and the bowels at this point, for at this stage of the illness these often cause considerable disability and distress.

Urinary frequency (especially at night) and urgency due to detrusor instability are a common part of Parkinson's disease,[100] and can be improved with levodopa treatment. In elderly men there is the common added problem of an enlarged prostate. Frequently, it is difficult to know whether the prostate or the Parkinson's disease is responsible for urinary problems in men. Referral to an expert uroneurologist may be essential, and careful investigation is often required to distinguish outflow obstruction from the bladder dysfunction inherent to Parkinson's disease. Careful selection of those suitable for prostatic resection is essential if incontinence is to be avoided. An anticholinergic may help urgency and frequency, but can precipitate urinary retention (and glaucoma) and can make constipation worse.

Constipation is a very common problem in Parkinson's disease,[99 101] caused by many factors including reduced mobility, anticholinergic drugs, dietary imbalance, and autonomic dysfunction. A high fibre diet with fruit, drinking more water, and bulk laxatives are useful.

Postural hypotension and syncope may sometimes be a problem in true Parkinson's disease, due partly to pathology in the autonomic nervous system and also to the effects of drug treatment. Head-up tilt of the bed at night, elastic stockings, and fludrocortisone may be required.

Cognitive and neuropsychiatric problems

Most patients with Parkinson's disease, early in their illness, have subtle changes on neuropsychological testing suggestive of frontal lobe dysfunction.[52 102 103] In the early stages these usually do not appear to cause obvious cognitive disability. With the passage of time, however, they may develop into a more disabling syndrome of abulia. Abulia refers to apathy, slowness of thought (bradyphrenia),[104] and blunting of drive and response to external stimuli. Such a syndrome may progress further with increasing impairments of memory to form a focal dementia of frontal lobe type. Around 20–30% of patients may go on to develop a more multifocal, pervasive dementia affecting many or all areas of cognitive function.[105] A particular characteristic of this syndrome, which predominantly affects elderly patients with Parkinson's disease, is a fluctuating, confusional state, often with visual, and even auditory, hallucinations.[106] Such patients may have good

193

days, when cognitive function seems to be relatively preserved, interspersed with periods of mental confusion, impairment of attention, and hallucinations.

There are many reasons for cognitive impairment in Parkinson's disease.[51] Drug treatment may be responsible, particularly anticholinergic agents in the elderly.[107] Undoubtedly some people may develop the coincidental pathology of Alzheimer's disease, which is common in the elderly. Some of the features of frontal lobe dysfunction may be attributed to increasing dopaminergic inactivation of frontocaudate cognitive systems. As the disease advances, not only is there greater involvement of nigrocaudate dopaminergic pathways but also dopaminergic innervation of the frontal cortex itself is probably impaired. Another factor that has emerged in recent years is the realisation that Lewy body pathology in the cerebral cortex is much more widespread than was hitherto envisaged. The advent of ubiquitin immunostaining for Lewy bodies has shown that these inclusions are present in cortical neurons to some extent in virtually every patient with Parkinson's disease. In many of those with severe cognitive impairment there is widespread cortical Lewy body pathology. Diffuse Lewy body disease was previously thought to be a rare condition, but it is now suggested that it may be a common cause of the confused dementia in elderly patients with Parkinson's disease.[106 108–110]

Along with cognitive impairment, a number of neuropsychiatric problems may also emerge associated with chronic disease. Isolated visual pseudo-hallucinations are not infrequent. Patients may see human or animal "familiars", which may or may not be threatening. Such hallucinations, which again are more common in elderly patients, and particularly at night, may be due in part to drug intake. Reducing dopaminergic drugs often leads to their disappearance. Some patients, however, go on to develop a frank confusional state and may even become psychotic.

The appearance of disabling cognitive impairment or of a confusional state in a patient with Parkinson's disease should prompt a search for some intercurrent illness, including chest and urinary infections and metabolic disturbances. In many cases drug treatment is likely to be the cause. All anticholinergic drugs should be withdrawn, including amantadine. If the confusion does not clear, the dose of dopaminergic drugs needs to be reduced. Unfortunately, however, though the confusional state may clear as drugs are withdrawn, mobility may deteriorate. Often, as drugs are manipulated, a state is reached in which the patient is either mobile but confused and hallucinating, or mentally clear but immobile. The balance between the extremes may be brittle and it is very difficult to achieve a satisfactory compromise. In this situation, a limited drug holiday, withdrawing dopaminergic drugs for one day each week, sometimes helps to dispel the psychotoxicity, allowing a reasonable dose of drugs to maintain mobility on other days. Prolonged drug holidays have been abandoned, as the patient may deteriorate to a severe state of immobility, with risks of pneumonia or deep vein thrombosis. Indeed, dopaminergic drug withdrawal may precipitate a state of intense rigidity, mental confusion, and unexplained pyrexia akin to the neuroleptic malignant syndrome.

If drug manipulation fails, it may be necessary to use the atypical neuroleptic, clozapine, to control the neuropsychiatric complications. Clozapine, which acts predominantly through D-4 dopamine receptors, has much less propensity to cause extrapyramidal side effects and to reduce mobility in Parkinson's disease. It is not devoid of this risk, but sometimes it can be used succesfully to control neuropsychiatric complications while maintaining an adequate dose of dopamine replacement therapy to maintain mobility.[111-113] There are, however, practical difficulties in using clozapine because of its tendency to produce agranulocytosis in a proportion of patients (perhaps 1–2%). This requires frequent and regular monitoring of blood counts and withdrawal of clozapine at the slightest hint of toxicity. An alternative strategy is to use a small dose of a conventional neuroleptic, such as thioridazine, at night.

Finally, mood changes are a major component of Parkinson's disease. Around two thirds of patients are appreciably depressed.[114 115] In part this is a natural reaction to the disabilities imposed by their illness but that may not be the only reason for depression in Parkinson's disease. It has been argued that pathology in serotonergic systems, and perhaps also in noradrenergic systems, known to occur in Parkinson's disease, may also contribute to depression. A nocturnal dose of tricyclic antidepressant such as imipramine or amitriptyline may be required. A sedative antidepressant with anticholinergic properties may also aid sleep and reduce nocturnal urinary frequency. Although a popular antidepressant drug, fluoxetine may increase parkinsonian disability.[116] Occasionally, electroconvulsive therapy (ECT) may be required to treat severe depression in Parkinson's disease. Not only does ECT relieve the depression, but the parkinsonism also can be reduced temporarily.

Anxiety and panic attacks also can be a disabling feature of Parkinson's disease, especially during "off" periods. A benzodiazepine such as diazepam or a β blocker such as propranolol may help such patients.

Role of neurosurgery in Parkinson's disease

Before the introduction of levodopa treatment around 1970, stereotaxic surgery was widely used to treat Parkinson's disease.[117] The preferred target in most centres was the ventrolateral nucleus of the thalamus, in particular the nucleus ventralis intermedius. A unilateral thalamotomy could successfully reduce or abolish contralateral tremor and rigidity in most patients, with an acceptably small (5–10%) risk of hemiparesis or hemiplegia. Bilateral thalamotomy, however, carried a higher (20% or so) risk of severe speech disturbance and other complications. Thalamotomy did not usually improve the various manifestations of akinesia, which often progressed to cause increasing disability.

Levodopa, for the first time, relieved akinesia, so the use of thalamotomy rapidly declined. It was reserved for the occasional patient with mainly unilateral drug resistant disabling tremor.[118 119]

As the long term complications of levodopa treatment emerged, and persisted in many patients despite every attempt at drug manipulation, stereotaxic surgery has begun to undergo a renaissance, in three forms.[120]

Laitinen and colleagues[121] had continued Leksell's practice of posteroventral pallidotomy and recently published evidence that this operation not only could improve tremor and rigidity, but also akinesia, gait, and speech. Furthermore, this lesion could reduce or abolish some disabling levodopa-induced dyskinesias. The role of posteroventral pallidotomy is being re-evaluated in many centres.

Benabid et al,[122] after the observation that suppression of tremor by electrical stimulation was a useful method of localising the target site for traditional thalamotomy, harnessed the technology of continuous electrical thalamic stimulation for suppression of tremor. The advantages of this method include a lower incidence of complications, and the opportunity for safe bilateral implantation. Furthermore, continuous thalamic stimulation also may suppress some levodopa-induced dyskinesias. Again, this technique is under clinical trial worldwide.

Finally, much has been written about brain grafting for Parkinson's disease. Initial enthusiastic reports on the use of adrenal autografts into the striatum have been subsequently tempered by the realisation that the method was not very successful and carried high risks.[123] Adrenal grafting, in its original form, has been discarded. The use of fetal substantia nigra grafts into striatum, using stereotaxic methods, however, holds greater promise. Such grafts have been shown by position emission tomography to survive and to exert some beneficial effects for years.[124-127] The method remains experimental at this stage, until the many practical problems surrounding it have been resolved.[128]

Standards of care and audit

Despite the large number of patients with Parkinson's disease in the community, the complications of its treatment, and the disability it produces, there has been little formal investigation of audit in this condition.

The Association of British Neurologists[129] noted that Parkinson's disease was the 12th commonest condition referred to neurologists in the United Kingdom. They recommended that all such patients should be referred to a neurologist (unless geriatric referral was most appropriate), and that they should have computed tomography of the brain (although many would not consider that computed tomography or magnetic resonance imaging of the brain to be necessary, unless there is another positive indication).

A Working Group of the Royal College of Physicians[130] provided a series of recommendations for the management of various neurological conditions, including Parkinson's disease. These could provide the standards against which quality of care may be audited. The working party of the Association of British Neurologists[4] document on neurological rehabilitation in the United Kingdom also provides a set of general standards of care for those with neurological disability, which can form the basis of audit of the management of disability in those with Parkinson's disease.

Management of Parkinson's disease

- The diagnosis is clinical; about 20% of those with parkinsonism will not have Parkinson's disease; drug-induced parkinsonism and the parkinsonian-plus syndromes (such as Steele–Richardson–Olszewski disease or multiple system atrophy) are alternative diagnoses
- No treatment is known to slow the rate of progression, but selegiline has mild antiparkinsonian actions and delays the need for levodopa
- Anticholinergic drugs and amantadine may give sufficient symptomatic benefit early in the illness, but should be avoided in elderly people because of psychotoxicity
- Eventually disability and handicap usually require levodopa or dopamine agonist therapy; levodopa (Sinemet or Madopar) relieves symptoms in nearly all patients, but many develop complications after long term treatment; dopamine agonists (bromocriptine or pergolide) provide adequate relief in about a third of cases, cause greater psychotoxicity (especially in elderly people), but may have fewer long term complications
- The decision to use levodopa or a dopamine agonist depends on the individual patient's handicaps, age, and expectations; low doses of levodopa combined with a dopamine agonist may be useful to reduce long term complications of treatment
- Fluctuations and dyskinesias are major long term problems of dopamine replacement treatment, especially in younger patients, occurring in about 10% of cases per year of treatment; psychotoxicity, falls, and gait problems are other major problems, especially in older patients
- Dyskinesias require a reduction in levodopa or dopamine agonist treatment; fluctuations (wearing-off and on-off phenomena) may be helped by selegiline, the use of delayed release levodopa preparations (Sinemet CR or Madopar CR), the addition of a dopamine agonist, or apomorphine rescue injections or infusions
- Psychotoxicity requires withdrawal of anticholinergic drugs or amantadine, reduction of levodopa or dopamine agonist dosage, or the addition of clozapine or other atypical neuroleptic drugs with a low incidence of extrapyramidal side effects
- Various surgical treatments are available for those with severe drug-resistant Parkinson disease; thalamic stimulation may help tremor; posteroventral pallidotomy may benefit those with uncontrolled dyskinesias; fetal nigral brain grafts are still experimental
- Physiotherapy, speech therapy, and disability aids help many patients; regular assessment is crucial
- Depression, swallowing difficulties, drooling of saliva, constipation, urinary frequency and urgency, and sexual problems are common and require special attention

1 Mutch WJ, Dingwall-Fordyce I, Downie AW, *et al.* Parkinson's disease in a Scottish city. *BMJ* 1986;**292**:534–6.

2 Office of Health Economics. *Parkinson's disease.* Luton: White Crescent 1974;**51**:1–23.

3 Harris AI. *Handicapped and impaired in Great Britain.* London: HMSO, 1971.

4 Association of British Neurologists. *Neurological rehabilitation in the United Kingdom.* Report of a working party, London: ABN, 1992.

5 Wade DT, Langton-Hewer R. Epidemiology of some neurological diseases with special reference to workload on the NHS. *Int Rehabil Med* 1987;**8**:129–37.

6 Rajput AH, Rozdilsky B, Rajput A. Accuracy of clinical diagnosis in parkinsonism—a prospective study. *Can J Neurol Sci* 1991;**18**:275–8.

7 Hughes AJ, Daniel SE, Kilford L, Lees AJ. Accuracy of clinical diagnosis of idiopathic Parkinson's disease—a clinico-pathological study of 100 cases. *J Neurol Neurosurg Psychiatry* 1992;**55**:181–4.

8 Brooks DJ. PET studies on the early and differential diagnosis of Parkinson's disease. *Neurology* 1993;**43**:Suppl 6:S6–16.

9 Hughes AJ, Daniel SE, Blankson S, Lees AJ. A clinico-pathologic study of 100 cases of Parkinson's disease. *Arch Neurol* 1993;**50**:140–8.

10 Palmer SS, Mortimer JA, Webster DD, *et al.* Exercise therapy for Parkinson's disease. *Arch Phys Med Rehabil* 1986;**67**:741–5.

11 Parkinson Study Group. Effect of deprenyl on the progression of disability in early Parkinson's disease. *N Engl J Med* 1989;**321**:1364–71.

12 Parkinson Study Group. Effects of tocopherol and deprenyl on the progression of disability in early Parkinson's disease. *N Engl J Med* 1993;**328**:176–83.

13 Lees A, Stern GM. Sustained bromocriptine therapy in previously untreated patients with Parkinson's disease. *J Neurol Neurosurg Psychiatry* 1981;**44**:1020–3.

14 Marsden CD, Parkes JD. Success and problems of long-term levodopa therapy in Parkinson's disease. *Lancet* 1977;**i**:345–9.

15 Hoehn MM. Parkinsonism treated with levodopa: progression and mortality. In: Birkmayer W, Duvoisin RC, eds. *Extrapyramidal disorders. J Neural Transm* Suppl 19. New York: Springer-Verlag, 1983:253–64.

16 Curtis L, Lees AJ, Stern GM, Marmot MG. Effect of L-dopa on the course of Parkinson's disease. *Lancet* 1984;**ii**:211–12.

17 Clarke CE. Mortality from Parkinson's disease in England and Wales 1921–89. *J Neurol Neurosurg Psychiatry* 1993;**56**:690–3.

18 Grimes JD, Delgado MR. Bromocriptine: problems with low-dose de novo therapy in Parkinson's disease. *Clin Neuropharmacol* 1985;**8**:73–7.

19 Rinne UK. Early dopamine agonist therapy in Parkinson's disease. *Mov Disord* 1989;**4** Suppl 1:S86–94.

20 Rinne UK. Lisuride, a dopamine agonist in the treatment of early Parkinson's disease. *Neurology* 1989;**39**:336–9.

21 Parkinson's Disease Research Group. Comparisons of therapeutic effects of levodopa, levodopa and selegiline, and bromocriptine in patients with early, mild Parkinson's disease: three year interim report. *BMJ* 1993;**307**:469–72.

22 Monastruc JL, Rascol O, Rascol A. A randomized controlled study of bromocriptine versus levodopa in previously untreated parkinsonian patients: a three year follow up. *J Neurol Neurosurg Psychiatry* 1989;**52**:773–5.

23 Blin J, Bonnet A-M, Agid Y. Does levodopa aggravate Parkinson's disease? *Neurology* 1988; **38**:1410–16.

24 Horstink MWIM, Zijlmans JCM, Pasman JW, *et al.* Which risk factors predict the levodopa response in fluctuating Parkinson's disease. *Ann Neurol* 1990;**27**:537–43.

25 Horstink MWIM, Zijlmans JCM, Pasman JW, Berger HJC, Vanthof MA. Severity of Parkinson's disease is a risk factor for peak-dose dyskinesia. *J Neurol Neurosurg Psychiatry* 1990;**53**:224–6.

26 Roos RAC, Vredevoogd CB, Vandervelde EA. Response fluctuations in Parkinson's disease. *Neurology* 1990;**40**:1344–6.

27 Chase TN, Baronti F, Fabbrini G, Heuser IJ, Juncos JL, Mouradian MM. Rationale for continuous dopaminomimetic therapy of Parkinson's disease. *Neurology* 1989;**39** suppl 2: 7–10.

28 Juncos JL, Engber TM, Raisman R, *et al.* Continuous and intermittent levodopa differentially affect basal ganglia function. *Ann Neurol* 1989;**25**:473–8.

29 Rinne UK. Combined bromocriptine-levodopa therapy early in Parkinson's disease. *Neurology* 1985;**35**:1196–8.

30 Rinne UK. Early combination of bromocriptine and levodopa in the treatment of Parkinson's disease: a 5 year follow-up. *Neurology* 1987;**37**:826–8.

31 Factor SA, Weiner WJ. Early combination therapy with bromocriptine and levodopa in Parkinson's disease. *Mov Disord* 1993;**8**:257–62.

32 Weiner WJ, Factor SA, Sanchez-Ramos JR, *et al.* Early combination therapy (bromocriptine and levodopa) does not prevent motor fluctuations in Parkinson's disease. *Neurology* 1993; **43**:21–7.

33 Fahn S. Adverse effects of levodopa. In: Olanow CW, Lieberman AN, eds. *The scientific basis for the treatment of Parkinson's disease.* Carnforth, Lancs: Parthenon, 1992:89–112.

34 Marsden CD, Parkes JD. 'On-off' effects in patients with Parkinson's disease on chronic levodopa therapy. *Lancet* 1976;**1**:292–6.

35 Lesser RP, Fahn S, Snider SR, *et al.* Analysis of the clinical problems in parkinsonism and the complications of long-term levodopa therapy. *Neurology* 1979;**29**:1253–60.

36 Shaw KM, Lees AJ, Stern GM. The impact of treatment with levodopa on Parkinson's disease. *Q J Med* 1980;**49**:283–93.

37 Poewe WH, Lees AJ, Stern GM. Low-dose L-dopa therapy in Parkinson's disease: a 6-year follow-up study. *Neurology* 1986;**36**:1528–30.

38 Quinn N, Critchley P, Marsden CD. Young onset Parkinson's disease. *Mov Disord* 1987; **2**:73–91.

39 Kostic V, Przedborski S, Flaster E, Sternic N. Early development of levodopa-induced dyskinesias and response fluctuations in young-onset Parkinson's disease. *Neurology* 1991; **41**:202–5.

40 Riley DE, Lang AE. The spectrum of levodopa-related fluctuations in Parkinson's disease. *Neurology* 1993;**43**:1459–64.

41 Quinn NP, Koller WC, Lange AE, Marsden CD. Painful Parkinson's disease. *Lancet* 1986; **i**:1366–9.

42 Goetz CG, Tanner CM, Levy M, Wilson RS, Garron DC. Pain in Parkinson's disease. *Mov Disord* 1986;**1**:45–9.

43 Lang AE, Johnson K. Akathisia in idiopathic Parkinson's disease. *Neurology* 1987;**37**: 477–81.

44 Ilson J, Braun N, Fahn S. Respiratory fluctuations in Parkinson's disease. *Neurology* 1983; **33** suppl 2:113.

45 Nissenbaum H, Quinn NP, Brown RG, *et al.* Mood swings associated with the "on-off" phenomenon in Parkinson's disease. *Psychol Med* 1987;**17**:899–904.

46 Cantello R, Gilli M, Riccio A, Bergamasco B. Mood changes associated with "end-of-dose deterioration" in Parkinson's disease: a controlled study. *J Neurol Neurosurg Psychiatry* 1986; **49**:1182–90.

47 Menza MA, Sage J, Marshall E, Cody R, Duvoisin R. Mood changes and "on-off" phenomena in Parkinson's disease. *Mov Disord* 1990;**5**:148–51.

48 Barbeau A. The clinical physiology of side effects in long-term L-dopa therapy. *Adv Neurol* 1974;**5**:347–65.

49 Stein MB, Heuser IJ, Juncos JL, Uhde TW. Anxiety disorders in patients with Parkinson's disease. *Am J Psychiatry* 1990;**147**:217–20.

50 Steiger MJ, Quinn NP, Toone B, Marsden CD. Off-period screaming accompanying motor fluctuations in Parkinson's disease. *Mov Disord* 1991;**6**:89–90.

51 Brown RG, Marsden CD, Quinn N, Wyke MA. Alterations in cognitive performance and affect-arousal state during fluctuations in motor function in Parkinson's disease. *J Neurol Neurosurg Psychiatry* 1984;**47**:454–65.

52 Gotham AM, Brown RG, Marsden CD. 'Frontal' cognitive function in patients with Parkinson's disease 'on' and 'off' levodopa. *Brain* 1988;**11**:299–321.

53 Nutt JG. On-off phenomenon: relation to levodopa pharmacokinetics and pharmacodynamics. *Ann Neurol* 1987;**22**:535–40.

54 Wooten GF. Progress in understanding the pathophysiology of treatment-related fluctuations in Parkinson's disease. *Ann Neurol* 1988;**24**:363–5.

55 Mouradian MM, Juncos JL, Fabbrini G, Chase TN. Motor fluctuations in Parkinson's disease. *Ann Neurol* 1989;**25**:633–4.

56 Fabbrini G, Juncos J, Mouradian MM, Serrati C, Chase TN. Levodopa pharmacokinetic mechanisms and motor fluctuations in Parkinson's disease. *Ann Neurol* 1987;**21**:370–6.

57 Mouradian MM, Juncos JL, Fabbrini G, et al. Motor fluctuations in Parkinson's disease: central pathophysiological mechanisms, part II. Ann Neurol 1988;24:372–8.

58 Melamed E, Bitton V, Zelig O. Episodic unresponsiveness to single doses of L-dopa in parkinsonian fluctuators. Neurology 1986;36:100–3.

59 Hardie RJ, Lees AJ, Stern GM. On-off fluctuations in Parkinson's disease: clinical and neuropharmacological study. Brain 1984;107:487–506.

60 Quinn N, Parkes JD, Marsden CD. Control of on/off phenomenon by continuous intravenous infusion of levodopa. Neurology 1984;34:113–16.

61 Sage JI, Trooskin S, Sonsalla PK, et al. Long-term duodenal infusion of levodopa for motor fluctuations in parkinsonism. Ann Neurol 1988;24:87–9.

62 Sage JI, McHale DM, Sonsalla P, Vitagliano D, Heikkila RE. Continuous levodopa infusions to treat complex dystonia in Parkinson's disease. Neurology 1989;39 suppl 2:60–3.

63 Frankel JP, Lees AJ, Kempster PA, Stern GM. Subcutaneous apomorphine in the treatment of Parkinson's disease. J Neurol Neurosurg Psychiatry 1990;53:96–101.

64 Lees AJ, Shaw KM, Kohout LJ, et al. Deprenyl in Parkinson's disease. Lancet 1977;ii: 791–5.

65 Golbe LI, Lieberman AN, Muenter MD, Ahlskog JE, Gopinathan G. Deprenyl in the treatment of symptom fluctuations in advanced Parkinson's disease. Clin Neuropharmacol 1988;11:45–55.

66 Poewe WH, Lees AJ, Stern GM. Treatment of motor fluctuations in Parkinson's disease with an oral sustained-release preparation of L-dopa: clinical and pharmacokinetic observations. Clin Neuropharmacol 1986;9:430–9.

67 Pezzoli G, Tesei S, Ferrante C, et al. Madopar HBS in fluctuating parkinsonian patients: two-year treatment. Mov Disord 1988;3:37–45.

68 Cedarbaum JM, Breck L, Kutt H, et al. Controlled-release levodopa/carbidopa. I. Sinemet CR-3 treatment of response fluctuations in Parkinson's disease. Neurology 1987;37:233–41.

69 Bush DF, Liss CL, Morton A, for the Multicenter Study Group. An open multicenter long-term treatment evaluation of Sinemet CR. Neurology 1989;39 suppl 2:101–4.

70 Goetz CG, Tanner CM, Gilley DW, Klawans HL. Development and progression of motor fluctuations and side effects in Parkinson's disease: comparison of Sinemet CR versus carbidopa/levodopa. Neurology 1989;39 suppl 2:63–6.

71 Hutton JT, Morris JL, Bush DF, et al. Multicenter controlled study of Sinemet CR vs Sinemet (25/100) in advanced Parkinson's disease. Neurology 1989;39 suppl 2:67–73.

72 Hutton JT, Morris JL. Long-acting carbidopa-levodopa in the management of moderate and advanced Parkinson's disease. Neurology 1992;42: suppl 1:51–60.

73 LeWitt PA, Ward CD, Larsen TA, et al. Comparison of pergolide and bromocriptine therapy in parkinsonism. Neurology 1983;33:1009–14.

74 Langtry HD, Clissold SP. Pergolide: a review of its pharmacological properties and therapeutic potential in Parkinson's disease. Drugs 1990;39:491–506.

75 Pezzoli G, Martignoni E, Pacchetti C, et al. Pergolide compared with bromocriptine in Parkinson's disease: a multicentre, crossover, controlled study. Mov Disord 1994. In press.

76 Kurth MC, Tetrud LW, Irwin I, Lyness WH, Langston JW. Oral levodopa/carbidopa solution versus tablets in Parkinson's patients with severe fluctuations—a pilot study. Neurology 1993;43:1036–9.

77 Berkowitz DM, McCallum RW. Interaction of levodopa and metoclopramide on gastric emptying. Clin Pharmacol Ther 1980;27:414–20.

78 Lau E, Waterman K, Glover R, et al. Effect of antacid on levodopa therapy. Clin Neuropharmacol 1986;9:477–9.

79 Pincus JH, Barry K. Protein redistribution diet restores motor function in patients with dopa-resistant "off" periods. Neurology 1987;38:481–3.

80 Hughes AJ, Bishop S, Kleedorfer B, et al. Subcutaneous apomorphine in Parkinson's disease: response to chronic administration for up to five years. Mov Disord 1993;8:165–70.

81 Luquin MR, Scipioni O, Vaamonde J, Gershanik O, Obeso JA. Levodopa-induced dyskinesias in Parkinson's disease: clinical and pharmacological classification. Mov Disord 1992;7:117–24.

82 Marconi R, Lefebvre-Caparros D, Bonnet A-M, et al. Levodopa-induced dyskinesias in Parkinson's disease phenomenology and pathophysiology. Mov Disord 1994;9:2–12.

83 Mouradian MM, Heuser IJE, Baronti F, et al. Pathogenesis of dyskinesias in Parkinson's disease. Ann Neurol 1989;25:523–6.

84 Nutt JG. Levodopa-induced dyskinesia: review, observations and speculations. Neurology 1990;40:340–5.

85 Muenter MD, Sharpless NS, Tyce GM, Darley FL. 'I-D-I' and 'D-I-D' in response to L-dopa therapy of Parkinson's disease. *Mayo Clin Proc* 1977;**46**:231–9.

86 Lhermitte F, Agid Y, Signoret JL. Onset and end-of-dose levodopa-induced dyskinesias. *Arch Neurol* 1978;**35**:261–2.

87 Giladi N, McMahon D, Przedborski S, *et al.* Motor blocks in Parkinson's disease. *Neurology* 1992;**42**:333–9.

88 Koller WC, Glatt S, Vetere-Overfield B, Hassanein R. Falls and Parkinson's disease. *Clin Neuropharmacol* 1989;**12**:98–105.

89 Critchley EMR. Speech disorders of parkinsonism: a review. *J Neurol Neurosurg Psychiatry* 1981;**44**:751–8.

90 Downie AW, Low JM, Lindsay DD. Speech disorder in parkinsonism. *J Neurol Neurosurg Psychiatry* 1981;**44**:52–3.

91 Bushmann M, Dobmeyer SM, Leeker L, Perlmutter JS. Swallowing abnormalities and their response to treatment in Parkinson's disease. *Neurology* 1989;**39**:1309–14.

92 Bonnet A-M, Loria Y, Saint- Hilaire M-H, Lhermitte F, Agid Y. Does long-term aggravation of Parkinson's disease result from nondopaminergic lesions? *Neurology* 1987;**37**:1539–42.

93 Durso R, Isaac K, Perry L, Saint-Hilaire M, Feldman RG. Age influences magnitude but not duration of response to levodopa. *J Neurol Neurosurg Psychiatry* 1993;**56**:65–8.

94 Oxtoby M. *Parkinson's disease patients and their social needs.* 36 Portland Place, London: Parkinson's Disease Society, 1982.

95 Beattie A, Caird FI. The occupational therapist and the patient with Parkinson's disease. *BMJ* 1980;**i**:1354–5.

96 Scott S, Caird FI. Speech therapy for Parkinson's disease. *J Neurol Neurosurg Psychiatry* 1983;**46**:140–4.

97 Robertson SJ, Thomson F. Speech therapy and Parkinson's disease. *Coll Speech Ther Bull* 1983;**1**:10–11.

98 Robertson SJ, Thomson F. Speech therapy in Parkinson's disease. *Br J Disord Commun* 1984;**19**:213–24.

99 Edwards LL, Quigley EMM, Pfeiffer RF. Gastrointestinal dysfunction in Parkinson's disease: frequency and pathophysiology. *Neurology* 1992;**42**:726–32.

100 Fitzmaurice H, Fowler CJ, Rickards D, *et al.* Micturition disturbance in Parkinson's disease. *Br J Urol* 1985;**57**:652–6.

101 Mathers SE, Kempster PA, Law PJ, *et al.* Anal sphincter dysfunction in Parkinson's disease. *Arch Neurol* 1989;**46**:1061–4.

102 Lees AJ, Smith E. Cognitive deficits in the early stages of Parkinson's disease. *Brain* 1983;**106**:257–70.

103 Taylor AE, Saint-Cyr JA, Lang AE. Frontal lobe dysfunction in Parkinson's disease. *Brain* **109**:845–53.

104 Rogers D, Lees AJ, Trimble A, *et al.* Bradyphrenia in Parkinson's disease and psychomotor retardation in depressive illness, an experimental study. *Brain* 1987;**110**:761–76.

105 Brown RG, Marsden CD. How common is dementia in Parkinson's disease? *Lancet* 1984;**ii**:1262–5.

106 McKeith IG, Perry RH, Fairbairn AF, Jabeen S, Perry EK. Operational criteria for senile dementia of Lewy body type (SDLT). *Psychol Med* 1992;**22**:911–22.

107 De Smet Y, Ruberg M, Serderai M, *et al.* Confusion, dementia and anticholinergics in Parkinson's disease. *J Neurol Neurosurg Psychiatry* 1982;**45**:1161–4.

108 Byrne EJ, Lennox G, Lowe J, Godwing-Austen RB. Diffuse Lewy body disease: clinical features in 15 cases. *J Neurol Neurosurg Psychiatry* 1989;**52**:709–17.

109 Perry RH, Irving D, Blessed G, Fairbairn A, Perry EH. Senile dementia of Lewy body type, a clinically and neuropathologically distinct form of Lewy body dementia in the elderly. *J Neurol Sci* 1990;**95**:119–39.

110 Crystal HA, Dickson DW, Lizardi JE, Davies P, Wolfson LI. Antemortem diagnosis of diffuse Lewy body disease. *Neurology* 1990;**40**:1523–8.

111 Scholz E, Dichgans J. Treatment of drug-induced exogenous psychosis in parkinsonism with clozapine and fluperlapine. *Eur Arch Psychiatry Neurol Sci* 1985;**235**:60–4.

112 Friedman JH, Lannon MC. Clozapine in the treatment of psychosis in Parkinson's disease. *Neurology* 1989;**39**:1219–21.

113 Wolters EC, Hurwitz TA, Mak E, *et al.* Clozapine in the treatment of parkinsonian patients with dopaminomimetic psychosis. *Neurology* 1990;**40**:832–4.

114 Gotham AM, Brown RG, Marsden CD. Depression in Parkinson's disease: a quantitative and qualitative analysis. *J Neurol Neurosurg Psychiatry* 1986;**49**:381–9.

115 Brown RG, MacCarthy B, Gotham AM, *et al.* Depression and disability in Parkinson's disease: a follow-up of 132 cases. *Psychol Med* 1988;**18**:49–55.

116 Steur ENHJ. Increase of Parkinson disability after fluoxetine medication. *Neurology* 1993; **43**:211–3.

117 Hoehn MM, Yahr MD. Evaluation of the long term results of surgical therapy. In: Gillingham FJ, Donaldson IML, eds. *Third symposium on Parkinson's disease.* Edinburgh: E&S Livingstone, 1969;274–80.

118 Fox MW, Ahlskog JR, Kelly PJ. Stereotactic ventrolateralis thalamotomy for medically refractory tremor in post-levodopa era Parkinson's disease patients. *J Neurosurg* 1991;**75**: 723–30.

119 Diederick N, Goetz CG, Stebbins GT, *et al.* Blinded evaluation confirms long-term asymmetric effect of unilateral thalamotomy or subthalamotomy on tremor in Parkinson's disease. *Neurology* 1992;**42**:1311–14.

120 Goetz CG, DeLong MR, Penn RD, Bakay RAE. Neurosurgical horizons in Parkinson's disease. *Neurology* 1993;**43**:1–7.

121 Laitinen LV, Bergenheim AT, Hariz MI. Leksell's posteroventral pallidotomy in the treatment of Parkinson's disease. *J Neurosurg* 1992;**76**:53–61.

122 Benabid AL, Pollak P, Gervason C, *et al.* Long-term suppression of tremor by chronic stimulation of the ventral intermediate thalamic nucleus. *Lancet* 1991;**337**:403–6.

123 Goetz CG, Stebbins GT III, Klawans HL, *et al.* United Parkinson Foundation Neurotransplantation Registry on adrenal medullary transplants: presurgical and 1- and 2-year follow-up. *Neurology* 1991;**41**:1719–22.

124 Lindvall O, Brundin P, Widner H, *et al.* Grafts of fetal dopamine neurons survive and improve motor function in Parkinson's disease. *Science* 1990;**247**:574–7.

125 Spencer DD, Robbins RJ, Naftolin F, *et al.* Unilateral transplantation of human fetal mesencephalic tissue into the caudate nucleus of patients with Parkinson's disease. *N Engl J Med* 1992;**327**:1541–8.

126 Freed CR, Breeze RE, Rosenberg NL, *et al.* Survival of implanted fetal dopamine cells and neurologic improvement 12 to 46 months after transplantation for Parkinson's disease. *N Engl J Med* 1992;**327**:1549–55.

127 Widner H, Tetrud J, Rehncrona S, *et al.* Bilateral fetal mesencephalic grafting in two patients with parkinsonism induced by MPTP. *N Engl J Med* 1992;**327**:1556–63.

128 Fahn S. Fetal-tissue transplants in Parkinson's disease [editorial]. *N Engl J Med* 1992; **327**:1589–90.

129 Association of British Neurologists. *Guidelines for the care of patients with common neurological disorders in the United Kingdom.* Fitzroy Square, London: Association of British Neurologists 1993.

130 Working Group. Standards of care for patients with neurological disease. A consensus. *J R Coll Phys* 1990;**24**:90–7.

8 Dementia

M N ROSSOR

Dementia is the clinical syndrome of impairment in multiple domains of cognitive function occurring in an alert patient. Some definitions of dementia demand that the cognitive impairment is progressive, but for the clinician the static cognitive impairment arising after an encephalitic illness or head injury shares many of the problems of management encountered with the progressive dementias such as Alzheimer's disease. The dementias as a group constitute one of the commonest problems presenting to neurologists and psychiatrists and comprise the fourth leading cause of death.

The commonest causes of dementia—namely, Alzheimer's disease and vascular dementia—are predominantly diseases of elderly people. Recent epidemiological studies suggest a low prevalence of dementia in populations below the age of 70, being in the region of 1% in those aged between 50 and 70 years with a dramatic rise to about 50% in very elderly people.[1-3] Because dementia by definition means that cognitive impairment is sufficient to result in a loss of previous skills to the extent that the patient's normal, social, or work activity is compromised, the dementing illnesses represent a major burden on society.

With an aging population the number of patients with dementia is expected to rise. Based on demographic trends of people aged over 80 in the United States it is anticipated that there may be 10–15 million people affected by Alzheimer's disease by the middle of the next century.[4] Estimates that include the rapidly aging population in Japan and other Asian countries give global figures that may exceed one hundred million.[5] The same trend can be anticipated in the United Kingdom; there are currently over half a million people predicted to have Alzheimer's disease and a larger total with dementia. It should, however, be recognised that about

18 000 people below the age of 65 are believed to have Alzheimer's disease or related dementia; and if one considers the number of neurological illnesses in which cognitive dysfunction may also feature, such as multiple sclerosis or the extrapyramidal diseases, then the figure is clearly far higher.

A recent systematic cost of illness analysis of Alzheimer's disease in England has been undertaken.[6] This included estimates of inpatient or outpatient day care as well as residential care costs and arrived at a total figure of £1144 million for 1992. Comparison with other burden of illness analyses and adjustment for overall United Kingdom costs makes Alzheimer's disease more expensive than epilepsy although less than stroke if community and non-NHS care costs are excluded. If these are included then the comparable figures are £1373 million for Alzheimer's disease and £838 million for stroke. Moreover, this analysis did not include the indirect costs to family carers over and above the benefits they received from Government agencies. The burden of informal care from family members is substantial.

Diagnosis

Published definitions of dementia all include the involvement of multiple domains of cognitive impairment with intact arousal mechanisms to distinguish the patient with dementia from one with a confusional state. Moreover, the cognitive impairment should be of sufficient severity to result in the loss of previously acquired skills such that this interferes with normal social or employment function.

The most widely used criteria are those of the American Psychiatric Association Diagnostic and Statistical Manual of which the latest edition (DSM IV) has just been published.[7] Such criteria can provide a useful guide to the identification of the syndrome but not to the cause. The syndrome of dementia is of grave significance, as it usually reflects progressive degenerative disease that threatens the very integrity of the patient. Moreover, dementia occurs in the setting of many neurological disorders necessitating a broad differential diagnosis and wide ranging investigations. In this group, the clues to the diagnosis and direction of subsequent investigations are usually provided by the additional neurological abnormalities, although some disorders—for example, multiple

---

Box 8.1   Differential diagnosis of degenerative dementia

Alzheimer's disease:

Sporadic	Early onset
	Late onset
Familial	Chromosome 14-linked
	Amyloid precursor protein mutations
	Apolipoprotein E4
	Non-chromosome 14, 19, 21
Cortical Lewy body disease	Pure
	With senile plaques
Prion disease	Sporadic
	Iatrogenic
	Familial—PrP gene mutations
Pick's disease	
Frontal lobe degeneration	With motor neuron disease
Focal degenerations, for example, primary progressive dysphasia	
Corticobasal degeneration	
Progressive subcortical gliosis	

Differential diagnosis of patients presenting with dementia or progressive isolated cognitive deficits on a degenerative basis. It is not exhaustive and does not include diseases in which dementia is not commonly the presenting feature.

---

sclerosis—can present as cognitive impairment with little else to find on examination.

Alzheimer's disease is the most common of the degenerative dementias (box 8.1). Characteristically, the disease starts with impairment of memory, at which time, if this is an isolated cognitive impairment, the patient would not fulfil the dementia criteria of multiple domains of cognitive dysfunction. Language impairment with both word finding and comprehension difficulties and visuospatial dysfunction, however, soon emerge. Neuropathologically, the disease is identified by senile plaques and neurofibrillary tangles (fig 8.1). The plaques consist of dystrophic neurites clustered around a core of β amyloid protein, which is derived from a larger precursor protein, the amyloid precursor protein (APP).[8] Neurofibrillary tangles are derived from the microtubule associated protein tau, which is in an abnormally

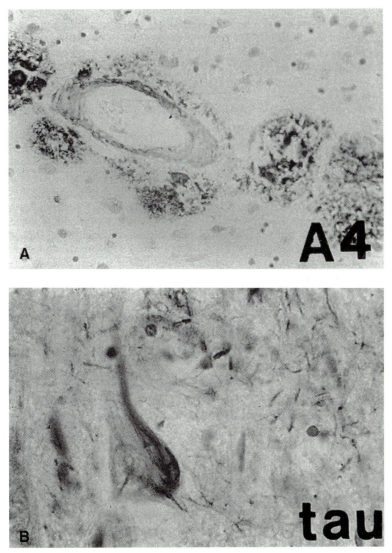

Figure 8.1 *(A) Beta A4 immunohistochemistry showing a senile plaque and vascular amyloid in a patient with Alzheimer's disease. (B) Anti-tau immunohistochemistry showing a neurofibrillary tangle in the same patient (courtesy of Dr T Revesz, Institute of Neurology, London).*

hyperphosphorylated state.[9] The definitive diagnosis of Alzheimer's disease depends on histological confirmation, usually at necropsy, although as the histological abnormalities of senile plaques and neurofibrillary tangles are also found to a lesser extent in normal old people, neuropathological quantitative criteria have been developed for the diagnosis.[10]

Criteria for the clinical diagnosis have been published by the National Institutes of Neurological and Communicative Disorders and Stroke and the Alzheimer's Disease and Related Disorders Association (NINCDS/ADRDA).[11] Three levels of diagnostic certainty are provided by these criteria: definite Alzheimer's disease requires histological confirmation in a patient who fulfils the criteria for dementia; probable Alzheimer's disease can be diagnosed without histology in the presence of a typical history and dementia; possible Alzheimer's disease is reserved for those patients with atypical features or in whom additional potential causes for dementia, such as vascular disease, are present. These criteria have been assessed against subsequent neuropathology and in some studies have provided very high rates of accuracy.[12 13] Tierney *et al* assessed the clinical criteria against various neuropathological criteria and derived figures of 0·64–0·86 for sensitivity (cases clinically diagnosed as Alzheimer's disease with histopathological confirmation as a proportion of all cases with histologically proved Alzheimer's disease) and of 0·89–0·9 for specificity (cases clinically diagnosed as *not* Alzheimer's disease without Alzheimer histopathology as a proportion of all non-Alzheimer cases).[14]

Within the degenerative dementia group clinical diagnoses are becoming more refined although there is still a poor correlation between histology and phenotype, particularly in non-Alzheimer dementias. Thus although identification of regional patterns of deficits can define a group of patients with frontal lobe dementia,[15] the underlying histology can include a non-specific mild cell loss with white matter change, Pick's disease, plaques and tangles, or spongiform change.

Similarly, the focal degenerations such as progressive dysphasia can be associated with a variety of histopathologies such as occur in Pick's disease, Alzheimer's disease, neuronal achromasia, and focal spongiform change.[16]

The other main dementia group is vascular disease, usually due either to multiple cortical infarcts, to small vessel disease, or both.[17] Occasionally, a discrete small infarct—for example, in the paramedial thalamus—can cause appreciable cognitive impairment.[18] The criteria developed by Hachinski et al[19] provide a relatively poor guide when assessed against neuropathology, with an accuracy of only about 60%.[20] Recently, more detailed criteria, which utilise additional information from neuroimaging, have been published.[20 21]

Diseases with subcortical pathology (such as Parkinson's disease, progressive supranuclear palsy, and hydrocephalus) are associated with cognitive slowing, referred to as subcortical dementia.[22] Although the concept has been challenged, the pattern of pronounced slowing of cognition is useful clinically to identify with relatively low error a group of patients, some of whom (for example, those with hydrocephalus) can be amenable to treatment.

History and examination

It is essential to obtain a history from an independent carer, usually the spouse, as well as from the patient, particularly as anosognosia for cognitive impairment occurs often in Alzheimer's disease and frontal lobe dementias. This should be done when the patient is not present as carers are often unwilling to be open in front of the patient. Details of the history that suggest deficits in specific areas of cognition should be explored, and enquiries about activities of daily living such as shopping, cooking, housework, and household administration must be included. A useful clue is a change in the role of a patient within the family although this may be due to factors other than cognitive impairment, and features of a depressive illness causing a pseudodementia should be excluded. Pseudodementia should be suspected if the patient complains more of the memory impairment than the spouse, although depressive symptoms are a common accompaniment to early Alzheimer's disease.[23] Changes in sexual behaviour should be sensitively discussed as this is an area that can cause considerable distress but is rarely mentioned by the spouse.

A general medical history must be obtained including current and previous medications. A family history of dementia is often present if carefully and specifically sought, as most of the degenerative dementias can occur as autosomal dominant as well as sporadic disease. With younger patients it is necessary to enquire about employment, and all patients should be asked about driving, not only because it gives a guide to cognitive function but also because of the medicological implications (see later). It is important to emphasise that whereas dementia is defined by the presence of multiple domains of cognitive impairment, patients will often start with a single deficit and this may not always be memory; Alzheimer's disease may occasionally present with visuospatial dysfunction, visual disorientation, dysphasia, or dyspraxia. A focal presentation may be characteristic of other dementias such as Pick's disease.

Examination should ensure adequate exploration of the major domains of cognitive function and must involve some simple tests of function of the non-dominant hemisphere. The mini mental state examination[24] is a brief bedside test of cognitive function that is now widely used and although not designed to provide any detail of neuropsychological function it is easy and rapid to give to outpatients.[25] The clinical dementia rating scale provides an overall staging of the functional deficit.[26] CAMDEX and its associated cognitive assessment, CAMCOG, provide a more comprehensive diagnostic assessment,[27] but take time and can be inflexible. The US Consortium to Establish a Registry of Alzheimer's disease (CERAD) has attempted to develop a battery of tests useful for the early diagnosis of Alzheimer's disease[28] but these are more appropriate to the detailed investigation of neuropsychological function than as simple bedside tests.

On general neurological examination the presence of pyramidal signs, extrapyramidal features, or peripheral neuropathy may suggest a diagnosis other than a simple degenerative dementia. Many patients with Alzheimer's disease may have extrapyramidal features, however, most commonly rigidity but occasionally bradykinesia, which may relate to additional Lewy body formation.[29 30] A careful general medical examination is essential as this may provide important clues to secondary causes of dementia—for example, cardiac murmurs in vascular dementia or cytomegalovirus retinitis in a patient with cognitive impairment due to HIV infection.

Investigation

Ideally all patients should undergo formal neuropsychological assessment to assess the extent and severity of the cognitive deficit. Routine haematology and biochemistry should also investigate treponemal serology, thyroid function, and vitamin B12 and red cell folate concentrations. Chest radiography and neuroimaging should be performed. Computed tomography will exclude space occupying lesions and hydrocephalus and may also indicate changes in white matter associated with demyelination or vascular disease. Special orientation of the plane of tomography can show medial temporal lobe atrophy in Alzheimer's disease.[31] Magnetic resonance imaging is of greater value than computed tomography, and regional volumetric studies may increasingly aid the diagnosis of specific degenerative dementias (fig 8.2).[32] It is recognised that in elderly demented patients routine neuropsychology and neuroimaging may not be practical; nevertheless, this is the ideal that should be sought. An electroencephalogram can be valuable; early slowing would favour Alzheimer's disease by contrast with a normal electroencephalogram commonly found with Pick's disease and other frontal lobe dementias; periodic complexes may be important in the diagnosis of prion disease.

In some patients a wider range of investigations is necessary. Specific blood tests might include screening for metabolic disorders such as Wilson's disease, metachromatic leucodystrophy, and GM_2 gangliosidoses; tests for HIV should always be considered in unexplained cognitive impairment, particularly in young patients. CSF is often examined in patients with presenile dementia but is usually normal in degenerative dementia: a raised protein or cell count would suggest the possibility of vasculitis or other inflammatory disorder and, in view of the potentially treatable nature of these diseases, may be an important finding. It is nevertheless uncommon to find abnormal CSF in the presence of a normal magnetic resonance image. Muscle biopsy may be indicated to look for ragged-red fibres in association with mitochondrial cytopathies. Very occasionally a brain biopsy may be indicated if a treatable cause such as cerebral vasculitis is suspected. In hereditary disease appropriate genetic screening for the Huntington mutation, amyloid precursor protein mutations, and prion protein gene mutations are all available; the extent to which apolipoprotein e4 allele genotyping might prove to be of use in diagnosis and management remains to be seen.[33] Functional imaging with positron emission tomography (PET) is still largely a research investigation, but single photon emission computed tomography (SPECT) is now more widely available and may be valuable in showing a posterior (common with Alzheimer's disease) as opposed to anterior pattern of hypometabolism.[34]

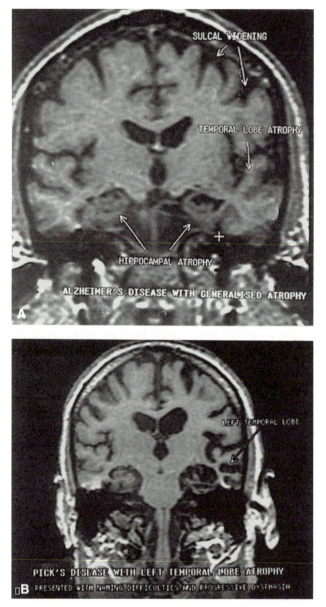

Figure 8.2 *Magnetic resonance imaging showing (A) bilateral hippocampal and temporal lobe atrophy in a patient with Alzheimer's disease and (B) asymmetrical anterior hippocampal, amygdala, and temporal lobe atrophy in a patient with Pick's disease (courtesy of Dr N Fox, St Mary's Hospital, London)*

212

Prevention

At present few causes of dementia are preventable. Control of hypertension may prevent some of the cases of vascular dementia although there is no simple relation between the development of dementia and vascular risk factors. With the discovery of the Huntington mutation, amyloid precursor protein mutation, and prion protein mutations, prenatal testing is likely to become more important in young onset dementias.

Prognosis

The diagnosis of dementia carries a grave prognosis. Prompt treatment of some underlying diseases such as neurosyphilis, cerebral vasculitis, and metabolic disturbances can result in stabilisation and even reversal. Unfortunately most cases follow a relentless progression. This may vary from the devastatingly rapid deterioration measured in months in some cases of sporadic Creutzfeldt-Jakob disease to a deterioration measured in 10–15 years for some of the focal degenerations. The median survival from diagnosis in Alzheimer's disease is in the range of seven to 10 years, although some patients may have a prolonged mild stage.[35] Average rates of decline are in the order of 3–4 points on the mini mental state examination per year.

Communication and counselling

Although grave and tragic information often has to be imparted, a frank discussion when the diagnosis and prognosis are known is essential. Commonly, however, the diagnosis may be unclear in the early stages. Thus when first seen the patient may show only mild changes in cognition and in the absence of a specific clinical test there is a natural reluctance to make a diagnosis such as Alzheimer's disease: inevitably there is a burden of uncertainty that has to be shared between the patient, the family, and the doctor. Nevertheless, there is still a reluctance to discuss Alzheimer's disease and its implications that is comparable with that associated with a diagnosis of cancer 10 to 20 years ago. Early discussion of the implications and how help can be offered, together with appropriate counselling, is vital. The disease affects not only the patient but the entire family: in young onset dementia the illness can be devastating for the children and in older patients disruption of the shared plans for retirement can present a considerable sense of loss.

Memory clinics can provide diagnosis, counselling, and advice but most longer term support is provided in the community by the social work and community psychiatric services. The Alzheimer's Disease Society provides additional information and support. Some smaller patient support groups are now being established for some of the rarer disorders such as Pick's disease and Creutzfeldt-Jakob disease (see appendix).

Neurological follow up of cases of dementia is indicated when the diagnosis is unclear or when specialist advice is needed for some of the rarer diseases. In general, however, management is shared between the general practitioner, hospital, and community psychiatric services.

Management

The specific treatment of dementia relates to the underlying condition. There are the rare instances of reversible dementia such as those associated with hydrocephalus, hypothyroidism, cerebral vasculitis, neurosarcoid, or neurosyphilis. For most, there are no specific treatments although there is now the emerging prospect of symptomatic treatment. When there is any doubt about the diagnosis or the presence of depressive symptoms, patients should be given a trial of an antidepressant, commonly one of the selective serotonin uptake inhibitors that avoid the anticholinergic side effects of tricyclic antidepressants and are better tolerated. This will help to identify patients with depressive pseudodementia and may also improve cognitive function in depressed patients early in the course of Alzheimer's disease.

Attention has recently been directed towards enhancing cholinergic transmission, which is reduced in Alzheimer's disease due to disruption of the subcorticocortical cholinergic projection. Most attention has been directed towards the acetylcholinesterase inhibitors after the report of a beneficial effect of tetra-hydroaminoacridine (tacrine). Recent studies have confirmed this. The study by Farlow et al using a parallel design with 468 Alzheimer patients given tacrine in doses of 20–80 mg or placebo for 12 weeks showed improvement both on a global clinical impression of change and the cognitive subset of the Alzheimer's disease assessment scale (ADAS-COG).[36] About half the patients taking the highest dose had an improvement of four points on the ADAS-COG, which is equivalent to about six months of normal spontaneous decline. The most recent study[37] comprised 653 patients given treatment for 30 weeks with doses of tacrine up to 160 mg a day, and improvement was seen at the higher dose in about 40% of patients who were able to complete the study, with an improvement of more than four points on the ADAS-COG; however, 43% withdrew due to cholinergic side effects. Changes in transaminases reflecting the hepatotoxicity of the drug are commonly seen, with 29% of patients developing abnormal transaminases of more than three times the upper limit of normal, and about half showing some abnormality. This is normally reversible on withdrawal of the drug and patients can often be successfully rechallenged.

Tacrine (Cognex) has received a licence for use in Alzheimer's disease in the United States and more recently in France, but not in the United Kingdom. Further acetylcholinesterase inhibitors are likely to become available over the next few years and there is intense activity within the pharmaceutical industry to develop other symptomatic treatments for Alzheimer's disease and, in the longer term, drugs that may alter the underlying disease process. Thus efforts are being directed towards drugs that might inhibit the hyperphosphorylation of the protein tau, which leads to neurofibrillary tangle formation and the deposition of β amyloid protein associated with senile plaques.

As well as these exciting developments in Alzheimer's disease, treatment of behavioural disturbance is important and is common to many of the dementias. Hallucinations, aggressive behaviour, and psychoses can be difficult to treat as many patients are very sensitive to the effects of neuroleptics, particularly patients with diffuse Lewy body disease in whom rapid deterioration in motor and cognitive function can occur. The judicious and closely monitored introduction of a neuroleptic drug, however, particularly one with less extrapyramidal side effects, may be beneficial. Sleep disturbance is also common but can respond to small doses of a rapidly acting benzodiazepine such as temazepam.

Liaison

In the United Kingdom neurologists tend to see younger patients presenting with presenile dementia or cases of dementia with additional neurological abnormalities. Most cases of dementia that occur in elderly people and which are due to Alzheimer's disease are seen by psychiatrists and geriatricians. By contrast, in the United States and in many European countries, Alzheimer's disease is predominantly seen by neurologists. Dementia encompasses many disciplines and good management will involve care by neurologists, psychiatrists, and geriatricians as appropriate, together with neuropsychologists and specialist nurse counsellers. Liaison with general physicians, surgeons, and other professionals is also important to ensure that the patient gets appropriate care for other medical problems. Untreated or inadequately managed conditions can often exacerbate confusion and behavioural disturbance, yet there is sometimes reluctance to treat if there has been a diagnosis of dementia.

As well as medical and paramedical liaison other agencies are important, particularly when patients are still in employment. We have clear guidelines for employment of those with epilepsy or cardiac disease who are airline pilots, public service vehicle drivers, etc. For those with cognitive impairment the opportunities for harm are far greater but the guidelines fewer. Even for driving the information is unclear.[38] Once a diagnosis of dementia has been made then the Driver and Vehicle Licensing Authority should be informed by the patient but there are few guidelines as to whether the patient is able to drive or not. Unfortunately for many patients driving is seen as important for maintaining independence in society and self esteem.

Although the ideal is for seamless care from the initial neurological assessment and diagnosis through the longer term management within the community and on to long term hospital care, this is often not achieved and one is faced with crisis management of the patient who is unable to be managed at home. This makes the early diagnosis, explanation, and prognosis all the more important.

Appendix

Alzheimer's Disease Society (Creutzfeldt-Jakob Group), Gordon House, 10 Greencoat Place, London, SW1P 1PH, UK.

Pick's Disease Self Help Group, National Hospital for Neurology and Neurosurgery, Queen Square, London, WC1N 3BG, UK.

Management of dementia

- Dementia is the clinical syndrome of impairment in multiple domains of cognitive function with intact arousal; by definition memory must be impaired
- The prevalence of dementia increases with age to about half of those approaching 90 years; Alzheimer's disease is the commonest cause
- Specific diagnosis is important for prognosis and identification of treatable diseases. Clinical criteria have been developed by the National Institutes of Neurological and Communicative Disorder and Stroke and the Alzheimer's Disease and Related Disorders Association (NINCDS/ADRDA) for Alzheimer's disease. Neuropsychometry defines the pattern of cognitive dysfunction. Neuroimaging will identify structural lesions, hydrocephalus, ischaemic damage, and regional atrophy. Genetic testing may identify some hereditary dementias
- Some dementias are treatable—for example, vasculitis, infections, hydrocephalus, and clinical depression presenting as pseudodementia
- Symptomatic treatment of Alzheimer's disease using the acetylcholinesterase inhibitor, tetrahydroaminoacridine (THA, tacrine), is available in the United States, Australia, and France: further cholinergic drugs show promise
- Treatment of depression and underlying systemic disorders is important; behavioural disturbance may require judicious neuroleptic treatment
- Management of all cases of dementia requires careful advice and counselling of patient and family; shared care will involve hospital specialist, general practitioner, and community psychiatric services
- Patients or caregivers should inform the Driver and Vehicle Licensing Agency of a diagnosis of dementia, and the ability to drive should be considered carefully

1 Evans DA, Funkenstein HH, Albert MS, *et al.* Prevalence of Alzheimer's disease in a community of older persons: higher than previously reported. *JAMA* 1989;**262**:2551–6.
2 Jorm AF. *The epidemiology of Alzheimer's disease and related disorders.* London: Chapman and Hall, 1990.
3 Skoog I, Nilsson L, Palmertz BO, Andreasson L-A, Svanborg A. A population-based study of dementia in 85-year-olds. *N Engl J Med* 1993;**328**:153–8.
4 Office of Technology Assessment, US Congress. *Losing a million minds: confronting the tragedy of Alzheimer's disease and other dementias.* Washington, DC: US Government Printing Office, 1987. Publ No OTA-BA-323.
5 Whitehouse PJ, ed. *Dementia.* Philadelphia: FA Davies Co, 1993.
6 Grey A, Fenn P. Alzheimer's Disease: the burden of the illness in England. *Health Trends* 1993;**25**:31–7.

7 American Psychiatric Association. *Diagnostic and statistical manual of mental disorders* 4th ed (DSM-IV). Washington DC: APA, 1994.

8 Selkoe DJ, Haass C. Cellular processing of beta-amyloid precursor protein and the genesis of amyloid beta-peptide. *Cell* 1993;**75**:1039–42.

9 Lee VM-Y, Balin BJ, Otvos L, Jr, Trojanowski JQ. A68: a major sub-unit of paired helical filaments and derivatized forms of normal tau. *Science* 1991;**251**:675–8.

10 Khachaturian ZS. Diagnosis of Alzheimer's disease. *Arch Neurol* 1985;**42**:1097–105.

11 McKhann G, Drachman D, Folstein M, *et al.* Clinical diagnosis of Alzheimer's disease: report of the NINCDS/ADRDA workgroup under the auspices of the Department of Health and Human Services Task Force on Alzheimer's disease. *Neurology* 1984;**34**:939–44.

12 Morris J, McKeel D, Fulling K, *et al.* Validation of clinical diagnostic criteria in senile dementia of the Alzheimer type. *Ann Neurol* 1987;**22**:122.

13 Kukull WA, Larson EB, Reifler BV, *et al.* Inter-rater reliability of Alzheimer's disease diagnosis. *Neurology* 1990;**40**:1364–9.

14 Tierney M, Fisher R, Lewis A, *et al.* The NINCDS/ADRDA workgroup criteria for the clinical diagnosis of probable Alzheimer's disease: a clinico–pathologic study of 57 cases. *Neurology* 1988;**38**:359–64.

15 Neary D, Snowden JS, Northen B, *et al.* Dementia of frontal type. *J Neurol Neurosurg Psychiatry* 1988;**51**:353–61.

16 Casselli RJ, Jack CR. Asymmetric cortical degeneration. A proposed clinical classification. *Arch Neurol* 1992;**49**:770–80.

17 Jellinger K, Danielcyzk W, Fisher P, Gabriel E. Clinicopathological analysis of dementia disorders in the elderly. *J Neurol Sci* 1990;**95**:239–58.

18 Katz D, Alexander MP, Mandell AM. Dementia following strokes in the mesencephalon and diencephalon. *Arch Neurol* 1987;**44**:1127–33.

19 Hachinski VC, Iliff LD, Zilkha E, *et al.* Cerebral blood flow in dementia. *Arch Neurol* 1975; **32**:632–7.

20 Chui HC, Victoroff JI, Margolin D, Jagust W, Shankle R, Katzman R. Criteria for the diagnosis of ischemic vascular dementia proposed by the State of California Alzheimer's Disease Diagnostic and Treatment Centers. *Neurology* 1992;**42**:437–80.

21 Roman GC, Tatemichi TK, Erkinjuntti T, *et al.* Vascular dementia: diagnostic criteria for research studies. Report of the NINDS-AIREN international workshop. *Neurology* 1993; **43**:250–60.

22 Albert ML, Feldman RG, Willis AL. The "subcortical dementia" of progressive supranuclear palsy. *J Neurol Neurosurg Psychiatry* 1974;**37**:121–30.

23 Burns A, Jacoby R, Levy R. Psychiatric phenomena in Alzheimer's disease. *Br J Psychiatry* 1990;**157**:72–94.

24 Folstein MF, Folstein SE, McHugh PR. "Mini-mental state": a practical method for grading the mental state of patients for the clinician. *J Psychiatr Res* 1975;**12**:189–98.

25 Dick JP, Guiloff RJ. Stewart A, Blackstock J, *et al.* Mini-mental state examination in neurological patients. *J Neurol Neurosurg Psychiatry* 1984;**47**:496–9.

26 Hughes CP, Berg L, Danziger W, Cogen LA, Martin RL. A new clinical scale for the staging of dementia. *Br J Psychiatry* 1972;**140**:566–72.

27 Roth M, Tym E, Mountjoy C, Huppert F, Hendrie H, Verma S, Goddard R. CAMDEX: a standardised instrument for the diagnosis of mental disorder in the elderly with special reference to the early detection of dementia. *Br J Psychiatry* 1986;**149**:698–709.

28 Mirra SS, Heyman A, McKeel D, *et al.* The Consortium to Establish a Registry for Alzheimer's Disease (CERAD). Part II. Standardization of the neuropathologic assessment of Alzheimer's disease. *Neurology* 1991;**41**:479–86.

29 Hansen LA, Galasko D. Lewy body disease. *Current Opinion in Neurology and Neurosurgery* 1992;**5**:889–94.

30 Tyrrell PJ, Sawle GV, Ibanez V, *et al.* Clinical and positron emission tomographic studies in the "extra-pyramidal syndrome" of dementia of the Alzheimer type. *Arch Neurol* 1990; **47**:1318–23.

31 Jobst KA, Smith AD, Szatmari M, *et al.* Detection in life of confirmed Alzheimer's disease using a simple measurement of medial temporal lobe atrophy by computed tomography. *Lancet* 1992;**340**:1179–83.

32 Kesslak JP, Nalcioglu O, Cotman CW. Quantification of magnetic resonance scans for hippocampal and parahippocampal atrophy in Alzheimer's disease. *Neurology* 1991;**41**: 51–4.

33 Corder EH, Saunders AM, Strittmatter WJ, *et al.* Gene dose of apolipoprotein E type 4 allele and the risk of Alzheimer's disease in late onset families. *Science* 1993;**261**:921–3.

34 Burns A, Philpot M, Coasta D, Ell PJ, Levy R. The investigation of Alzheimer's disease with single photon emission tomography. *J Neurol Neurosurg Psychiatry* 1989;**52**:248–53.

35 Botwinick J, Storandt M, Berg L, Boland S. Senile dementia of the Alzheimer type. Subject attrition and testability in research. *Arch Neurol* 1988;**45**:493–6.

36 Farlow M, Gracon SI, Hershey LA, *et al.* A controlled trial of tacrine in Alzheimer's disease. *JAMA* 1992;**268**:2523–9.

37 Knapp MJ, Knopman DS, Solomon PR, *et al.* A 30 week randomised controlled trial of high-dose tacrine in patients with Alzheimer's disease. *JAMA* 1994;**271**:985–91.

38 O'Neil D. The doctors dilemma: the elderly driver and dementia. *International Journal of Geriatric Psychiatry* 1992;**7**:237–41.

9 Multiple sclerosis

D BATES

Definitions

Multiple sclerosis is the most common demyelinating disease and the main cause of neurological disability in young and middle aged adults. Its prevalence in Northern Europe and North America is greater than 1 per 1000, and the disease process is characterised by areas of demyelination within the central nervous system.[1] It most commonly presents with a relapsing and remitting course, exacerbations being assumed to be related to new areas of demyelination or "plaques". Recovery is possible after an episode of demyelination but, with repeated attacks, disability tends to accrue. The disease affects women more often than men, with ratios variously reported between 1·5 and 2:1 and, though there are reported cases in the first decade of life, the incidence rises during the second decade to a peak at the beginning of the fourth decade; rarely does the disease begin in patients aged over 65.

Diagnosis

The diagnosis of multiple sclerosis is essentially clinical, supported by imaging, biochemical, and electrophysiological investigations. It is a prerequisite that the symptoms and signs are disseminated in time and anatomical space and explicable on the basis of damage to the white matter pathways. The practical difficulties of making the diagnosis at the time of the first symptom or in patients with the primary progressive form of the disease should not be overlooked, but the widespread availability of magnetic resonance imaging and the improvements in CSF examination for oligoclonal bands, together with the use of evoked potential recording, means that the diagnosis is nearly always correctly established in patients investigated in modern neurological centres. One of the most useful agencies in identifying the diagnosis of multiple sclerosis remains that of a clinician skilled and experienced in recognising the symptoms or signs that are likely to indicate the disease.

Several series of guidelines have been published to establish the diagnosis of multiple sclerosis, most of which are intended for the identification of patients in epidemiological or therapeutic studies and many of which have been surpassed by the development of biochemical tests and magnetic resonance imaging. The most useful and widely used of the diagnostic criteria are those propounded by Poser *et al* which weight historical and clinical evidence most highly but allow for paraclinical evidence including magnetic resonance imaging, evoked potentials, and the identification of oligoclonal bands in the CSF.[2] The grading allows for patients to be identified as having clinically definite multiple sclerosis, laboratory supported definite multiple sclerosis, or clinically probable multiple sclerosis which may also be laboratory supported.

Patients who have, or fear that they may have, multiple sclerosis understandably expect the diagnosis to be "confirmed" by a clinical neurologist, ideally one with expertise and interest in the disease, but it is important that both the neurologist and the patient remain aware of the fact that the diagnosis is made with a greater or lesser degree of confidence and that the diagnosis may be mistaken. Multiple sclerosis, despite the advent of newer investigative techniques, remains a diagnosis of exclusion.

The problem of diagnosis is complicated further by the recognition that there are different forms of the illness; the most typical is the relapsing and remitting form with well defined exacerbations and remissions. It is more easily identified than the primary progressive form, which is seen typically but not solely in older patients. The relapsing and remitting form of the disease will often become progressive secondarily, but the timing of evolution into a progressive illness and the recognition of the development of progression may be difficult to identify and earlier, and often forgotten, episodes of blurred vision, minor sensory symptoms, or dizziness may create difficulties in individual cases.

History and examination

In taking a history a doctor will attempt to define episodes of neurological dysfunction explicable on the basis of white matter disease which have been scattered in time and anatomical place. Most studies of the presentation of patients with multiple sclerosis record motor and visual disturbances, specifically weakness and optic neuritis, as being the most common initial symptoms. Altered sensation, disturbance of equilibrium, and paroxysmal phenomena, such as Lhermitte's symptom, are probably often overlooked by both patient and doctor and may be more common than usually reported. Fatigue has certainly been underrecognised and underreported commonly by patients in the early phases of the illness.[3] None the less, visual blurring or loss, double vision, weakness, and unsteadiness and, less commonly, anaesthesia, neuralgia, or sphincter disturbance in young adults should raise suspicion of the diagnosis. It is worthwhile asking specifically about visual disturbance such as double vision; symptoms believed to be caused by "ephaptic transmission" such as tonic spasms, transient diplopia, dysarthria, and disequilibrium; and neuralgic pains, periods of fatigue, and disturbance of memory because, although these symptoms may occur in other conditions, they may give a clue to the dissemination of the disease process.[4]

One particularly useful symptom is that relating to fluctuation of symptoms, particularly motor and visual, in response to exercise or temperature. Weakness is often most evident after exertion, and it is not uncommon for patients with some degree of weakness in the legs to identify that, after having a hot bath or shower, their weakness becomes more profound. Similar worsening of symptoms may be seen in the visual system in relation to exercise and temperature.

Examination should be directed to detecting disseminated clinical signs, in particular optic pallor on fundoscopy, asymptomatic internuclear ophthalmoplegia or phasic nystagmus on eye movements, mild and sometimes unrecognised dysarthria, or a pathologically brisk jaw jerk. In the limbs, evidence for a spastic increase in tone, loss of power or difficulty in coordination, altered sensation or brisk reflexes with clonus, extensor plantar responses, and absent abdominal reflexes are all relevant in helping to identify scattered lesions. It must be remembered that finding numerous signs simply identifies a multiplicity of lesions and does not necessarily prove that they all have the same pathology or that the pathology is due to inflammatory demyelination. The relevance of these findings will vary; optic atrophy is more relevant in a patient with leg weakness or unsteadiness than in a patient whose primary complaint is of visual loss, whereas the finding of ankle clonus and an extensor plantar may be more significant in a patient presenting with retrobulbar neuritis than in one complaining of weakness in the legs.

Symptoms and signs that may be of particular help in the diagnosis of multiple sclerosis include those of deafferentation of the hands (the useless hands of Oppenheim) which are common in multiple sclerosis though which require differentiation from a high cervical compressive myelopathy; Lhermitte's phenomenon of tingling dysaesthesiae extending down the spine and often into the legs and occasionally into the arms on neck movement, may indicate a compressive cervical myelopathy but is much more likely to indicate demyelinating disease; trigeminal neuralgia occurring in a young patient and the occasional finding of sheathing of the retinal veins which, though not confined to the condition of multiple sclerosis, may be seen in up to 40% of cases. Facial myokymia may also indicate multiple sclerosis, as may episodes of facial palsy, particularly if occurring bilaterally.

Mental symptoms are not common at the beginning of the disease, and euphoria should not be regarded as a common symptom; depression is more often seen.[5] Disturbances of memory and of intellect occur most commonly in the context of more longstanding and severe disease, but occasionally such problems may occur relatively early in the illness.[6]

Investigations

The investigations needed for an individual patient with multiple sclerosis will depend, to a large extent, on the certainty of the diagnosis clinically, the concern and requirements of the patient, and the planning of future treatment and management. In some respects the main purpose of investigation in the patient suspected of having multiple sclerosis is to exclude other diagnoses.

Magnetic resonance imaging

Ideally all patients suspected of having multiple sclerosis should be subjected to magnetic resonance imaging with T2 weighted images of the cerebrum and possibly the cervical spinal cord. If there is uncertainty about activity of the disease, or if the patient is to be included in a clinical trial, a T1 gadolinium enhanced scan may also be indicated to identify activity of the lesions. High signal lesions, classically periventricular in site and scattered throughout the supratentorial and infratentorial regions, are strongly supportive of the diagnosis of multiple sclerosis. It should be appreciated that white matter lesions occur in vascular (including hypertensive) disease and other inflammatory or infective conditions: although they have been associated in younger patients with migraine, non-specific white matter lesions occur coincidently with age-related frequency in the young or middle aged adults who may be at risk of multiple sclerosis. Magnetic resonance imaging criteria for multiple sclerosis have been defined, and scans should fulfil these criteria to be thought diagnostic of multiple sclerosis, and figures for specificity and sensitivity of these tests have been produced.[7–9]

In patients in whom the diagnosis is considered clinically definite such an expensive investigation may be thought unnecessary, but magnetic resonance imaging adds considerable certainty to the diagnosis and, as we move into an era of increasing therapeutic intervention in multiple sclerosis, it will help to establish which patients should be given the newer treatments and may help in monitoring them. In patients in whom the diagnosis is in doubt, particularly those with predominantly spinal multiple sclerosis, magnetic resonance imaging of the cervical and dorsal spine is obligatory. In such patients the spinal scan may show high signal lesions on T2 weighted images within the cord or, more frequently, thinning of the spinal cord, but it must exclude structural pathology such as disc prolapse and extrinsic or intrinsic tumours. A proportion of patients will be shown to have cervical spine disease, in which case the finding of cerebral lesions indicates an inflammatory demyelinating condition rather than a compressive or ischaemic pathology.

Magnetic resonance imaging is particularly valuable in investigating monosyptomatic patients because there is some evidence that the finding of high signal lesions within the cerebrum on T_2 weighted images not only helps to establish the diagnosis of multiple sclerosis before other clinical symptoms develop but also correlates with the prognosis of the disease process. It is inevitable that, as more information accumulates relating to the scans of patients with multiple sclerosis, their value as predictors of outcome in individual patients will increase.[10 11] The possible role of newer magnetic resonance imaging techniques and the value of magnetic resonance spectroscopy in diagnosis require further studies.

CSF examination

Examination of the CSF by lumbar puncture should be obligatory in investigating patients suspected of having multiple sclerosis, even if the clinical and magnetic resonance imaging evidence strongly supports the diagnosis. Assessment of the CSF cell count, the concentrations of total protein and immunoglobulin and, most importantly, oligoclonal banding of immunoglobulin that is not matched in a simultaneous specimen of serum will help to identify patients who have an inflammatory disease like multiple sclerosis.[12] A Venereal Disease Research Laboratory test is commonly undertaken to exclude neurosyphilis. A cell count of more than $5 \times 10^6/l$, a protein concentration of more than 1 g/l, or the absence of oligoclonal bands should raise doubts about the diagnosis and suggest alternative diagnoses such as sarcoidosis, borrelliosis, lymphoma, systemic lupus erythematosus, primary Sjogren's syndrome, polyarteritis nodosa, Behçet's syndrome, HIV infection, or mitochondrial cytopathy. Though not part of a routine investigation, if concern regarding metabolic disease persists, the measurement of lactic acid in the CSF is a useful screening test.

Evoked potentials

The role of evoked potentials in investigating patients with multiple sclerosis is now less clearly defined. Visual evoked potentials are well established and reproducible as a means of studying conduction and radiation within the optic nerve and tract. When they can be shown to be abnormal in a patient with symptoms suggesting a brain stem or spinal cord lesion they can be taken as good evidence of a "second" lesion but when there is clinical evidence of that second lesion, such as reduced visual acuity or the presence of optic atrophy, their value is necessarily lessened. Somatosensory evoked potentials and brain stem evoked potentials

225

are less standardised, and their value is consequently lessened. The value of evoked potentials in investigating multiple sclerosis was undoubtedly reduced after the advent of magnetic resonance imaging and, although still routine in many neurological units, the investigation, except for visual evoked responses in patients with monosymptomatic non-retrobulbar neuritis, now has limited value and should be questioned.

Other investigations

Serum should always be taken at the time of the lumbar puncture to allow interpretation of oligoclonal bands in CSF. Other specific investigations may be required as part of the exclusion of other diagnoses. There is no indication at present for routine measurement of T-cell subsets, cytokines, or myelin basic protein fragments and, although the search for a serum marker continues, it has so far been fruitless. In certain specific instances, such as the need to differentiate from other demyelinating conditions, it may be necessary to measure the level of hexosaminidase A and very long chain fatty acids in the serum.

One of the most important aspects of the investigation of a patient suspected of having multiple sclerosis is the timing of the various investigations. Many patients who present with fears of multiple sclerosis but relatively benign or mild symptoms of a sensory or visual nature do not warrant formal investigation. None the less, the social circumstances of the patient, their fears, their understanding, and their need to have a defined diagnosis may, in individual cases, cause the doctor to pursue investigations at a relatively early phase. In general the two most useful investigations are magnetic resonance imaging and examination of the CSF; however, particularly in patients with early symptoms, it should be recognised that the normality of results of these two investigations does not necessarily exclude the diagnosis, and it may be appropriate to repeat the tests later in the course of the disease.

Prevention

Primary

Although there is increasing evidence from epidemiological studies that multiple sclerosis has a genetic basis, there is not yet a suggestion that this will lead to any form of prevention. The way in which this genetic basis might relate to the development of demyelination is probably in terms of immunomodulation, and much evidence now points to a central role for immune mediated events in the genesis of multiple sclerosis. The precipitant for the attacks is not recognised and, although an environmental agent such as a virus has been hypothesised, there is no evidence that a single virus is incriminated and therefore consideration of immunisation is not appropriate. At present the most likely and recognised pathogenesis of multiple sclerosis lies in the topic of autoimmunity, but it seems unlikely that this will be susceptible to primary prevention.

Secondary prevention

No therapeutic agent has yet been shown to alter significantly the outcome for patients with multiple sclerosis. The single published trial with one of the beta interferons and the currently ongoing and recently completed trials with beta interferon, Copolymer-I, and other immunomodulating agents including antibody to CD4 are designed to try to show an effect in terms of reducing exacerbations of the disease thereby affecting the development of disability in the long term. No agent has yet been shown to be clinically effective in reducing the onset of disability, and correlation between the information relating to magnetic resonance imaging changes and clinical outcome is awaited. There is some suggestion, from older trials, that when the diagnosis has been established patients who consume diets that are relatively low in animals fats and relatively high in polyunsaturates from vegetables and fish body oils have a better prognosis.

Prognosis

Multiple sclerosis may, rarely, cause death in the first attack or, alternatively, may be discovered coincidentally at autopsy without having been suspected during life. Between these two extremes lies a continuous range of severity of the disease, which makes it difficult to provide information about prognosis in an individual patient. The mean survival of patients from diagnosis is approximately 30 years which, with the mean age of onset being 32 years, implies only a slight reduction in life expectation. The

25 year survival rate has been estimated at 74% compared with an expected 86% in a control population. Factors that identify poor prognosis regarding survival include advanced age at onset of the disease, progressive course from onset, and severe disability within five years of diagnosis.[13] The cause of death is usually related to complications of inanition, infections, or decubitus ulceration. Respiratory paralysis and choking are relatively rare causes of death.

The prognosis regarding disability is less well defined and depends, to an extent, on the population from which the figures are derived. It has been suggested that about 10% of patients are severely disabled within five years, 25% within 10 years, and 50% of patients within 18 years.[14] The proportion of patients who remain in work reduces constantly for about 15 years and is then about 15%, which figure remains reasonably static. The main cause of disability relates to mobility, but severe ataxia of the arms, loss of sphincter control, and impaired mental capacity are also important features.

Communication and counselling

The diagnosis

It is suggested that simply being given the diagnosis of multiple sclerosis is regarded by patients to be equivalent, in terms of emotional effect, to a moderate disability. It should therefore be recognised that the patient interview, when this news is given, is an important "life event". There are practical problems in that the diagnosis is usually only suspected at the first encounter, the patient will have concerns and fears about the diagnosis of multiple sclerosis but also about other possible conditions, and therefore a discussion of the various diagnoses may be appropriate at this time. There will then be a period of testing, often undertaken as an outpatient, followed by an invariable delay before the results of the investigations are available and the important and definitive interview can take place. All too often this important interview may occur in a busy outpatient clinic where both the patient and the doctor will be conscious of the constriction of time and of other patients waiting outside. Ideally, therefore, a separate time should be allocated for the patient and relative or carer to see the doctor, hear the diagnosis, ask and have answered the relevant questions, and express their fears. A further interview is often of benefit to enable the patient and carer to broach subjects that had not been discussed on the first occasion and also to allow them time to think about the diagnosis and to phrase their worries and concerns most appropriately. To provide this sort of information to an individual takes time and may be difficult to identify as being "cost effective" in health care terms, but patients are very conscious of the need to talk to a doctor who understands their disease and recognise that, because of the relative rarity of multiple sclerosis, most general practitioners do not have the requisite knowledge or interest to be able to answer all of the questions. Consideration might be given to paramedical staff discussing matters with the patient, and certainly a nurse dedicated to the care of people with multiple sclerosis can often be invaluable at this stage of the interview process.

The prognosis

The most important advice at diagnosis that the doctor can provide is that, in many cases, multiple sclerosis is a benign condition. The possibility of disability must not be dismissed lightly, however, and patients should have their questions answered appropriately but with the explanation that precise prediction of the disease process is impossible in individual patients and that abrupt changes may occur. Advice should be given about the various symptoms, the problem of fatigue explained, and advice given on how best to avoid and limit it. Patients should be advised of the potential effect of acute febrile infections and be given an explanation of factors, such as exercise and heat, that might make symptoms worse. They should be reassured that treatments are available for the acute exacerbations though be informed realistically of the lack of a cure.

Support and external agencies

The way in which patients are advised of the availability of support from external agencies will vary. It is neither appropriate nor necessary to describe in great detail to a mildly affected patient the various services which are available. None the less, it is important that information about help from social services, physiotherapy, and other aspects of rehabilitation is available when required; an appropriate system is to have a liaison worker in the clinic who will deal with these aspects of care when necessary.

Support organisations

Most countries have multiple sclerosis societies which are devoted to the support of patients and the genesis of monies for research. Not all patients want to be associated with the multiple sclerosis society or with the local branch or chapter meetings. It is, none the less, appropriate that the patient and carer are made aware of the existence of the organisation at the time of diagnosis and possibly provided with some of the publications from the society. Many of the local branches or chapters have welfare officers and counsellers available who will spend time talking to newly diagnosed patients and to their carers, and all have access to national information and advice resources.

Medical follow up

For most patients with early disease follow up at hospital is neither necessary nor practical. In most instances the follow up may be left to the general practitioner and increasingly to some aspect of "care in the community". It is important, however, that referral back to the neurological unit is made if new symptoms develop or if the patient or carer have specific questions or problems. In the United Kingdom the average general practitioner will only have two or three patients with multiple sclerosis in a list of about 2000 patients and therefore help and support from the neurological centre in terms of information and advice will be required. If patients, or their general practitioners, feel that they would like continuing neurological supervision it should be made available on a three to six monthly basis. Any patients who are to be involved in trials of new treatments or to be given treatments that are potentially injurious will necessarily be seen more often, may well be subjected to repeated magnetic resonance imaging, and will need to remain under hospital care. Patients who have more active disease (such as exacerbations) or continuing and increasing disability may need neurological follow up.

At present most supportive treatment is prescribed by general practitioners with hospital advice, and increasingly methyl prednisolone for acute exacerbations may be given by the general practitioner or, on a day case basis, at the outpatient unit of the local hospital. These provisions of services in the local environment are of considerable advantage to the patient and can potentially be linked with rehabilitation facilities in the local community.

Specific treatment

Acute exacerbations of multiple sclerosis are most commonly treated with intravenous or oral corticosteroids, which have been shown to improve the speed of recovery from an exacerbation. Long term use of steroids does not, however, alter the natural course and the side effects outweigh any possible benefits. The use of intramuscular corticotrophin has declined considerably in recent years, and the medication most commonly used acutely is intravenous methyl prednisolone, which probably has fewer side effects and possibly better long term preventative effects than oral prednisone alone.[15] The precise doses of courses of methyl prednisolone vary considerably but patients are usually given a total of 1·5 to 2·5g in saline intravenously over three to five consecutive days. In most instances this is followed for a 6–8 week period by a reducing dose of oral prednisone, often given on alternate days.

Over the past three decades there has been considerable interest in the use of possible immunomodulating therapy. Azathioprine, which has been shown to be effective in myasthenia gravis and polymyositis, was initially suggested after incompletely controlled and unblinded studies to reduce progression and relapse rate. A recent meta-analysis has suggested that it gives some reduction in attack rate and a possible benefit on progression, but it is doubtful whether this benefit significantly outweighs the possibility of an increased risk of malignancy and other side effects.[16] The agent is still used, particularly in patients who seem to have a progressing form of the illness. A dose of 2·0–2·5 mg/kg body weight is used, haematological and biochemical variables are monitored, and six months must elapse for the immunosuppressant effect to start.

Cyclophosphamide has also been used in multiple sclerosis and is commonly used in some parts of Europe, though placebo controlled double blind studies have failed to confirm that there is any appreciable effect upon disease progress or exacerbation rate. A recent trial in North America suggested that patients given repeated courses of cyclophosphamide with prednisone and plasma exchange gained benefit, but there are problems in interpreting that particular study because of the behaviour of the placebo group.[17] Cyclosporin A has also been subjected to double blind controlled trials but has been shown to be ineffective in the management of multiple sclerosis.[18]

A recent study of Cladribine, which was planned to run for two years, was discontinued when an interim analysis suggested that the agent decreased the speed of chronic progressive multiple sclerosis.[19] Cladribine is a lymphocyte specific nucleotide that had been used in hairy cell leukaemia and which results in a profound reduction in CD-4 lymphocyte counts. Several patients developed pancytopenia and there have been other reports of aplastic anaemia, so further research will be required before this can be recommended. There have been controlled trials of plasma exchange, total lymphoid irradiation, and the anthracene dione anti-neoplastic agent mitoxantrone, which have been ineffective in the treatment of multiple sclerosis.[20-22]

Trials are in progress using antibodies to CD4, soluble tumour necrosis factor (TNF) receptor, and other cytokine and immunomodulating agents. A recently completed trial of Copolymer-I has apparently shown fewer relapses in the treated group in a double blind placebo controlled trial, though the results are yet to appear in print.

A trial of interferon beta 1b in patients with acute remitting disease has been published.[23] High doses of the agent reduced clinical attacks of multiple sclerosis by about a third over two years compared with placebo, and magnetic resonance imaging showed an appreciable reduction in evidence of disease activity, both on active scans with gadolinium enhancement and overall accumulation of high signal lesions on T2 weighted images. These results have apparently been supported by continued follow up of the group of patients; more recent trials with lower doses of recombinant interferon beta are reported to have given similar results, though again the figures have not yet been published.[24]

At present, apart from the long recognised use of corticosteroids for acute exacerbations and the possible use of interferon beta in patients with acute remitting relapsing disease, there are no specific treatments available for managing patients with multiple sclerosis.

Supportive treatment

The most common symptom of multiple sclerosis that requires some form of assistance is that of spasticity and cramps, more commonly in the legs than the arms. There are various ways in which patients who suffer from such cramps and spasms may be helped. Oral medication with the gaba-receptor agonist baclofen, the alpha 2 receptor agonist tizanidine, or the peripherally acting dantrolene sodium (which has its effect on the sarcoplasmic reticulum) may all be used, either alone or in combination, to reduce muscle tone and stiffness. Benzodiazepines may also have a part to play in the management of such symptoms, though they are more likely than the other agents to result in drowsiness. If such agents are not helpful or not appropriate the use of peripheral chemical blocks with phenol, alcohol, or intramuscular botulinum toxin can also be considered and are particularly useful for patients with focal spasticity that is disabling. For those with more severe and diffuse spasticity either dorsal column electrical stimulation or intrathecal baclofen provided by an implanted pump can be considered, and ultimately the non-reversible invasive procedures of intrathecal chemical blocks with phenol or alcohol or surgery can be considered. With all treatments for spasticity there is the possibility of unmasking weakness as one reduces the spasticity and prevents the spasms.

The second most common symptom requiring treatment is that of pain. On occasions the pain relates to episodes of spasms and is then treated appropriately with spasmolytic agents, but pain may also occur as a lancinating paroxysmal discomfort, most typically as seen in trigeminal neuralgia, when it may be helped by centrally acting analgesics such as carbamazepine, phenytoin, or sodium valproate or by surgical procedures. More chronic pain may occur, presumably due to demyelination of ascending pathways, and often consists of dysaesthesiae in the feet or legs. It will occasionally respond to the use of a tricyclic antidepressant such as amitriptyline and is sometimes helped by agents such as baclofen; electrostimulation either by transcutaneous nerve stimulator or by dorsal column stimulation may be considered. Patients may also complain of chronic back pain, which is most reasonably helped by the use of physiotherapy and non-steroidal anti-inflammatory agents. Pain that is related to an acute episode of demyelination, as in retrobulbar neuritis, is most usually helped by corticosteroids.

233

Sometimes tremor in multiple sclerosis requires treatment. When minor, it may occasionally be helped by the use of non-selective β blockers such as propranolol or a low dose of barbiturates such as primidone. There are, however, few pharmacological agents which help patients with intention tremor though there are published reports of benefit with clonazepam, carbamazepine, and isoniazid. Some authors have recommended a trial of choline chloride. Occasionally an intention tremor may be improved in patients with multiple sclerosis by fastening weights to the wrists to reduce the amplitude of the tremor. Thalamic surgery has, in the past, been attempted to reduce the tremor in multiple sclerosis, but results have been disappointing and both clinical and histopathological evidence of deterioration due to demyelinating lesions arising at the site of the stereotaxis have been reported. More recently, thalamic electro-stimulation shows promise for the management of this infrequent but extremely disabling symptom.[25]

The uncommon but important paroxysmal symptoms in multiple sclerosis such as epileptic seizures, tonic seizures, dysarthria, ataxia, diplopia, dyskinesia syndrome, hemifacial spasm, kinesogenic choreoathetosis, and acute sensory disturbances are frequently helped by the use of agents such as carbamazepine and valproate.

Recently there has been increasing recognition of the importance of the symptom of fatigue in multiple sclerosis. Virtually all patients with multiple sclerosis will, at some time, complain of this symptom and in about 75% of cases it is regarded as being one of the most important of their disabilities. Various agents have been tried. Non-pharmacological treatments have included emotional support, reassurance, and graded exercise programmes. Pharmacological treatments have included the CNS stimulants pemoline and methyl phenidate; the potentially dopaminergic agents amantadine and selegiline have been recommended, and amantadine has been subjected to placebo controlled trials which seem to show benefits.[26] Antidepressants have also been used with varying effects. There have been recent trials of the agent 4 aminopyridine, which seems to have a notable effect in reducing fatigue in patients with multiple sclerosis and is more effective than 3:4 diaminopyridine in crossing the blood brain barrier.

One of the aspects of symptomatic management for patients with multiple sclerosis, which has been changed and considerably improved recently, is that relating to the management of bladder and bowel dysfunction. The most effective form of treatment for the incomplete bladder emptying often seen in patients with multiple sclerosis is intermittent self catheterisation. Once patients can undertake this technique they have to assess the frequency at which it is required. This will depend on their bladder storage capacity but is usually between three and six times a day.[27] For those patients who show detrusor hyperreflexia, oral or intravesical anticholinergics may be used. Desmopressin spray at night will reduce the problems of night time frequency and enuresis, and the recent suggestion that the use of intravesical capsaicin may help is of interest and requires further evaluation. Bowel dysfunction is less commonly reported as a problem than bladder dysfunction. Constipation is most common and is best treated by aperients; faecal incontinence is probably underrecorded and is occasionally helped by advice relating to diet.

Sexual dysfunction is also a problem for patients with multiple sclerosis. Men with erectile dysfunction may be given oral yohimbine, intracorporeal injections of papaverine or prostaglandin E1, or surgical implanted protheses. For those with ejaculatory dysfunction there is, unfortunately, no treatment available. In women the most common problems are in relation to leg spasticity, bladder problems, and fatigue which requires separate advice and help.

Psychological symptoms occurring in multiple sclerosis also require specific help. Depression is probably the most common symptom and can be treated with tricyclic antidepressants or 5HT reuptake inhibitors. Euphoria is rare and not susceptible to treatment. Pathological laughing and crying occurs occasionally and may also respond to a tricyclic antidepressant, though there are anecdotal reports of levodopa being effective. Cognitive impairment may need help and advice from a psychologist and always requires the understanding of the carer or relative.

Rehabilitation

For patients who have disability caused by their multiple sclerosis, rehabilitation services are of vital importance. Advice from physiotherapists, occupational therapists, speech therapists, and dietitians is important and should be part of the package that is available for patients with multiple sclerosis. Not everyone who is given the diagnosis of multiple sclerosis needs to be involved with a rehabilitation team but the availability of such a facility within the local district is important, and the provision of various aids ranging from simple household appliances and a walking stick to environmental control equipment may be of great importance in maintaining a degree of independence.[28]

Complications

The most important complications relating to multiple sclerosis are the development of contractures due to spasticity, decubitus ulceration in relation to lack of sensation, bladder infection, and the possible development of bladder stones in patients who have long term indwelling catheters. The management of bladder disturbances has improved so much that few patients need indwelling catheters and those who do more commonly have suprapubic catheters than urethral catheters, but all who have long term catheters ought to be given at least yearly investigation for bladder stones. It is rare for patients with multiple sclerosis to develop upper urinary tract infections, though the possibility of septicaemia arising from a bladder infection must not be overlooked and may be the explanation for a sudden deterioration.

In a severely disabled patient the use of physiotherapy and splinting to prevent deformity and contracture, together with the judicious use of botulinum toxin, may avoid complications. For those patients who do develop decubitus ulceration adequate nursing in hospital on low airflow beds and plastic surgery may be considered. It is to be hoped that more accessible advice and help in the community will reduce the rate of development of decubitus ulceration, though it should be recognised that many bed sores develop in patients in hospital.

Discharge from hospital

The initial investigation at the time of diagnosis is now often performed on an outpatient basis, so the discharge from hospital is handled through the outpatient clinic. When patients are admitted for a complication or exacerbation of multiple sclerosis arrangements need to be made from the hospital for their continued follow up at home, and a prepared discharge package and plan ought to be provided for the general practitioner.

Monitoring and follow up

Follow up depends to an extent on the individual patient, but in patients who have significant disabilities or active and progressing disease it is probably most appropriate that their attendance in the neurological outpatients is guaranteed so that they may be exposed to new treatments that become available and have access to the information and help they may require.

Outcome

There are many outcome measures of use in multiple sclerosis. The most widely applied is the Kurtzke expanded disability status scale which assesses the individual disability of the patient.[27] It is useful in the long term follow up of patients with multiple sclerosis for some grading to be made on each occasion that the patient is seen so that changes in the pattern of the disease may be recognised easily. The greatest use of outcome scales is in the monitoring of therapeutic trials, though they will be increasingly important in the performance of audit.

Liaison

Relatives and carers

The provision of information, explanation, and access to help and advice for relatives and carers of patients with multiple sclerosis is vital. An appreciable proportion of patients may show some degree of psychological disturbance during the course of their illness, and therefore adequate advice to the relative or carer is important.

General practitioner

The general practitioner will remain the primary doctor for a patient with multiple sclerosis. The incidence of the disease is such that the average general practitioner will only expect to have two or three patients with multiple sclerosis and therefore his or her expertise is bound to be limited. It is appropriate and important that easy access to the hospital consultant, and advice regarding services, is provided. In addition to nursing services, physiotherapy, occupational therapy, speech therapy, and other advice services will be available increasingly to the general practitioner.

Hospital medical staff

Although it is impracticable for hospital medical staff to provide domiciliary services to patients with multiple sclerosis, it would be useful for nursing staff with a dedicated interest in multiple sclerosis to be available to travel between the hospital and the patient and to be on hand at the time of outpatient consultations.

Other agencies

The Multiple Sclerosis Society provides an important link and advice about employment, insurance, information regarding driving, and other helplines. In this role it can be of extreme importance in terms of continuing the independence of the individual patient.

Audit

Several aspects of the management of patients with multiple sclerosis are susceptible to audit. Perhaps one of the most relevant is for an audit of the investigations undertaken to establish and confirm the diagnosis. It would be reasonable to analyse the value of the various investigations, including CSF examination, magnetic resonance imaging, and evoked potentials and their relative values in assisting and confirming the diagnosis.

In terms of treatment, the dose and practical arrangements required for intravenous courses of methyl prednisolone, and for the length of treatment with oral prednisone after its intravenous administration, should be audited to try to assess which is the most effective form. Audit is also important in helping to establish whether the most cost effective forms of management for patients with multiple sclerosis are practicable in the community, rather than through the hospital service, and in this instance it would be very important to undertake an audit of patients' satisfaction with the various alternative measures of management.

Management of multiple sclerosis

- Diagnosis is essentially clinical, made by excluding other disorders, anddifficult to make because there are several forms of the disease and patients probably overlook many early symptoms; it can only be made after extensive investigations, and is therefore open to revision
- Investigations to support diagnosis include magnetic resonance imaging for evidence of multiple white matter lesions and to exclude structural pathology, biochemical tests of CSF and serum for evidence of inflammatory disease and to exclude alternative diagnoses, and (less important now) electrophysiological (evoked potentials)
- Disease does not greatly reduce life expectancy; mean survival from diagnosis is 30 years (onset at mean age of 32); main causes of death (except for patients who die during the first attack) relate to complications of inanition, infection, or decubitus ulceration
- Disability, particularly reduced mobility from spasticity, is the main outcome; is progressive; and may also include arm ataxia, loss of sphincter control, and impaired mental capacity
- Treatment (with intravenous methyl prednisolone followed by oral prednisone) is only effective in reducing exacerbations and thus delaying disability; trials of antibodies to CD4, soluble tumour necrosis factor, and other cytokine and immunomodulating agents are in progress; trials of Copolymer-I and interferon beta have shown fewer relapses and reduced attacks but few results have yet been published
- Supportive treatments include: baclofen, tizanidine, or dantrolene sodium to reduce muscle tone and stiffness of spasticity and cramps; centrally acting analgesics, tricyclic antidepressants, baclofen, corticosteroids, non-steroidal anti-inflammatory agents, physiotherapy, transcutaneous nerve or dorsal column electrostimulation, or operation to reduce pain; β blockers or barbiturates for tremor; carbamazepine and valproate for paroxysmal symptoms; intermittent self-catheterisation for bladder control; aperients for constipation; dietary advice for faecal incontinence; oral yohimbine, intracorporeal injections of papaverine or prostaglandin E1, or implanted prostheses for erectile dysfunction in men; tricyclic antidepressants for 5HT reuptake inhibitors for depression; and various agents for fatigue
- Rehabilitation is vital and is provided by physiotherapists, occupational therapists, speech therapists, and dietitians; other support agencies include (in the United Kingdom) social services and the Multiple Sclerosis Society; in addition, emotional support and counselling is essential for patients and carers; liaison between neurologists, rehabilitation and support agencies, and general practitioners is also important

1 Kurtzke JF. Multiple sclerosis: changing times. *Neuroepidemiology* 1991;**10**:1–8.
2 Poser CM, Paty DW, Scheinberg L, *et al.* New diagnostic criteria for multiple sclerosis: guidelines for research proposals. *Ann Neurol* 1983;**13**:227–31.
3 Krupp LB, Alvarez LA, LaRocca NG, *et al.* Fatigue in multiple sclerosis. *Arch Neurol* 1988; **45**:435–7.
4 Matthews WB. Paroxysmal symptoms in multiple sclerosis. *J Neurol Neurosurg Psychiatry* 1975;**38**:617–23.
5 Whitlock FA, Siskind MM. Depression as a major symptom of multiple sclerosis. *J Neurol Neurosurg Psychiatry* 1980;**43**:861–5.
6 Rao SM, Glatt S, Hammeke TA, *et al.* Chronic progressive multiple sclerosis: relationship between cerebral ventricular size and neuropsychological impairment. *Arch Neurol* 1985; **42**:678–82.
7 Paty DW, Oger JJF, Kastrukoff LF, *et al.* Magnetic resonance imaging in the diagnosis of multiple sclerosis: a prospective study of comparison with clinical evaluation, evoked potentials, oligo clonal banding and CT. *Neurology* 1988;**38**:180–5.
8 Fazekas F, Offenbacher H, Fuchs S, *et al.* Criteria for an increased specificity of MRI interpretation in elderly subjects with suspected multiple sclerosis. *Neurology* 1988;**38**: 1822–5.
9 Offenbacher H, Fazeckas F, Schmidt R, *et al.* Assessment of MRI criteria for a diagnosis of MS. *Neurology* 1993;**43**:905–9.
10 Ormerod IEC, McDonald WI, duBoulay GH, *et al.* Disseminated lesions at presentation in patients with optic neuritis. *J Neurol Neurosurg Psychiatry* 1986;**49**:124–7.
11 Miller DH, Ormerod IEC, McDonald WI, *et al.* The early risk of multiple sclerosis after optic neuritis. *J Neurol Neurosurg Psychiatry* 1988;**52**:1569–71.
12 Kostulas V, Link H, Lefvert AK. Oligo clonal IgG bands in cerebrospinal fluid: principles for demonstration and interpretation based on findings in 1,114 neurological patients. *Arch Neurol* 1987;**44**:1041–4.
13 Phadke JG. Survival pattern and cause of death in patients with multiuple sclerosis: results from an epidemiological survey in north-east Scotland. *J Neurol Neurosurg Psychiatry* 1987; **50**:523–31.
14 Confavreux C, Aimard G, Devic M. Course and prognosis of multiple sclerosis assessed by the computerised data processing of 349 patients. *Brain* 1980;**103**:281–300.
15 Milligan NM, Newcombe R, Compston DAS. A double blind controlled trial of high dose methyl prednisolone in patients with multiple sclerosis: clinical effects. *J Neurol Neurosurg Psychiatry* 1987;**50**:511–6.
16 Yudkin PL, Ellison GW, Ghezzi A, *et al.* Overview of azathioprine treatment in multiple sclerosis. *Lancet* 1991;**338**:1051–5.
17 Weiner HL, Mackin GA, Orav EJ, *et al.* Intermittent cyclophosphamide pulse therapy in progressive multiple sclerosis: final report of the North-East Cooperative Multiple Sclerosis Treatment Group. *Neurology* 1993;**43**:910–8.
18 Rudge P, Koetsier JC, Mertin J, *et al.* Randomised double blind controlled trial of cyclosporin in multiple sclerosis. *J Neurol Neurosurg Psychiatry* 1989;**52**:559–65.
19 Sipe JC, Romine JS, Koziol JA, *et al.* Cladribine in treatment of chronic progressive multiple sclerosis. *Lancet* 1994;**344**:9–13.
20 Rodriguez M, Karnes WE, Bartleson JD, Pineda AA. Plasmaphoresis in acute episodes of fullmen and CNS inflammatory demyelation. *Neurology* 1993;**43**:1100–4.
21 Wiles CM, Omar L, Swan AV, *et al.* Total lymphoid irradiation in multiple sclerosis. *J Neurol Neurosurg Psychiatry* 1994;**57**:154–63.
22 Noseworthy JH, Hopkins MB, Vandervoorte MK, *et al.* An open trial evaluation of mitoxantrone in the treatment of progressive MS. *Neurology* 1993;**43**:1401–6.
23 The IFNB Multiple Sclerosis Study Group. Interferon-β 1b is effective in relapsing–remitting multiple sclerosis. *Neurology* 1993;**43**:655–61.
24 McDonald WI. New treatments for multiple sclerosis. *BMJ* 1995;**318**:345–6.
25 Nguyen JP, Dagos JD. Thalamic stimulation and proximal tremor: a specific target in the nucleus ventro-intermedius thalami. *Arch Neurol* 1993;**50**:498–500.
26 Krupp LB, Coyle PK, Docher C, *et al.* A comparison of amantidine, pemoline and placebo in the treatment of MS fatigue. *Neurology* 1993;**43**:A281.
27 Betts CD, D'Mellow MT, Fowler CJ, *et al.* Urinary symptoms and the neurological features of bladder dysfunction in multiple sclerosis. *J Neurol Neurosurg Psychiatry* 1992;**55**:245–50.
28 Working Party Report of the British Society of Rehabilitation Medicine. *Multiple sclerosis.* 1993. Copies from BSRM, Royal College of Physicians, 11 St Andrews Place, Regents Park, London.
29 Kurtzke JF. Rating neurologic impairment in multiple sclerosis: an expanded disability status scale (EDSS). *Neurology* 1983;**33**:1444–52.

240

10 Motor neuron disease

P N LEIGH, C M LLOYD, K RAY-CHAUDHURI

For neurologists, the management of motor neuron disease involves prompt and accurate diagnosis; an understanding of the clinical course, prognosis, and of the physical and psychological consequences of the disease for the individual and for carers; familiarity with the techniques, philosophies, and ethical aspects of symptomatic treatment, rehabilitation medicine, and palliative care; and awareness of the new opportunities for research into the causes and treatment of motor neuron disease and other motor neuron disorders. Because motor neuron disease is a relatively rare condition for most health workers, the neurologist can make an important contribution to effective multidisciplinary management. Underprovision of neurology services militates against this in the United Kingdom. Nevertheless, an argument can be made that the disease be treated as a "special case" and that health districts should develop appropriate models of interdisciplinary care, not necessarily led, but advised and supported, by local neurologists.

Definitions and terminology

The disease is a progressive disorder in which degeneration of upper and lower motor neurons leads to progressive weakness of bulbar, limb, thoracic, and abdominal muscles with relative sparing of oculomotor muscles and sphincter function. Death from ventilatory failure usually follows within five years of onset. Most (90–95%) cases are sporadic, whereas 5–10% are familial,[1][2] usually with autosomal dominant transmission. Many other motor system and anterior horn cell disorders are recognised (box 10.1). An

241

Box 10.1 Some rare disorders showing features of anterior horn cell degeneration

Disorder	Associated neurological features	Diagnostic pointers
X linked recessive bulbar and spinal muscular atrophy	Postural tremor; prominent facial fasciculations	Male gender; gynaecomastia; diabetes; infertility
Hereditary spastic paraparesis with distal amyotrophy	Pes cavus; vibration sense loss; dementia; dystonia	Absent sensory action potentials; androgen receptor gene mutation
Juvenile spinal muscular atrophy of the distal upper extremity	Exacerbation of weakness by cold; minipolymyoclonus of fingers	Family history; early age at onset; slow progression; ethnic origin (Amish; Tunisian; Lebanese)
"Madras" pattern motor neuron disease	Sensorineural hearing loss; minipolymyoclonus of fingers	Young Japanese males; vasomotor disturbances; benign course; structural abnormality of cervical cord
Western Pacific amyotrophic lateral sclerosis	Parkinsonism; dementia	Ethnic origin (southern Indian); young age at onset
Adult GM_2 gangliosidosis	Intellectual impairment; psychiatric disturbances; ataxia; stutter-dysarthria; pyramidal tract signs; dystonia; dyskinesias; supranuclear ophthalmoplegia	Ethnic origin (Guam, Western New Guinea, Kii peninsula of Japan)
Azorean disease (Machado-Joseph disease)	Cerebellar syndrome; parkinsonism; supranuclear ophthalmoplegia; pseudobulbar palsy; dystonia	Ethnic origin (Ashkenazi Jews) White cell/skin fibroblast hexosaminidase A deficiency; electron microscopy of rectal biopsy
Multiple system atrophy and olivopontocerebellar atrophy	Orthostatic hypotension; parkinsonism; cerebellar ataxia; nystagmus; urinary incontinence; impotence; dementia; involuntary movements; dysphagia; supranuclear ophthalmoplegia	Ethnic origin (Portuguese; Azorean); family history; diabetes
		Family history (some cases); infratentorial atrophy on computed tomography or magnetic resonance imaging

unusual form of the disease occurs in the Western Pacific associated with parkinsonism and dementia.[3]

In the United Kingdom the term motor neuron disease (MND) is used generically to include the complete range of the disease, including Charcot-type amyotrophic lateral sclerosis (ALS) with typical upper and lower motor neuron involvement, progressive muscular atrophy with only lower motor neuron involvement, and progressive bulbar palsy with bulbar and pseudobulbar palsy. Commonly the terms MND and ALS are used interchangeably. The relation between primary lateral sclerosis (in which progressive upper motor neuron degeneration is not accompanied by anterior horn cell degeneration) and other forms of motor neuron disease remains uncertain. Although most cases do not progress to typical motor neuron disease,[4] some undoubtedly do.

Diagnostic criteria

At a World Federation of Neurology consensus conference in 1990 at El Escorial, Spain, research diagnostic criteria for amyotrophic lateral sclerosis were suggested (box 10.2).[5] These criteria are based on clinical evidence of a progressive disorder with the characteristic combination of upper and lower motor neuron involvement in the same body regions and with certain exclusion criteria. Validation of these criteria is needed, but the predictive power of the definite and probable categories is high, judged by neuropathological correlations[6] and by experience in clinical trials that have used these categories as inclusion criteria. The diagnostic accuracy of the category of possible amyotrophic lateral sclerosis remains to be defined by long term follow up and neuropathology. Although valuable as research criteria, the El Escorial criteria do not take account of the vagaries of clinical practice. Patients with motor neuron disease sometimes have bladder dysfunction. Dementia and parkinsonism are rare features of otherwise pathologically typical motor neuron disease.[7-9] Other disorders, such as spondylotic myelopathy, often coexist with the disease. Thus for clinical rather than research purposes the exclusion criteria should be interpreted flexibly and used to alert clinicians to rare and potentially treatable disorders.

These research diagnostic criteria have been applied to sporadic and familial forms of the disease.[5] The familial motor neuron disorders of adult onset are rare, and only the milder forms

---

Box 10.2 Diagnostic criteria for amyotrophic lateral sclerosis/motor neuron disease

The diagnosis of ALS requires the presence of:
- Lower motor neuron signs (including electromyographic features in clinically normal muscles)
- Upper motor neuron signs
- Progression of the disorder

Diagnostic categories:
- *Definite ALS:* Upper motor neuron plus lower motor neuron signs in three regions
- *Probable ALS:* Upper motor neuron plus lower motor neuron signs in two regions with upper motor neuron signs rostral to lower motor neuron signs
- *Possible ALS:* Upper motor neuron plus lower motor neuron signs in one region, or upper motor neuron signs in two or three regions, such as in monomelic ALS, progressive bulbar palsy, and primary lateral sclerosis
- *Suspected ALS:* Lower motor neuron signs in two or three regions, such as in progressive muscular atrophy, and other motor syndromes

The diagnosis of ALS requires the absence of:
- Sensory signs
- Sphincter disturbances
- Visual disturbances
- Autonomic dysfunction
- Parkinson's disease
- Alzheimer-type dementia
- ALS "mimic" syndromes (see boxes 10.1 and 10.3)

The diagnosis of ALS is supported by:
- Fasciculation in one or more regions
- Neurogenic change in electromyography studies
- Normal motor and sensory nerve conduction (distal motor latencies may be increased)
- Absence of conduction block

Regions are defined as follows: brain stem, brachial, thorax and trunk, crural.

---

of spinal muscular atrophy, Kennedy's disease, and autosomal dominant familial motor neuron disease are seen regularly in adult neurological practice. Nevertheless these disorders offer new possibilities for understanding the mechanisms of motor neuron degeneration.[10][11] The diversity and genetic heterogeneity of motor neuron disorders are exemplified by the World Federation of Neurology classification which includes 28 autosomal dominant syndromes, 37 autosomal recessive syndromes, and 7 X linked syndromes, with an additional 16 different types of motor neuron disease dementia syndrome.[12]

Clinical features and differential diagnosis

Symptoms and signs

In 75% of patients the first symptoms are in the limbs; 25% present with bulbar symptoms[13-15] The earliest symptom is usually asymmetrical weakness of one extremity or, with bulbar onset disease, slurring of speech. The latter is often noted first by family or friends. Specific symptoms with limb onset disease depend on the anatomical area involved. In the arms, weakness may start around one shoulder, and sometimes is noticed after a minor local injury, or progresses after what has been considered to be a "frozen shoulder". Distal weakness is often manifested as increasing difficulty turning a key in a lock or car ignition, unscrewing bottle tops, holding a pen, or gripping objects. Arms are affected first in about 35% of cases, whereas the disease begins in the lumbosacral region of the spinal cord in about 40% of patients. Such patients begin to trip or stumble due to a unilateral foot drop, or may have difficulty rising from a chair if weakness starts proximally. Rarely patients note stiffness and flexor spasms in the legs, resulting from spasticity. Fatigue is not a particularly prominent early symptom, but muscle cramps are common, mostly in the legs, in which proximal and distal muscles are affected. Fasciculations may attract attention, and cramps and fasciculations sometimes precede weakness and wasting by several months. Sensory symptoms, usually variable distal paraesthesiae or numbness, are present in about 10% of patients, and pain may be a prominent symptom in up to 50% of patients with advanced motor neuron disease.

With time, weakness progresses but fasciculations often become less obvious. The majority of patients with limb onset eventually develop bulbar symptoms, and conversely, patients with bulbar onset disease ultimately develop symptoms in the limbs. Orthopnoea, due to diaphragmatic weakness, is common. In bulbar onset disease, dysarthria progresses until speech is incomprehensible; many patients become anarthric. Dysphagia usually begins as difficulty

245

clearing a bolus of solids, proceeds to difficulty even with liquified foods and fluids, and eventually becomes total. Drooling of saliva may be a constant irritation. These symptoms, with limb weakness, ultimately render such people dependent on others for every form of comfort, sustenance, and care. Fortunately, pressure sores are rare, and urinary and faecal incontinence seldom occur.

Although ventilatory muscle weakness occurs in almost all patients and, with or without pneumonia, is usually responsible for death, dyspnoea is not always a prominent symptom. It may however be present early in the course of the disease when limb weakness is negligible, and rarely patients present with dyspnoea or even ventilatory failure.

The physical signs of motor neuron disease stem from upper motor neuron involvement causing weakness, spasticity, hyperreflexia, and the Babinski sign (although the latter is present only in half)[15] and from lower motor neuron involvement causing weakness, muscular atrophy, and fasciculation. Dysphagia and dysarthria may be due to upper or lower motor neuron involvement or, in most cases, combined lesions. Emotional lability is usually associated with pseudobulbar palsy and is a sign of upper motor neuron involvement. Both upper and lower motor neuron signs are often evident at presentation in 65% of patients.[14 15] Fasciculation can occur in the absence of other lower motor neuron signs. Ten per cent of patients present with lower motor neuron features only, but some develop upper motor neuron signs and only about 5% show the phenotype of progressive muscular atrophy throughout the course of the disease.[15]

Objective sensory signs exclude a diagnosis of motor neuron disease unless there is a clear alternative explanation, such as carpal tunnel syndrome. Detailed testing with measurement of, for example, thermal threshold may show impaired sensation, and sural nerve biopsies have shown evidence of axonal degeneration in some cases of the disease.[16 17] In end stage motor neuron disease there may be multisystem involvement with degeneration of the spinocerebellar tracts, posterior columns, and brain stem reticular formation, although clinically this is of little importance.[18]

Dementia, which may be associated with parkinsonism, is seen in less than 5% of patients,[7–9] but subtle cognitive changes indicative of frontal and temporal lobe dysfunction can be detected in 25–50% of patients, and positron emission tomography activation studies show noticeably impaired responses in the medial frontal region and anterior thalamus in these patients.[19] Dementia associated with motor neuron disease is usually of frontal lobe type, and patients present typically with changes in conduct and character, although memory impairment may predominate. A family history of dementia with or without motor neuron disease, suggestive of autosomal dominant transmission, is present in some cases.[7 20]

The Western Pacific ALS-parkinsonism-dementia complex occurs on the island of Guam, the Kii peninsula in Japan, and in parts of New Guinea. In this syndrome features of amyotrophic lateral sclerosis coexist with extrapyramidal signs and dementia. The spinal cord pathology is that of typical motor neuron disease, but in addition there is neurofibrillary degeneration in cerebral cortex and brain stem and, to a lesser extent, in the spinal cord.[21] Current indications are that amyotrophic lateral sclerosis on Guam is declining in frequency.

Although many disorders should be considered in the differential diagnosis of motor neuron disease (boxes 10.1 and 10.3), in practice the diagnosis is usually straightforward by the time the patient is referred to a neurologist. Because the early symptoms may be ill defined or may be mistaken for localised lesions it is common for patients to be referred first to rheumatological, orthopaedic, ENT, or psychiatric departments. In the very elderly the diagnosis may be especially difficult in the early stages. In 62 consecutive patients referred with a diagnosis of motor neuron disease to a research clinic for clinical trials we found six who were judged not to have the disease: two with Kennedy's syndrome, one with cerebrovascular disease and cervical spondylosis, two with motor neuronopathy and multifocal conduction block, and one with inclusion body myositis. It is difficult to know what the diagnostic error rate would be in a less selected group of patients.

Investigations

The purpose of laboratory investigations is to exclude other diagnoses and to support the diagnosis of motor neuron disease. At present there are no specific biochemical or pathological markers of the disease.

Essential investigations

Erythrocyte sedimentation rate testing, haematological and biochemical screening, chest radiography, and electrocardiography

---

Box 10.3   Conditions that should always be considered in the differential diagnosis of motor neuron disease

- Cervical spondylotic myelopathy and other cervical and lumbosacral radiculopathies
- Disorders associated with autoimmune processes:
  (a) Dysimmune lower motor neuron syndromes (GM_1, GD_{1b} and asialo-GM_1 antibodies)
  (b) Monoclonal gammopathy with conduction block and motor neuropathy
  (c) Lymphoma
  (d) Paraneoplastic syndrome (encephalomyelitis with anterior horn cell involvement)
- Thyrotoxicosis
- Hyperparathyroidism
- Diabetic "amyotrophy"
- Radiation-induced neurogenic disorders
- Post-poliomyelitis progressive muscular atrophy
- Genetic enzyme defects: hexosaminidase A and (rarely) B deficiency (particularly in young patients)
- Exogenous toxin disorders (lead, mercury, manganese toxicity)
- "Prion" disorders (amyotrophic forms of Creutzfeldt-Jakob disease)
- Certain myopathies, such as inclusion body myositis

---

should be undertaken for all patients with suspected motor neuron disease. It is advisable to request tests of antinuclear antibody, thyroid function, and vitamin B12 and folate concentrations and Venereal Disease Research Laboratory tests and protein electrophoresis. These tests are done mainly to exclude coincidental disease that may influence management, but also to exclude thyroid and parathyroid disorders and autoimmune disorders that may be associated with motor neuronopathy or atypical spinal cord syndromes. Serum creatinine kinase activities may be high, particularly in people with predominantly lower motor neuron involvement and slow progression, but also in Kennedy's disease. Kennedy's disease can be excluded by testing for the androgen receptor gene mutation in all male patients if there is a suggestion of X linked inheritance or, if there is no clear family history, when the clinical picture raises the possibility.[10 22] The patient and family should receive appropriate counselling before testing. Key features

---

Box 10.4   Electromyographic criteria for diagnosis of motor neuron disease (from ref[23], with permission)

- Fibrillation and fasciculation in muscles of the lower and the upper extremities, or in the extremities and the head
- Reduction in number and increase in amplitude and duration of motor unit action potentials
- Normal electrical excitability of remaining fibres of motor nerves, and motor fibre conduction velocity within the normal range in nerves of relatively unaffected muscles and not less than 70% of the average normal value according to age in nerves of more severely affected muscles
- Normal excitability and conduction velocity of sensory nerve fibres even in severely affected extremities

---

of Kennedy's disease are early onset (which can be in the teens, although it may be as late as the sixth or seventh decades), slow progression of mainly proximal lower motor neuron weakness associated with facial and tongue weakness and fasciculation, gynaecomastia, and tremor of the hands. Depressed reflexes and reduced sensory nerve action potentials may also be potential clues to Kennedy's syndrome.

Electromyography and nerve conduction studies are important aids to the diagnosis of motor neuron disease and can exclude other neuromuscular disorders such as myopathy and motor neuronopathy. In essence, electromyography furnishes evidence of widespread anterior horn cell damage that cannot be explained on the basis of a localised disease process. Thus it is necessary to show denervation and reinnervation outside the distribution of a single peripheral nerve or nerve root. Although the examination depends largely on analysis of potentials detected by concentric needle electrodes, recording fasciculation potentials using surface electrodes is a useful non-invasive adjunct that allows many muscles to be examined. Box 10.4 summarises the criteria used to support a diagnosis of motor neuron disease.[23] These criteria cannot always be satisfied in early stages of motor neuron disease. Fibrillation potentials are often absent, particularly in patients with slower disease progression. Unstable motor units and increased jitter are an essential part of electrophysiological diagnosis, but are not

249

specific for the disease. Likewise, reduced recruitment and large motor unit potentials are non-specific, but in motor neuron disease larger motor unit amplitudes are seen in relation to duration of disease than in any other condition. The balance between the features of rapidly advancing denervation with little reinnervation (frequent fibrillations and fasciculations, highly unstable complex potentials of only moderately increased amplitude) and those of more slowly progressive disease (scanty fibrillations, with complex very high amplitude but relatively stable motor units) differs from case to case and even between different muscles in one patient. Fasciculations in motor neuron disease are of a lower frequency (0·3 Hz) than in the benign fasciculation syndrome (1·25 Hz). In the latter, fasciculations are not associated with abnormal voluntary motor unit potentials.

Several other points are worth considering. Firstly, motor conduction velocity is seldom low enough to suggest demyelination, although conduction studies may be unreliable when the compound muscle action potential amplitudes are very low.[24] Secondly, a mild reduction in sural nerve action potential amplitude does not exclude the diagnosis of motor neuron disease. Thirdly, low amplitude of compound muscle action potentials and a decremental response to repetitive nerve stimulation may indicate rapid progression.[25] Finally, conduction block is not a feature typical of the disease and, when present, raises the possibility of multifocal motor neuronopathy or other demyelinating neuronopathy. On the other hand, conduction block is not by itself diagnostic of multifocal motor neuronopathy, particularly if it is only present at common sites of nerve compression. Motor conduction block should therefore be sought in nerves not usually liable to pressure palsies. Conduction block implies a more than halved compound muscle action potential amplitude and negative peak area, and a less than 15% longer negative peak, after proximal, compared with distal, nerve stimulation.

Single fibre electromyography, macro-electromyography, and central motor conduction using magnetic stimulation are useful techniques for research into motor system and motor unit physiology. Abnormal jitter and blocking of neuromuscular transmission and increased fibre density detected by single fibre electromyography reflect early reinnervation and collateral sprouting and may provide evidence of anterior horn cell damage in otherwise normal muscles. These techniques are not mandatory for clinical diagnosis and seldom add critical information beyond what can be obtained with the more conventional approaches described above.

Desirable investigations

Many neurologists would now regard magnetic resonance imaging as mandatory in patients with possible motor neuron disease; that is, when there is any possibility that the signs might be caused by a single lesion. Imaging may be focused on the head, neck, or thoracolumbar region, depending on the presenting symptoms and signs. It not only helps to exclude common disorders such as spondylotic myelopathy or neoplasm but may show that the corticospinal tract is affected extensively, with high intensity white matter lesions in the cortex, internal capsule, brain stem, and spinal cord.[26 27] Bilateral T2 shortening in the precentral cortex and hyperintensity of the spinal cord corticospinal tracts on nuclear magnetic resonance imaging have been reported in motor neuron disease.[28]

Lumbar puncture and analysis of CSF should be undertaken in atypical cases but, in most cases, CSF analysis adds little and in many centres it is not done routinely. A high protein concentration (>0·75 g/l), the presence of oligoclonal bands, or increased numbers of leucocytes indicate other causes. In a group of nine patients in whom motor neuron disease was associated with lymphoma, most had high CSF protein concentrations, and oligoclonal bands were present in three.[29]

Occasional investigations

Various conditions may mimic the clinical features of motor neuron disease (boxes 10.2 and 10.3), and occasionally the following investigations may be relevant: a search for antibodies against gangliosides[30 31] and, occasionally, antibodies against Hu antigen[32]; leucocyte or fibroblast hexosaminidase A and B activity; HIV and HTLV1 assay; or blood lead and 24 hour urinary lead excretion.

Single photon emission tomography studies may show reduced cerebral blood flow in the frontal regions in patients with motor neuron disease and dementia,[9] but this investigation is not helpful in most cases of motor neuron disease.

251

Patients with familial motor neuron disease may now be screened for point mutations in the Cu/Zn superoxide dismutase (SOD 1) gene on the long arm of chromosome 21 (21q22.1–22.2), but this should not be undertaken without proper counselling.[11] Mutations in the SOD 1 gene account for 10–20% of all familial cases with autosomal dominant inheritance. Thus the genetic basis is still unknown in 80–90% of patients with a family history of motor neuron disease.

Epidemiology, risk factors, and prevention

The incidence of motor neuron disease is about 2–3 per 100 000 and the prevalence 4–7 per 100 000 in most parts of the world except the Western Pacific foci.[33 34] In Guam the incidence of the disease fell from 87 per 100 000 in 1962 to 5 per 100 000 in 1985.[21] The incidence elsewhere may be rising, although this could be due to improved ascertainment and demographic factors.[35–37] The average general practitioner might expect to see a new case only once every 25 years. Most surveys have found that the incidence of the disease increases with age to a peak between 60 and 70 years.[34 36] In almost all studies, men are more commonly affected than women, with a ratio of around 1·5:1.[34–36] In brief, proved risk factors for the disease include increasing age, male sex, and residence for many years in certain parts of the Western Pacific.

As the cause of motor neuron disease is unknown, and modifiable risk factors have yet to be defined with certainty, there are at present no known primary or secondary prevention options. Trauma of many types, exposure to a variety of toxins (cyanide, lead, or aluminium) and farming, particularly heavy manual activity, are possible but unproved risk factors.[34 36] In the small community of Two Rivers in Wisconsin, United States, a cluster of six cases occurring over a period of 7·5 years was detected.[38] Generally the evidence for clustering is weak. Physical trauma, freshly caught fish from Lake Michigan, and family history of cancer were implicated as risk factors in this group. Previous infection with polio virus is probably not a risk factor.[39]

A factor implicated in causing the Guam MND-parkinsonism-dementia-complex syndrome has been a dietary excitotoxin, β-N-methylamino-L-alanine (L-BMAA), which is found in cycad flour obtained from false sago palm (*Cycas circinalis*).[40] L-BMAA now seems to be an unlikely factor, however, because insufficient amounts exist in cooked food for it to be a neurotoxin.[41]

Mortality from motor neuron disease has been reported to be different in various ethnic communities. Asian immigrants (Indian and Pakistani) to England have less than half the mortality from the disease than the general population of England and Wales. Mortality from it may also be low in white South Africans (particularly in the Afrikaans-speaking group) and in Mexican patients.[42-44]

Prognosis

Known outcomes

Median survival for all patients with sporadic motor neuron disease is about 3·5 years from onset of symptoms.[15 45] In a recent prospective study of 229 patients with the disease, however, Chancellor *et al* reported that, overall, 50% survival from symptom onset was 2·5 years, and five year survival was 28%.[46] Benign or long duration motor neuron disease is recognised, and comprises about 5% of all cases.[15] Early onset (below 50 years) is associated with longer survival. It has been reported that 10–16% of patients with the disease may live longer than 10 years.[47] Tucker *et al* reported four patients with an MND-like syndrome who recovered completely 5–12 months after disease onset.[48] Complete recovery from motor neuron disease was not confirmed, however, in a follow up study of 708 cases.[15]

Bulbar onset is associated with appreciably reduced survival, median survival being about 2·2 years. It is the single most important indicator of poor prognosis. People presenting with progressive bulbar palsy rarely survive beyond five years.[15] Older age and female sex are adverse risk factors; progressive bulbar palsy occurs more often in women.

Communication and counselling

Increasingly, the neurologist is part of a multidisciplinary team, and a team approach is probably most satisfactory for coping with the changing needs of people with motor neuron disease.

Telling the diagnosis

Once the diagnosis has been established by clinical examination and supported by the appropriate investigations, the patient and spouse or close carer should be informed of the diagnosis and should be allowed time to explore the implications. "Telling" should take place with privacy, and a provisional plan for early follow up and support should be agreed. Most people register only a fraction of the information imparted at such interviews, and leaflets can alarm more than reassure at this early stage. Our practice is to explain the diagnosis with a chosen carer (usually a spouse) and with our care team coordinator present. Follow up is then arranged within two weeks. Close liaison with the general practitioner is important. The patient is given the local contact telephone numbers for the motor neuron disease care team and for the Motor Neuron Disease Association, which funds regional care advisers to provide advice and practical support. With the permission of the patient and family, we inform the regional care adviser about the newly diagnosed patient.

In our experience, support from the local and national Motor Neuron Disease Association forms a key part of an effective care strategy. Although a few people prefer not to have contact with the Motor Neuron Disease Association, most patients benefit from early referral.

Support and external agencies: the role of the key worker

Models of care through team work will differ according to local circumstances, but the concept that each patient should be allocated a key worker has much to recommend it. A key worker is likely to be a health professional who agrees to coordinate the activities of the many services that must work efficiently together to support patients with the disease and their families. The key worker might be the general practitioner, community occupational or speech therapist, practice nurse, or the hospital based team coordinator.

Follow up and support

Patients may know little about motor neuron disease or may have preconceived and erroneous ideas. They can be reassured that generally the intellect, sexual, and sphincter functions will remain intact. The patient should be encouraged to lead a normal life for as long as possible, but practical difficulties should be foreseen so that appropriate action can be taken to prevent crises. Patients may benefit from a visit to a disabled living centre or to a specialised neurological rehabilitation centre. Referral to a "mobility centre" for advice on driving can be helpful. This theme of coordinating care to minimise delays in providing aids and appliances and other forms of support is fundamental to the good management of the disease. Advice about employment, finance, and family matters should be available from the team and from expert counsellors. People with the disease often feel abandoned by doctors, but regular outpatient attendances may be of little value unless there is a positive care plan and both the patient and doctor have a clear idea of what clinic visits can achieve. Continued support from a key worker, close links with the general practitioner, a telephone hotline for advice and help in crises, hospital admission for respite care or crises, and access to hospice care are all important components of the management of the disease. Depression is common, as are frustration, anger, and irritability, the last most often directed against spouse or carer but also against health professionals.[49]

Treatment strategies

Specific therapy

Box 10.5 summarises the various treatments that have been tried and found wanting for motor neuron disease, but there are a number of promising strategies that might yield treatments to influence the course of the disease.

Trials in progress

Branched chain amino acids

Plaitakis *et al* reported significant benefit in terms of maintenance of muscle strength and walking ability in 22 patients with the disease treated with branched chain amino acids (L-leucine/L-isoleucine/L-valine).[50] This trial was based on the hypothesis that partial glutamate dehydrogenase deficiency can occur in atypical motor neuron disease and forms of multiple system atrophy. Branched chain amino aids activate glutamate dehydrogenase and

---

Box 10.5   Various therapeutic trials undertaken or in progress in motor neuron disease

Immunotherapy:
  Steroids
  Immunosuppression
  Whole body lymphoid
    irradiation
  Plasma exchange
  Interferon

Vitamin and anti-free radical
therapy:
  Vitamin E
  Vitamin B12
  Selegiline
  N-acetylcysteine

Agents thought to modulate
glutaminergic transmission:
  Dextromethorphan
  Lamotrigine
  Branched chain amino acids
  Riluzole

Miscellaneous:
  Chelating agents
  Thyrotrophin releasing
    hormone
  Levodopa
  Amantadine
  Guanidine
  Naloxone
  Cytosine arabinoside
  Bovine gangliosides
  Testosterone
  Pancreatic extracts

Current trials:
  Riluzole
  N-acetylcysteine
  Branched chain amino acids
  Motor neuron neurotrophic
  factors:
  (a) Ciliary neurotrophic factor
  (b) Insulin-like growth factor 1
  (c) Brain-derived neurotrophic
      factor

---

may modify glutamate metabolism and glutaminergic transmission. A double blind placebo controlled trial of 126 patients found a higher mortality in the group randomised to active treatment, but patients in this group were slightly older than the placebo group and had a lower forced vital capacity.[51] A recent European multicentre, double blind, placebo controlled trial of branched chain amino acids recruited over 400 patients who were treated for one year. No difference in outcome, measured by survival or by various functional scales, was found.

Glutamate inhibition

Inhibition of glutamate has been tried with dextromethorphan, lamotrigine, MK-801, and more recently riluzole.[52] Riluzole modulates glutaminergic transmissions by presynaptic inhibition of glutamate release and postsynaptic interference with the effects of excitatory amino acids. Riluzole may also act by inactivating voltage-dependent sodium channels and the cytotoxic factor, GP 120, which releases macrophagic toxic factors.[53 54] Bensimon *et al* reported the results of a prospective, randomised, double blind, placebo controlled trial of riluzole in 155 patients with definite or probable motor neuron disease.[51] The primary end points were survival and rates of change of functional status, and at the end of one year survival was significantly greater in the riluzole group (74%) than in the placebo group (58%). The apparent effect of riluzole was greater in patients with bulbar onset than with limb onset disease. In those with bulbar onset the survival rate at 12 months was 73% with riluzole compared with 35% with placebo ($p = 0.014$), whereas in the patients with limb onset the difference was not significant. Decline in muscle strength was appreciably slower in the riluzole than the placebo group. Randomisation was stratified according to the site of onset of the disease (bulbar *v* limb onset, by first symptoms), the numbers in the bulbar onset group were small (32; 17 receiving placebo and 15 riluzole), and there were minor advantages for the riluzole group in terms of age and bulbar function scores, although these differences were not statistically significant. Twenty four of the 155 patients randomised did not meet all the entry criteria, but nonetheless all were considered to have amyotrophic lateral sclerosis and were included in the analysis. Withdrawals due to adverse drug reactions were more common in the riluzole than the placebo group. These results cannot be taken as proof of the efficacy of riluzole, and it is not clear why patients with bulbar onset should respond better than those with limb onset—although such patients might receive the drug earlier in the course of lower motor neuron degeneration. On the other hand, ventilatory function was worse in patients with bulbar onset than in those with limb onset disease. Only a larger trial can answer these questions, and a multicentre trial of riluzole in Europe and North America has recruited over 950 patients. Preliminary indications are that this trial also shows a beneficial effect of riluzole on survival in both those with bulbar onset and those with limb onset disease.

N-acetylcysteine

N-acetylcysteine is a free radical scavenger and is a direct and indirect precursor of glutathione, a major intracellular oxidant defence system. Louwerse *et al* reported the results of a randomised, double blind, placebo controlled trial in 110 patients with motor neuron disease.[55] After one year, the treated group showed a 29% (non-significant) reduction in mortality from motor neuron disease of spinal onset but not of bulbar onset. Further studies are needed to decide whether N-acetylcysteine has any place in the treatment of the disease.

Neurotrophic factors

Ciliary neurotrophic factor is a neuroactive cytokine made in Schwann cells of peripheral nerve, which initiates repair process. It promotes survival of rat and human motor neurons in tissue culture, promotes sprouting of motor axon terminals, and slows progression of motor neuron degeneration in murine models.[56] Recombinant human ciliary neurotrophic factor has been tested in subjects with motor neuron disease; systemic side effects due to the cytokine-like actions of the factor were problematic and there was no evidence of benefit.[57]

Insulin-like growth factor is a 70 amino acid polypeptide that mediates the action of growth hormone. It enhances motor neuron sprouting in vivo and increases muscle end plate size in rats.[58 59] Multicentre trials are now under way.

Brain derived neurotrophic factor enhances the survival of motor neurons after axotomy and can rescue motor neurons from death during development.[60 61] Trials of recombinant human factor have started in North America.

Future prospects

Although multifocal motor neuronopathies may respond to immunosuppressive treatment, including intravenous infusion of immune globulin,[62] aggressive immunomodulation does not improve classical motor neuron disease.[63] If antibodies against calcium channels[64 65] are found to play a part in pathogenesis, there may be further attempts to treat the disease as an autoimmune disorder, but present indications are that this approach has failed. Future strategies for neuroprotection in motor neuron disease are likely to focus on new glutamate antagonists, agents protecting against free radical damage, neurotrophic factors, and on combinations of these.

A major difficulty with the human recombinant neurotrophic factors is that they have to be administered by subcutaneous, intravenous, or even intrathecal routes, and access to the brain and spinal cord is limited. Thus research is likely to focus on signal transduction mechanisms to identify compounds that activate intracellular systems that respond to neurotrophic factors.

Supportive treatment and treatment of complications

Dysarthria and communication problems

Dysarthria occurs in most patients before death.[66] In a hospice only 25% had normal speech on admission.[67 68] Early referral to a speech therapist and access to a communication aids centre are important. Management measures include encouraging the patient to decrease the speed of speech. Application of local ice, or the use of baclofen, may help to reduce tongue spasticity. Other measures include a palatal loop or palatal lift (for hypernasality caused by nasal escape of air). For patients with anarthria, communication aids may be useful. These include computerised type-in speech devices (Canon Communicator), and Lightwriters or Memowriter (equipped with memory). In cases of severe physical impairment, scanning aids such as the Possum Communicator, in which a switch-operated cursor light or pointer identifies each item, letter, or symbol, can be invaluable.

Salivation

Drooling or salivary dribbling is often a problem in people with severe bulbar symptoms. Two to three litres of saliva are produced and swallowed each day normally.[69] Loss of automatic swallowing and of erect head posture cause drooling of saliva, and persistent dribbling is a major source of distress to patients. Family and friends should be aware that dribbling is not a sign of mental impairment. Helpful interventions include neck support and correction of the head position; treatment of mouth infections (usually fungal); and application of local ice in the mouth. The lip seal may be strengthened by simple lip exercises (closing lips against finger resistance). Anticholinergic drugs, including atropine or more usually hyoscine hydrobromide tablets, elixir, or skin patches may prove effective. Hyoscine can be used sublingually (1–2 mg two or three times a day). Benzhexol or benztropine can also be tried; benzhexol can be used in tablet or elixir formulation, and benztropine may be useful given in the injectable form (1–2 mg two or three times a day) via a gastrostomy tube. Amitriptyline or impramine is sometimes helpful, and has the added benefit of improving sleep, mood, and probably emotional lability. A portable suction device may be of great value, provided that carers and patients are taught how to use it by an experienced professional. Accounts have been published of surgical approaches such as transtympanic neurectomy (section of chorda tympani in the middle ear)[70] and salivary gland denervation, but we have never resorted to these. Our preferred option, if the drug treatments mentioned above fail to control drooling of saliva, is to refer patients for salivary gland irradiation.

Swallowing

Dysphagia is a major problem in 50–70% of patients with motor neuron disease, and this may lead to choking, dehydration, weight loss, salivary dribbling, and aspiration pneumonia.[71] Investigation of dysphagia in the disease may include cine-videofluroscopy, which involves swallowing a barium suspension of varying consistency and analysis of the various stages of swallowing. Patients should be encouraged to eat where they feel relaxed and comfortable, as slowness of eating and dribbling may cause severe social embarrassment. It may be possible to improve head posture and head support, as well as lip closure. Again, application of ice in the mouth may reduce spasticity of the tongue. Dietary measures may include avoidance of food and drink that precipitates coughing and choking, such as highly spiced foods or spirits. Dairy foods (milk and cream) or proprietary thickeners may increase volume and tenacity of mouth secretions.[66] If the automatic swallow reflex becomes depressed in motor neuron disease it may be triggered by chewing sweets or gum.

Some drugs may help with swallowing problems: baclofen reduces spasticity and is sometimes helpful in doses up to 80–90 mg. L-threonine may help. Anticholinesterase drugs, however, are usually unhelpful and increase salivation. Division of the fibres of the cricopharyngeus muscle may help in cases of cricopharyngeal spasm due to demonstrable pseudobulbar incoordination. Postoperative mortality appears to be high (6%–30%) in some published series, and this procedure is not practised widely. Nasogastric feeding may be useful for temporary feeding when dysphagia is made worse by oral or upper respiratory tract infection.

The definitive procedure is percutaneous endoscopic gastrostomy, which is helpful in patients with advanced dysphagia and involves inserting a small bore catheter under local anaesthesia.[71 72] It is helpful to broach the idea relatively early in the course of the disease in people with bulbar symptoms. Percutaneous endoscopic gastrostomy requires careful dietetic advice on calorific and nutritional intake and food selection. Indications for percutaneous endoscopic gastrostomy include severe dehydration, frequent choking, aspiration pneumonia, progressive weight loss, and exhaustion caused by laboured feeding. Percutaneous endoscopic gastrostomy is particularly helpful in patients with severe bulbar symptoms but with relatively good limb function. It relieves the burden of laboured attempts to take adequate nourishment and often improves wellbeing and quality of life, at least for some months. The option of percutaneous endoscopic gastrostomy should be discussed with patients and carers early rather than late in the disease. For patients who refuse percutaneous endoscopic gastrostomy but who can swallow some fluids, oral morphine elixir given every four hours (or every 12 hours as a slow release preparation) relieves hunger and thirst to some extent. Oral morphine should not, however, prevent due attention to hydration and nutrition, and a fine bore nasogastric tube may be acceptable for some patients in the short term, although (in our experience) this is seldom satisfactory in the longer term.

Choking, principally with fluids, accompanies dysphagia, and patients are often anxious that they will choke to death. In fact, this rarely happens.[67 68] A home suction device may be helpful, at least to provide reassurance. Postural advice—for example, asking patients to lean forward—can be offered, and it may be necessary to teach carers the Heimlich manoeuvre so that foreign bodies may be dislodged in case of obstruction.

Ventilatory failure

Most patients with motor neuron disease die of ventilatory failure, predominantly because of diaphragmatic weakness, although weakness of intercostal muscle contributes to the breathing difficulty. Symptoms of ventilatory failure such as orthopnea or dyspnoea on exertion or at rest may be accompanied by daytime sleepiness, morning headaches, and excessive fatigue. Patients may complain that they do not feel refreshed by sleep.

Such symptoms may make life a misery, and their origin in ventilatory failure may not always be obvious. Respiratory failure may be precipitated by an upper respiratory tract infection associated with bronchitis or by an aspiration pneumonia, particularly when there is bulbar muscle weakness. Patients with weakness of the ventilatory muscles have difficulty clearing sputum from the bronchi and trachea. Pulmonary embolism is common, and attention should be paid to preventing deep vein thrombosis; in some patients the use of low molecular weight heparin or warfarin may be appropriate.

Important physical signs that indicate ventilatory failure include the use of the accessory muscles of respiration and the paradoxical movement of the abdominal muscles on inspiration.

The best measure of ventilatory function is the vital capacity, which will typically fall to less than half the predicted normal value before symptoms of ventilatory failure ensue. Vital capacity should fall by less than 20% when measured with the patient lying flat, compared with standing. Other measures include: respiratory rate, cough strength, diaphragmatic excursion, and the ability to count up to 20 in one breath. Chest radiography is important to exclude pneumonia or evidence of a pulmonary embolus, particularly if there is a sudden deterioration in ventilatory function. If assisted ventilation is being considered, nocturnal oximetry and carbon dioxide studies are valuable.[73] Arterial blood gases may show abnormalities, but are often normal until very late in the course of the disease.

The symptoms caused by ventilatory failure are often ameliorated if patients can be positioned upright rather than flat. If unable to move themselves they should be turned often to prevent pneumonia. Even mild chest infections should be treated early with antibiotics and physiotherapy. Influenza vaccine should be offered to patients and carers each year. As mentioned above, a portable suction machine should be provided, and the care team should ensure that carers and health professionals are confident about how to use it. If a patient is distressed by dyspnoea or symptoms of hyperventilation then assisted ventilation should be considered. This can certainly relieve symptoms and improve the quality of life, without necessarily committing the patient to long term assisted ventilation via tracheostomy. The decision to start assisted ventilation depends on whether symptoms of hypoventilation are present and sleep studies show evidence of hypoxaemia or hypercapnia, or both. Technically, several approaches are possible; the options include nasal ventilation using either a bi-level positive airway pressure ventilator, which permits a higher pressure (20–40 cm of water) during inspiration and a lower pressure (2–25 cm of water) during expiration, or a nasal intermittent positive pressure ventilator.[74-76] It is usual to admit patients to hospital for several days so that the use of the ventilator can be explored with the patient and carers, anxieties of both allayed, and confidence in the pulmonary care team established. Response to emergencies must be prompt, and technical support with 24 hour cover should be arranged, usually through the company providing the ventilator. Initially patients tend to use the ventilator at night, but often this extends to the day time as the disease progresses. Initial complications include discomfort or even ulceration of the skin (resulting from the mask being applied too tightly) and anxiety, either of the patient or the carer.

At present in the United Kingdom, tracheostomy with intermittent positive pressure ventilation is undertaken only in exceptional circumstances, partly because little counselling is provided about these issues in most centres. This practice may change, and patients and carers will become more aware of the options available. The decision to embark upon tracheostomy and long term intermittent positive pressure ventilation should be taken in the light of the "advanced directives" of the patient; detailed discussion with the neurology and pulmonary care teams; consultations with psychiatrists or psychologists; and consideration of both legal and, perhaps more important, "spiritual" issues. Several centres have set up teams to deal with these issues. In North America, where long term intermittent positive pressure ventilation with tracheostomy is more widely available for patients with motor neuron disease, a "living will" is necessary for dealing with potential complications and progression of the disease, so that the caring physicians and the family have a clear idea of what should be done should the patient become unable to communicate. It is not always possible to foresee tracheostomy, because about 2% of patients are admitted direct to intensive care units with ventilatory failure before a formal diagnosis of motor neuron disease is made. In summary, provision of non-invasive ventilatory support is likely to become more widespread, and as awareness of the options increases, some patients will opt for long term intermittent positive pressure ventilation with tracheostomy. In northern Illinois, only 8·6% of patients with the disease chose home ventilation.[77] Home ventilation is expensive, and imposes severe burdens on families.

Other forms of assisted ventilation that may suit a few patients are the negative pressure cuirass (which increases the risk of aspiration), the Tunnicliffe jacket, or the rocking bed.[78]

Many doctors in the United Kingdom have taken the view that a better approach is to control distressing dyspnoea with oral opiates, titrated to avoid drowsiness and confusion. This approach does not necessarily shorten life, and can appreciably reduce distress.

Spasticity

Spasticity may be treated with benzodiazepines, baclofen, or dantrolene. Severe contractures may be reduced by surgical lengthening or division of tendons. Although resort to operation is seldom indicated, correction of fixed plantar flexion of the feet may restore the ability to stand, and this alone may permit easier transfer from chair to bed or toilet and may reduce the difficulty encountered in dressing and undressing. Such operations can be performed under local anaesthesia but, because such patients often have diaphragmatic weakness, general anaesthesia is usually safer than spinal anaesthesia.

Pain

Pain may occur in 45%–64% patients with motor neuron disease and arises from muscle cramps, stiff joints, spasticity, abdominal colic caused by constipation, and skin pressure.[68 79] Pain may be controlled by correct positioning of the patient and use of a turning bed at night; physiotherapy (changing position, etc); and drugs, including muscle relaxants (benzodiazepines or baclofen), non-steroidal anti-inflammatory drugs, and opioids (in advanced stages of the disease).

Constipation

Constipation may occur because of weakness of pelvic muscles, improper diet, spasticity, and drugs such as anticholinergics and opioids. Management options include increase of dietary fibre and maintenance of fluid intake, bulk-forming laxatives such as methyl cellulose, osmotic laxatives such as lactulose, suppositories, and enemas.

Peripheral oedema

Dependent pedal oedema occurs in virtually all patients with motor neuron disease. This can be counteracted by raising the patient's legs, using elastic stockings, and the cautious use of diuretics.

Sleep disturbances

Disturbed sleep and poor nights may occur because of pain, depression and anxiety, immobility, or sleep apnoea. A suitable bed is of utmost importance to make the nights more comfortable for patients. Beds should be of correct height and have a firm mattress; turning beds with a powered elevator are an added advantage. Nocturnal hypoxia due to weakness of ventilatory muscles should always be considered when patients complain of undue fatigue, lassitude, morning headaches, or nocturnal confusion or anxiety.

Emotional problems

Depression and anxiety can be partially helped by effective management of the other disabilities described above and by antidepressant drugs in selected cases. Emotional lability may respond to imipramine or other antidepressants.

The final stages of motor neuron disease

Severe physical disability may require the use of an electronic scanning device whereby each item, letter, or symbol is identified by switch operated cursor or pointer. The Possum Communicator is such a device, and environmental control devices operated by the same method are available. Sophisticated communication aids are available, and with this and support from home care teams, many people with motor neuron disease can remain at home until death. In the United Kingdom, support from a local hospice is often the key factor that allows this to happen.

Patients with the disease usually die from respiratory failure, inhalation and aspiration pneumonia, or other infections. Pulmonary embolism is not uncommon. The various strategies available to manage these problems have already been discussed. In the last stage it is important to maintain symptomatic relief and avoid distress to patient and family as far as practicable. Narcotic

265

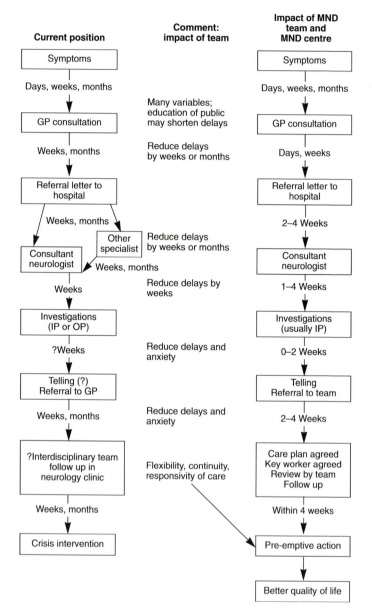

Figure 10.1 *Motor neuron disease: a patient's perspective (suggested framework for audit). (IP = inpatient; OP = outpatient).*

analgesics (morphine or diamorphine) are useful, and may be given as a suppository, intramuscular or subcutaneous injection, or by continuous subcutaneous infusion.

The consultant and general practitioner should be available for consultation, and the key worker should stay in close contact with the family. Hospital or hospice admission should be offered if appropriate, to ensure the stress-free death of the patient whenever possible.

After the death of the patient a letter of condolence should be sent to the partner or family, and the spouse should be offered counselling if necessary.

Audit issues

Provision for motor neuron disease support services has not been adequately audited in the past. In 1990 the Royal College of Physicians held a consensus conference on managing chronic neurological disorders and identified several topics in the management of motor neuron disease which can be audited. These include accessibility to specialist care (with information regarding waiting list period and travelling distance for neurologcal consultation) and multidisciplinary care (counselling, community physiotherapy, speech therapists, day hospitals, and provision of aids).

Provision should be made for continuing care (outpatient visit when the patient is seen by the consultant) and for full information and liaison (information given to patients about the Motor Neuron Disease Association, consultations to explain properly the diagnosis and its implications, and liaison between the hospital neurology team and the general practitioner). The role of the key worker should be defined. Other areas of patient care that can be audited include managing symptoms such as pain, dysphagia, salivary drooling, and insomnia; patient satisfaction with multidisciplinary care and general practitioner; support services for specialist help with problems such as dysphagia and availability of percutaneous endoscopic gastrostomy; and provision for managing respiratory failure, including assisted ventilation. Figure 10.1 shows a scheme for auditing the disease care team used by the motor neuron disease care and research centre at the Maudsley and King's College Hospitals.

Management of motor neuron disease

- People in whom motor neuron disease is suspected should undergo thorough investigations, including electrophysiological studies and appropriate imaging to exclude a focal lesion (such as cervical radiculomyelopathy) or a more generalised disorder (such as motor neuropathy or myasthenia gravis) that may, in the early stages, mimic features of motor neuron disease. The El Escorial criteria should be used to alert clinicians to atypical features indicating an alternative diagnosis
- The person with motor neuron disease and the carers should be told the diagnosis by a consultant neurologist, in a suitable setting, with adequate time for discussion. Ideally, another member of the motor neuron disease care team (such as the team coordinator) should be present. A provisional care strategy should be agreed, and follow up arranged within 2–4 weeks. Contact with the regional care adviser or other representative of a voluntary organisation (in the UK, the Motor Neuron Disease Association) should also be offered, and the role of the voluntary organisation explained
- As soon as possible a key worker should be identified. The team approach to management should be positive, emphasising autonomy, dignity, and quality of life
- As symptoms progress, links between the care team and community services must adapt and respond flexibly to pre-empt crises. Good communication between care providers is of paramount importance
- Counselling on the emotional and physical aspects of motor neuron disease should be available. Options for dealing with the final stage of the disease should be discussed early rather than late, but the timing of such discussion will vary from case to case. Some patients will wish to make advance directives, and if ventilatory support is considered, a "living will" may be appropriate
- Patients with dysarthria should have access to specialist advice on communication aids. Percutaneous endoscopic gastrostomy should be considered before severe swallowing difficulties impair hydration or nutrition. Only rarely should a nasogastric tube be considered. Control of symptoms such as cramps, spasticity, musculoskeletal pain, constipation, drooling of saliva, and depression require effective management. Nocturnal hypopnoea and daytime dyspnoea should prompt consideration of non-invasive ventilatory support (with bi-level positive airway pressure or nasal intermittent positive pressure ventilation) after assessment by a pulmonary physician experienced in the management of motor neuron disease patients. Unplanned tracheostomy and ventilation should be avoided if at all possible. The final stages of the disease should be managed at home or in a hospice experienced in the management of motor neuron disease

1 Mulder DW, Kurland LT, Offord KP, Beard CM. Familial adult motor neuron disease: amyotrophic lateral sclerosis. *Neurology* 1986;**36**:511–7.

2 Veltema AN, Roos RAC, Bruyn GW. Autosomal dominant adult amyotrophic lateral sclerosis. *J Neurol Sci* 1990;**97**:93–115.

3 Hirano A, Kurland LT, Krooth RS, Lessel S. Parkinsonism-dementia complex, an endemic disease on the island of Guam. *Brain* 1961;**84**:642–61.

4 Pringle CE, Hudson AJ, Munoz DG, Kiernan JA, Brown WF, Ebers GC. Primary lateral sclerosis. Clinical features, neuropathology and diagnostic criteria. *Brain* 1992;**115**:495–520.

5 Swash M, Leigh PN. Criteria for diagnosis of familial amyotrophic lateral sclerosis. *Neuromusc Disord* 1992;**2**:7–9.

6 Gaffney JS, Sufit RL, Hartmann H, *et al*. Clinical diagnosis of amyotrophic lateral sclerosis (ALS): a clinicopathological study of 'El Escorial' Working Group criteria in 36 autopsied patients [abstract]. *Neurology* 1992;**42**:455.

7 Hudson AJ. Amyotrophic lateral sclerosis and its association with dementia, parkinsonism and other neurological disorders: a review. *Brain* 1981;**104**:217–47.

8 Kew JJM, Leigh PN. Dementia with motor neuron disease. In: Rossor MN, ed. *Baillière's clinical neurology: unusual dementias*, vol 1(3). London: Ballière Tindall, 1992:611–26.

9 Neary D, Snowden JS, Mann DMA, Northern B, Boulding PJ, MacDermott N. Frontal lobe dementia and motor neurone disease. *J Neurol Neurosurg Psychiatry* 1990;**53**:23–32.

10 La Spada AR, Wilson EM, Lubahn DE, Harding AE, Fischbeck KH. Androgen receptor gene mutations in X-linked spinal and bulbar muscular atrophy. *Nature* 1991;**352**:77–9.

11 Rosen DR, Siddique T, Patterson D, Figlewicz D, Sapp P, Hentati A, *et al*. Mutations in Cu/Zn superoxide dismutase gene are associated with familial amyotrophic lateral sclerosis. *Nature* 1993;**362**:59–62.

12 De Jong JMBV. The World Federation of Neurology classification of spinal muscular atrophies and other disorders of the motor neurons. In: Vinken PJ, Bruyn GW, Klawans HL eds. *Handbook of clinical neurology*, vol 15(9). *Diseases of the motor system*. Amsterdam: Elsevier Science Publishers, 1991:1–12.

13 Jokelainen M. Amyotrophic lateral sclerosis in Finland. 2. Clinical characteristics. *Acta Neurol Scand* 1977;**56**:194–204.

14 Li T-M, Alberman E, Swash M. Clinical associations of 560 cases of motor neurone disease. *J Neurol Neurosurg Psychiatry* 1990;**53**:1043–5.

15 Norris F, Shepherd R, Denys E, Kwei U, Mukai E, Elias L, *et al*. Onset, natural history and outcome in idiopathic motor neuron disease. *J Neurol Sci* 1993;**118**:48–55.

16 Jamal GA, Weir AI, Hansen S, Ballantyne JP. Sensory involvement in motor neurone disease: further evidence from automated thermal threshold determination. *J Neurol Neurosurg Psychiatry* 1985;**48**:906–10.

17 Bradley WG. Recent views on anyotrophic lateral sclerosis with emphasis on electrophysiological studies. *Muscle Nerve* 1987;**10**:490–502.

18 Swash M, Scholtz CL, Vowles GH, Ingram DA. Selective asymmetrical vulnerability of corticospinal and spinocerebellar tracts in motor neurone disease. *J Neurol Neurosurg Psychiatry* 1988;**51**:785–9.

19 Kew JJM, Goldstein LH, Leigh PN, Abrahams S, Cosgrave N, Passingham RE, *et al*. The relationship between abnormalities of cognitive function and cerebral activation in amyotrophic lateral sclerosis. *Brain* 1993;**116**:1399–424.

20 Gunnarsson L-G, Dahlborn K, Strandman E. Motor neuron disease and dementia reported among 13 members of a single family. *Acta Neurol Scand* 1991;**84**:429–33.

21 Rodgers-Johnson P, Garruto RM, Yanagihara R, Chen K-M, Gajdusek DC, Gibbs CJ. Amyotrophic lateral sclerosis and parkinsonism-dementia on Guam: a 30 year evaluation and neuropathologic trends. *Neurology* 1986;**36**:7–13.

22 Harding AE, Thomas PK, Baraitser M, Bradbury PC, Morgan-Hughes JA, Ponsford JR. X-linked recessive bulbospinal neuronopathy: a report of ten cases. *J Neurol Neurosurg Psychiatry* 1982;**45**:1012–9.

23 Lambert EH, Mulder DW. Electromyographic studies in amyotrophic lateral sclerosis. *Mayo Clinic Proc* 1957;**32**:441–6.

24 Behnia M, Kelly JJ. Role of electromyography in amyotrophic lateral sclerosis. *Muscle Nerve* 1991;**14**:1236–341.

25 Kelly JJ, Thibodeau L, Andres PL, Finison LJ. Use of electrophysiologic tests to measure disease progression in ALS therapeutic trials. *Muscle Nerve* 1990;**13**:471–9.

26 Friedman DP, Taraglino LM. Amyotrophic lateral sclerosis: hyperintensity of the corticospinal tracts on MR images of the spinal cord. *AJR* 1993;**160**:604–6.

269

27 Goodin DS, Rowley HA, Olney RK. Magnetic resonance imaging in amyotrophic lateral sclerosis. *Ann Neurol* 1988;**23**:418–20.

28 Oba H, Araki T, Ohtomo K, Monzawa S, Uchiyama G, Koizumi K, *et al.* Amyotrophic lateral sclerosis: T2 shortening in motor cortex at MR imaging. *Radiology* 1993;**189**:843–6.

29 Younger DS, Rowland LP, Latov N, *et al.* Lymphoma, motor neuron diseases, and amyotrophic lateral sclerosis. *Ann Neurol* 1991;**29**:78–86.

30 Sadiq SA, Thomas FP, Kilidirias K, *et al.* The spectrum of neurological disease associated with anti-GM1 antibodies. *Neurology* 1990;**40**:1067–92.

31 Pestronk A. Invited review: motor neuropathies, motor neuron disorders and anti-glycolipid antibodies. *Muscle Nerve* 1991;**14**:927–36.

32 Szabo A, Dalmau J, Manly G, *et al.* HuD, a paraneoplastic encephalomyelitis antigen, contains RNA-binding domains and is homologous to Elav and Sex-lethal. *Cell* 1991;**67**: 325–33.

33 Leigh PN. Amyotrophic lateral sclerosis and other motor neuron disorders. *Curr Opinion Neurol Neurosurg* 1991;**4**:586–96.

34 Kurtzke JF. Risk factors in amyotrophic lateral sclerosis. In: Rowland LP, ed. *Amyotrophic lateral sclerosis and other motor neuron diseases, advances in neurology*, vol 56. New York: Raven Press, 1991:245–70.

35 Lilienfield DE, Chan E, Ehland J, Goobold J, Landrigan PJ, Marsh G, *et al.* Rising mortality from motor neuron disease in the USA, 1962–1984. *Lancet* 1989;**i**:710–3.

36 Chancellor AM, Warlow CP. Adult onset motor neuron disease: worldwide mortality, incidence, and distribution since 1950. *J Neurol Neurosurg Psychiatry* 1992;**55**:1106–15.

37 Neilson S, Robinson I, Rose FC, Hunter M. Rising mortality from motor neuron disease: an explanation. *Acta Neurol Scand* 1993;**87**:184–91.

38 Sienko DG, Davis JP, Taylor JA, Brooks BR. Amyotrophic lateral sclerosis. A case-control study following detection of a cluster in a small Wisconsin community. *Arch Neurol* 1990; **47**:38–41.

39 Swingler RJ, Fraser H, Warlow CP. Motor neuron disease and polio in Scotland. *J Neurol Neurosurg Psychiatry* 1992;**55**:1116–20.

40 Spencer PS, Nunn PB, Hugon J, *et al.* Linkage of Guam amyotrophic lateral sclerosis—parkinsonism-dementia to a plant excitotoxin. *Science* 1987;**237**:517–22.

41 Duncan MW, Steel JC, Kopin IJ, Markey SP. 2-amino-3-(methylamino)-propanoic acid (BMAA) in cycad flour: an unlikely cause of amyotrophic lateral sclerosis and parkinsonism-dementia of Guam. *Neurology* 1990;**40**:767–72.

42 Elian M, Dean G. The changing pattern of motor neuron disease and multiple sclerosis in England and Wales and the Republic of Ireland. *Neuroepidemiology* 1992;**11**:236–43.

43 Dean G, Elian M. Motor neuron disease and multiple sclerosis mortality in Australia, New Zealand, and South Africa compared with England and Wales. *J Neurol Neurosurg Psychiatry* 1993;**56**:633–7.

44 Olivares L, San Esteban E, Alter M. Mexican "resistance" to amyotrophic lateral sclerosis. *Arch Neurol* 1972;**27**:397–402.

45 Caroscio JT, Calhoun WF, Yahr MD. Prognostic factors in motor neuron disease: a prospective study of longevity. In: FC Rose, ed. *Research progress in motor neuron disease.* London: Pitman Books, 1984:34–43.

46 Chancellor AM, Slattery JM, Fraser H, Swingler RJ, Holloway SM, Warlow CP. The prognosis of adult onset motor neuron disease: a prospective study based on the Scottish motor neuron disease register. *J Neurol* 1993;**240**:339–46.

47 Mulder DW, Howard FM. Patient resistance and prognosis in amyotrophic lateral sclerosis. *Mayo Clin Proc* 1976;**51**:532–41.

48 Tucker T, Layzer RB, Miller RG, Chad D. Subacute reversible motor neuron disease. *Neurology* 1991;**41**:1541–4.

49 Hogg KE, Goldstein LH, Leigh PN. The psychological impact of motor neuron disease. *Psychol Med* 1994;**24**:625–32.

50 Plaitakis A, Berl S, Yahr MD. Abnormal glutamate metabolism in adult-onset neurological disorder. *Science* 1982;**215**:193–6.

51 The Italian ALS Study Group. Branched-chain amino acids and amyotrophic lateral sclerosis: a treatment failure? *Neurology* 1993;**53**:2466–70.

52 Bensimon G, Lacomblez V, Meininger V and the ALS/riluzole study group. A controlled trial of riluzole in amyotrophic lateral sclerosis. *N Engl J Med* 1994;**330**:585–91.

53 Benoit E, Escande D. Riluzole specifically blocks inactivated Na channels in myelinated nerve fibre. *Pflügers Arch* 1991;**419**:603–9.

54 Doble A, Hubert JP, Blanchard JC. Pertussis toxin pretreatment abolishes the inhibitory effect of riluzole and carbachol on D-[³H]aspartate release from cultured cerebellar granule cells. *Neurosci Lett* 1992;**140**:251–4.

55 Louwerse ES, Weverling GJ, Tijssen J-GP, Meyjes FEP, de Jong JMBV. The efficacy of N-acetylcysteine in amyotrophic lateral sclerosis. [Abstract] *4th International Symposium on ALS/MND, Neuroprotection and Clinical Trials*, Paris, 1993.

56 Dittrich F, Thoenen H, Sendtner M. Ciliary neurotrophic factor: pharmacokinetics and acute phase response in rat. *Ann Neurol* 1994;**35**:151–63.

57 Rowland LP. Amyotrophic lateral sclerosis: theories and therapies. *Ann Neurol* 1994;**35**: 129–30.

58 Caroni P, Grandes P. Nerve sprouting in innervated adult skeletal muscle induced by exposure to elevated levels of insulin-like growth factors. *J Cell Biol* 1990;**110**:1307–17.

59 Yu E, Callison KV, Roberts-Lewis JM, Grebow P. The effect of insulin-like growth factor-1 on the neuromuscular junction in adult rat skeletal muscle. *Soc Neurosci Abstr* 1991;**17**: 225A [abstract].

60 Yan Q, Elliott J, Snider WD. Brain-derived neurotrophic factor rescues spinal motor neurons from axotomy-induced cell death. *Nature* 1992;**360**:753–5.

61 Oppenheim RW, Qin-Wei Y, Prevette D, Yan Q. Brain-derived neurotrophic factor rescues developing avian motoneurons from cell death. *Nature* 1992;**360**:755–7.

62 Chaudhry V, Corse AM, Cornblath DR, *et al.* Multifocal motor neuropathy: response to human immune globulin. *Ann Neurol* 1993;**33**:237–42.

63 Drachman DB, Chaudhry V, Cornblath D, *et al.* Trial of immunosuppression in amyotrophic lateral sclerosis using total lymphoid irradiation. *Ann Neurol* 1994;**35**:142–50.

64 Glenn Smith R, Hamilton S, Hofmann F, *et al.* Serum antibodies to L-type calcium channels in patients with amyotrophic lateral sclerosis. *N Engl J Med* 1992;**327**:1721–8.

65 Kimura F, Smith RG, Delbono O, *et al.* Amyotrophic lateral sclerosis patient antibodies label CA²⁺ channel α_1 subunit. *Ann Neurol* 1994;**35**:164–71.

66 Enderby PM, Langton Hewer R. *Management of motor neuron disease.* Edinburgh: Churchill Livingstone, 1987:22–47.

67 Saunders CM, Walsh TD, Smith M. Hospice care in motor neuron disease. In: CM Saunders, ed. *Hospice: the living idea.* London: Edward Arnold, 1981:126–55.

68 O'Brien T. Kelly M, Saunders C. Motor neuron disease: a hospice perspective. *BMJ* 1992; **304**:471–3.

69 Crossner CG. Salivary flow rate in children and adolescents. *Swed Dent J* 1984;**8**:271–6.

70 Zalin H, Cooney TC. Chorda tympani neurectomy—a new approach to submandibular salivary obstruction. *Br J Surg* 1974;**61**:391–4.

71 Langton Hewer R, Enderby PM. Bulbar dysfunction. In: Clifford F, Rose F, eds. *Amyotrophics lateral sclerosis*, vol 1 New York: Demos, 1990:99–107.

72 Norris FH, Smith RA, Denys EH. Motor neuron disease: towards better care. *BMJ* 1985; **291**:259–62.

73 Simmonds AK. Sleep studies of respiratory function and home respiratory support. *BMJ* 1994;**309**:35–40.

74 Kerby GR, Mayer LS, Pingleton SK. Nocturnal positive pressure ventilation via nasal mask. *Am Rev Resp Dis* 1987;**135**:738–40.

75 Sullivan CE, Issa FG, Berthon-Jones M, Eves L. Reversal of obstructive sleep apnoea by controlled positive airway pressure applied through the nares. *Lancet* 1981;i:862–5.

76 Howard RS, Wiles GM, Loh L. Respiratory complications and their management in motor neuron disease. *Brain* 1989;**112**:1155–70.

77 Moss AH, Casey P, Stocking CB, Roos RP, Brooks BR, Siegler M. Home ventilation for amyotrophic lateral sclerosis patients: outcomes, costs, and patient, family and physician attitudes. *Neurology* 1993;**43**:438–43.

78 Chalmers RM, Howard RS, Wiles CM, Spencer GT. Use of the rocking bed in the treatment of neurogenic respiratory insufficiency. *Q J Med* 1994;**87**:423–9.

79 Newrick PG, Langton Hewer R. Pain in motor neuron disease. *J Neurol Neurosurg Psychiatry* 1985;**48**:838–40.

11 Resources and facilities

R LANGTON HEWER, I M S WILKINSON

In discussing the resources and facilities available to neurological patients it is useful to define an abitrary boundary between the diagnostic and therapeutic aspects of neurology as traditionally practised on one hand, and the later management of chronic disability on the other. Patients with tremor and rigidity of the limbs may be diagnosed as having Parkinson's disease. They will require appropriate medication which may need to be modified as time passes. This requires the skill and experience of the type usually available from a neurologist. As the years pass, however, medication becomes progressively less effective. Eventually, patients may become immobile and develop other problems relating to speech, cognition, bladder control, and posture. At this later stage disability problems predominate, and a different set of treatment or management skills are required—those of a neurorehabilitationist.

This chapter is written by two authors in two sections. The first looks at the resources and facilities currently available for diagnosing and managing patients with neurological disorders, the second with neurological disability. Both relate to the United Kingdom.

DIAGNOSING AND MANAGING PATIENTS WITH NEUROLOGICAL DISORDERS

Patients in the United Kingdom who develop neurological problems might reasonably expect to be able to consult a neurologist without undue delay, in a hospital near where they live. They would like to be sure that the neurologist is up to date, well informed, and able to make available all appropriate investigations necessary to confirm the diagnosis. Patients would also expect every treatment method to be readily available. They would welcome adequate time for them and members of their families to discuss their condition and its management with the neurologist, supported by written information if they want it. If the condition is a chronic one, they would expect some sort of continued monitoring by the neurologist.

These modest expectations have been the subject of three working papers recently produced by the Association of British Neurologists (*UK National Audit of the Care of Common Neurological Disorders* (1992) (see appendix 11.1, *Good Neurological Practice* (1993), and *Guidelines for the Care of Patients with Common Neurological Disorders in the UK* (1993)) available from their office at 9 Fitzroy Square, London W1P 5AH. The data used in the first section of this chapter, discussing the expectations compared with the reality for patients with neurological disorders in the United Kingdom, are derived from these three papers. The issues are discussed under the following headings: access to consultant neurologists, quality of consultant neurologists, access to neurological investigations, access to neurological treatment methods, time for discussion, and monitoring chronic neurological disorders.

Access to consultant neurologists

Box 11.1 shows the current pattern of referral of patients with neurological disorders to British neurologists. Table 11.1 lists in rank order the 16 disorders that accounted for 74% of the new patients referred to neurologists in the large audit study group. The remaining 26% of new referrals was largely composed of patients with less common neurological disorders, many of whom require a disproportionate amount of time and resources (just as the more rare complex disorders within any specialty do).

Waiting lists

The mean interval between the date of referral and the date of initial neurological consultation throughout the United Kingdom is currently about eight weeks. If the patients first seen as ward referrals or as emergency admissions in hospital are excluded, the mean interval between referral and initial consultation for patients who are first seen in outpatients is roughly 10 weeks. Patients with

---

Box 11.1   Current pattern of referral of patients to British neurologists

Referred by general practitioners—60%
Referred by hospital specialists—40%

First seen as outpatients—80%, of which:
   49% are discharged after one visit
   23% are requested to re-attend outpatients,
   8% are requested to be admitted
First seen as inpatients—20%, of which:
   13% are seen as ward referrals
   7% are seen as emergency admissions

First seen in a district general hospital—50%
First seen in a regional neuroscience centre—50%

Table 11.1   Rank order of common neurological disorders referred to British neurologists

Diagnosis	Percentage of patients seen	Cumulative %	
Epilepsy	12·6		
Headache (not migraine)	9·0		
Migraine	8·3		
Cerebrovascular disease (not transient ischaemic attack)	6·7	36·6	36·6
Faint, syncope, collapse	5·0		
Cervical disc disease	4·3		
Peripheral nerve palsy	3·9		
Transient ischaemic attack	3·6		
Multiple sclerosis (possible/probable)	3·2	20·0	56·6
Multiple sclerosis (definite)			
Dizziness, giddiness			
Parkinson's disease			
Lumbosacral disc disease			
Cranial nerve palsy			
Peripheral neuropathy			
Facial pain			
Dementia		17·4	74·0

neurological disorders must find the delayed access to neurologists unacceptable. Mean figures indicate variation, and there is considerable regional variation in outpatient waiting times. The expectations of patients with neurological complaints to be able to see a neurologist without undue delay, in a hospital near their homes, may be further frustrated for several further reasons.

Sources of referral

A general practitioner may not initiate a referral. Variation has always been recognised in the rates of referral between general practitioners. This variation had had nothing to do with the financial consequences of patient referral, but this is now an additional factor to be borne in mind. The general practitioner may refer the patient to a consultant other than a neurologist, such as a general physician, geriatrician, orthopaedic surgeon, or neurosurgeon. (The Association of British Neurologists has responded to these factors by writing its own set of guidelines for the referral and care of patients with the 16 common neurological disorders identified above).

Outpatient clinic doctors

Patients may be seen by a neurological trainee in the outpatient clinic (registrar or senior registrar grade, of varying degrees of experience, and under varying closeness of supervision by the neurological consultant) rather than by the neurological consultant.

Teaching role of consultants

Neurological consultants may have the additional role of teaching clinical medical students as well as attending to patients' care in outpatient clinics. This should in no way impair the quality of service offered to the patient, but it may add to the experience an element that the patients had not anticipated.

Numbers of consultants

Not all district general hospitals employ a consultant neurologist (see appendix 2), though this is improving gradually. General practitioners may therefore refer patients to a non-neurological consultant at the local hospital or further afield to a neuroscience unit.

Not all parts of the country have the recommended establishment of neurologists—one full time equivalent neurologist per 200 000 population (see appendix 2). The present evidence is that the United Kingdom has fewer neurological specialists per head of population than virtually any country in the Western world. Most countries in Europe have at least six times as many specialists pro rata.

Access to neurologists proves most difficult in the parts of the United Kingdom where the establishment falls seriously below the recommended figure. The patients requiring neurological consultation most urgently—that is, those with neurological emergencies—are often cared for by non-neurologists, being admitted to hospital as emergencies under the care of general physicians or geriatricians. Subsequent review by neurologists over the next few days, as ward referrals, may or may not occur depending on the views of the generalist in charge and on the availability of neurological consultants.

Quality of neurologists

Recruitment to clinical neurology is competitive, and the postgraduate training of clinical neurologists in the United Kingdom is, in general, strong. The exposure of young neurologists in training to several consultant neurologists, and to consultants in associated neurological disciplines at the neuroscience centres within the United Kingdom, is a strength of the country's system which must remain highly valued.

British neurologists are in three broad categories. Firstly, academic neurologists who are based at teaching hospitals and neuroscience centres; secondly, NHS neurologists who are based at neuroscience centres and go out to provide neurological services at one or two district general hospitals; and thirdly, NHS neurologists who are based at a district general hospital and spend some time each week at the neuroscience centre.

The main factor that maintains the quality of each of the three types of neurologist is the weekly educational activity occurring at the regional neuroscience centre. Interaction with colleagues within all the clinical neuroscience disciplines, educational and audit sessions, participation in the training of young neurologists and

---

Box 11.2   Investigations most commonly used by British neurologists in their management of patients with common neurological disorders, in rank order of frequency

Computerised tomography of the head or spine
Electroencephalography
Electromyography or nerve conduction studies
Other neurophysiological investigations
    for example, evoked potentials and special
    electroencephalographic techniques
Magnetic resonance imaging of the head or spine
Non-invasive arterial imaging
    for example, doppler studies and magnetic resonance
    angiography
Inpatient investigation
    for example, lumbar puncture
    myelogram with or without computed tomography
    angiogram involving intra-arterial injection
    biopsy of brain, muscle, or nerve

---

clinical students, and clinical research activity abound at such centres. The maintenance of the quality of British neurologists depends heavily on the continued strength of the neuroscience centres and the full and regular involvement of neurologists of all types therein.

As with all consultants in the United Kingdom, protected time in the week for continuing education and audit, and freedom to take study leave, are important contractual requirements for the maintenance of high quality neurologists.

Access to neurological investigations

Box 11.2 lists, in rank order as found by the 1992 audit study, the investigations used by neurologists in their management of patients with common neurological disorders. Since 1992 there have been changes in the use of investigations by neurologists. The benefits of carotid endarterectomy have increased the referral of patients with transient ischaemic attacks and minor stroke and thus the requirement for non-invasive and invasive arterial imaging. Magnetic resonance imaging facilities are developing, increasing

277

their use and decreasing the requirement for other more invasive investigations such as myelography. Some observations about each of the commonly used investigations follow.

Computed tomography of the head and spine

Computed tomographic scanners are widely distributed now to nearly all district general hospitals, mainly as a result of local charity appeals rather than by NHS provision. Availability is therefore good. For the neurologist and neurological patient there is a difference in confidence between the result of a scan reported by a consultant neuroradiologist and by a general radiologist. The availability of the scanner is one thing, the quality of reporting is another. This would be a topic for useful clinical audit.

Electroencephalography, electromyography, and other neurophysiological investigations

Such facilities are likely to be sited at the neuroscience centres and larger district general hospitals only. The patient is likely to wait, and to travel, to have these investigations performed. Availability is therefore still a factor. The distribution of consultant neurophysiologists in the United Kingdom is uneven, with many parts of the country still underprovided. This results in neurophysiological investigations being carried out and reported by non-specialist neurophysiologists, usually neurologists or rheumatologists, which undoubtedly raises the issue of quality of service.

Magnetic resonance imaging of the head and spine

Major problems of availability and quality still abound regarding magnetic resonance technology for patients with neurological disorders. Though facilities are slowly increasing, they are still far behind requirements. The difference in value of an investigation selected after consultation and carried out by an informed neuroradiologist checking a clinical neurological disorder using a first class scanner, compared with a report from a general radiologist on scans produced by a mobile scanning unit visiting a district general hospital, is appreciable. Neuroradiologists at neuroscience centres are commonly put in the invidious position of being asked

278

to make confident conclusions about magnetic resonance scans of inferior quality carried out elsewhere on patients seen by neurologists in district general hospitals. Neurologists working at district general hospitals may well have to use the magnetic resonance facility contracted by the district general hospital, rather than the magnetic resonance facility run by the neuroradiologists at the neuroscience unit. It is in neurological patients' interest that the use of magnetic resonance technology to investigate neurological diagnostic problems should always involve neuroradiologists.

Non-invasive arterial imaging

Non-invasive arterial imaging of both extracranial and intracranial arteries is a rapidly improving specialty. Magnetic resonance angiography will probably diminish the need for conventional invasive angiography over the next few years. Such sophisticated facilities are likely to be sited at the neuroscience centres. Meanwhile, any wait for doppler studies or magnetic resonance angiography by patients who have had transient ischaemic attacks is of concern, because time is important in these patients as critical carotid artery disease should be identified and treated before stroke develops. A "fast track" service for this group of patients is proving difficult to provide.

Inpatient investigation

Inpatient investigation means a wait from the time of contact between patient and neurologist in the outpatient clinic and the patient's subsequent admission; the mean wait is currently five weeks in the United Kingdom. Neurological units are not always able to coordinate a prebooked date for an investigation with the patient's admission date. Inefficiency, for the patient and for hospital bed use, results while the patient waits after admission for the investigation ordered. Neuroradiology units may require this inbuilt inefficiency to restrict investigations to numbers that their staff and equipment can manage.

Quality is an issue again here; myelographic investigations carried out by neuroradiologists in neuroscience centres differ from those that can be accomplished by general radiologists in district general hospitals. Similarly, central or peripheral nervous tissue biopsies

279

should not be carried out unless the tissue will be processed and examined by a proper neuropathological service. This means that these investigations need to be carried out at a neuroscience centre, and that each centre must have the service of trained specialist pathologists.

Access to neurological treatment methods

Drugs

No problems exist in providing routine pharmacological treatment of patients with the common neurological disorders such as epilepsy, migraine, stroke, spasticity, bladder problems, Parkinson's disease, and pain. Providing current and developing pharmacological treatments that are expensive, however, is much more problematic. The expense of intravenous methylprednisolone for patients with multiple sclerosis in relapse, which is a common clinical problem for neurologists, has been absorbed. The possible regular use of beta interferon for patients with multiple sclerosis presents a formidable problem of expense. Plasma exchange treatment, immunoglobulin therapy, and botulinum toxin therapy are not available at the level required for patients with peripheral nerve and neuromuscular disorders or with focal dystonias—purely on the grounds of expense. Developing budgets to provide such expensive treatments for uncommon conditions is extremely difficult in today's provider and user health care system in the United Kingdom.

Surgery

Surgical treatment of urgent neurological problems, such as subarachnoid haemorrhage caused by berry aneurysm, intracranial mass lesion, or spinal cord compression, is available at regional neuroscience centres. Surgical treatment of non-urgent problems, such as peripheral nerve entrapment or cervical or lumbar nerve root compression by intervertebral disc disease, may entail long waiting lists for patients who may be appreciably disabled. Evolving surgical treatments, such as neurosurgery for epilepsy and carotid endarterectomy, are held back by inadequate investment in the necessary investigation facilities to identify the patients who will benefit from the surgery. Referring patients to pain clinics often entails long waiting lists.

Occupational, physiotherapy, and speech therapy

The quality of paramedical therapists is high but their numbers for the work to be done are lamentably small in most areas. Their organisational fragmentation into caring for hospital inpatients, hospital outpatients, and patients at home in the community creates great practical and funding difficulties for patients with neurological disability who need their services.

Neurological disability is less hidden than a decade ago, but facilities and specialists (both medical and paramedical) require massive development. Coordination of care for neurologically disabled people in the community has undoubtedly improved in terms of daily living requirements, but so far targeted paramedical therapy organised by neurorehabilitation specialists exists in only small pockets of the country.

Genetic advice

Access for neurological patients to advice and diagnostic services by clinical genetics units is important now that knowledge of inherited disease is growing fast. Good units with the necessary counselling teams are developing, and this should be encouraged.

Time for discussion

Inpatient

There is usually adequate time and privacy for neurological inpatients and their relatives to discuss fully with the neurologist their illness and its management. Inpatients are, however, a small minority—about 10% of new patients currently requiring admission—of patients seen by neurologists.

281

Outpatient

Time for discussion in outpatient clinics is very much more scarce. Most neurologists in the United Kingdom need to keep an eye firmly on the clock throughout each clinic as they are working in the face of inexorable time pressure. There are several reasons for this. Rates of referral to the neurological outpatient clinic by general practitioners and by other hospital specialists, have increased. Discussions with neurological patients about their diagnosis and management have shifted from neurological wards to neurological outpatient clinics. This shift is the result of the increased sophistication of neuroradiological and neurophysiological diagnostic technology, allowing a definitive diagnosis to be established on an outpatient basis, or after an overnight stay on a programmed investigation unit, where no opportunity exists to discuss the result of investigations with the patient.

Full explanations of conditions like multiple sclerosis or motor neuron disease to patients and their families in outpatient clinics will increase considerably the delays for the rest of the patients due to see the neurologist in the same clinic. This cannot be corrected by better planning and organisation of clinics because so many patients need to be seen in each outpatient session. Neurologists will probably have junior staff to supervise and clinical medical students to educate in some of their outpatient clinics each week. Furthermore, the government's *Patient's Charter* has given publicity to waiting times in outpatient clinics, and the right of all patients to be seen by consultants. Recommendations regarding duration of consultations for new and follow up patients are easy for the Association of British Neurologists to make but difficult to apply in the face of current referral rates to neurological outpatient clinics.

Trust philosophies regarding the care of patients, emphasising their need to be treated as individuals, and highlighting dignity, respect, independence, compassion, understanding, time, patience, honesty, reassurance, encouragement, information, and involvement, are praiseworthy. In busy neurological outpatient clinics, however, compromise is occurring. Here, neurologists are perhaps feeling more hypocritical than Hippocratic, especially because they know that length of discussion time is the essential difference between the service that they can offer within the NHS compared with the service they offer to private patients.

Lack of proper time for explanation and discussion is a fertile source for patient dissatisfaction and misunderstanding, which has unfortunate practical consequences in patients' understanding of their illnesses and of their correct management. Attitudes of families towards patients' illnesses may also suffer.

Monitoring of neurological disorders

Short term, or acute, episodes

Many of the common neurological disorders identified earlier (such as an epileptic fit, many forms of headache, transient ischaemic attack or stroke, a faint, dizziness, a peripheral nerve palsy, or a problem with cervical or lumbar disc disease) are not chronic but acute or transient episodes. Patients with them often need to be seen once only by a neurologist, and investigation results and treatment recommendations are posted to the general practitioner and patient.

Some of the other common neurological disorders (such as epilepsy, migraine, multiple sclerosis, Parkinson's disease, peripheral neuropathy, and dementia) are chronic, but the patients do not need long term regular follow up care from neurologists because the conditions are mild and can be managed perfectly satisfactorily by most general practitioners after some initial diagnostic activity and suggested management plans by a neurologist.

Long term, or chronic, disorders

Of patients with one of the common neurological disorders who consult a neurologist in the United Kingdom, currently 60% are seen once only. Their subsequent care, if needed, is in the hands of the referring doctor. Patients who should be followed up long term by the neurologist are mostly in two broad categories: (1) those with severe manifestations of common disorders, or (2) those with rare disorders.

Patients who have severe manifestations of one of the common neurological disorders have appreciable long term disabilities and expect specialist advice, and their general practitioners expect specialist support. Both expectations are reasonable. Severe epilepsy, severe Parkinson's disease, and active multiple sclerosis are the main disorders in this category. Longer term care of patients with dementia, on the other hand, tends to be organised by the psychiatric and psychogeriatric services.

The more rare chronic neurological disorders, about which general practitioners need not expect to feel competent and informed, include narcolepsy, some neurological manifestations of arteritis or vasculitis, benign intracranial hypertension, extrapyramidal syndromes other than Parkinson's disease, syringomyelia, motor neuron disease, rare forms of peripheral neuropathy, myasthenia gravis, muscle disease, and neurological manifestations of AIDS or immune deficiency from other causes. Some aspects of the long term care of patients with these disorders can probably be attempted by neurologists only because only they are sufficiently informed.

Long term care of patients in each of these two groups by neurologists in outpatient clinics is compromised. Chronically ill patients generally have to share outpatient clinic time with new referrals to the clinic, and inadequate consultant time in the clinic remains the overriding restriction. Follow up consultations are often hurried, incomplete, and ineffective because of this time pressure. Patients who should receive consultant attention may be seen by junior staff who may be suboptimally supervised, and who change often during the treatment of patients with chronic neurological disorders. To reduce overall patient numbers attending a clinic, patients may be discharged despite needing longer term support. Full implementation of help from paramedical therapists, and from agencies provided by the neurological charities, often suffers because of insufficient time to consider all aspects of patients' care.

MANAGING PATIENTS WITH NEUROLOGICAL DISABILITY

Background

Disorders of the nervous system are responsible for a large proportion of severe disability in all age groups.[1 2] Such disability is associated with many different symptoms and problems such as ataxia, weakness, incontinence, and pain. This section presents some of the background facts and identifies what resources and

284

facilities are currently available or likely to become available soon.

This section is written against the background of important recent developments. Firstly, the new purchaser and provider arrangements, which entail separating the purchasing from the providing functions and then constructing business plans and contracts between the two parties. Much power is now placed in the hands of the purchasers, who are in the district health authorities and fundholding general practitioners. Secondly, the government document, *Health of the Nation*[3] identifies several priorities, such as stroke and coronary artery disease, and emphasises preventing disease (for example, by detecting and treating hypertension). Thirdly, emphasis is being placed upon audit—the setting and monitoring of standards. Many groups are involved with standard setting, including the government (*Patient's Charter*),[4] consumer organisations (such as neurological charities),[5] and professional bodies (for example, the Royal College of Physicians[6] and the Association of British Neurologists[7]). Fourthly, there is an ever increasing demand for evidence about the cost effectiveness of interventions such as stroke wards and epilepsy clinics. Lastly, there is the issue of geography, with greater emphasis being placed on care being provided as near to the patient's home as possible and district health authorities increasingly unwilling to purchase services from outside their own boundaries. This has obvious implications for centre-based services, which include neuroscience facilities such as neurosurgery, neurophysiology, and (to a considerable extent) clinical neurology. Furthermore, there is an intention to reduce hospital-based activity in favour of community provision in health centres and patients' homes.

This is a time of great change but also of opportunity. Traditional ways of providing services are being questioned and, in some instances, modified or even abandoned. Such changes may eventually be of benefit, but need careful evaluation after the collection and presentation of evidence. The changes have major implications for all involved in the delivery of neurological services.

Epidemiology

For the purpose of this review a neurological disorder is defined as one that has a recognisable structural or physiological (or both) basis involving the nervous system or one that is usually included, whether by convention or practice, within the purview of clinical neurology. This definition therefore covers Alzheimer's disease and sciatica but not schizophrenia or manic depressive psychosis. There are obviously many important interfaces with other disciplines, including general practice, general medicine, psychiatry, paediatrics, and orthopaedics. Neurological disability is defined as disability arising from a neurological disorder.

An average health district of 250 000 people will contain 4000–5000 with a disabling neurological disorder. Of these, up to 1500 will require daily help to enable them to remain out of institutional care.[1] Most disabled people are elderly—suffering disorders such as Alzheimer's disease, Parkinson's disease, or stroke. Experience indicates that 200–250 people aged 16–65 will be severely physically disabled and require help during much of a 24 hour period. At least 90% of these will have a neurological disorder.

Four major categories of disabling neurological disorders may be recognised: (1) those that cause major physical disability affecting mobility, self care, and everyday activities (for example, multiple sclerosis and Parkinson's disease); (2) those that cause disturbance of cognition or behaviour, or both (for example, head injury and Huntington's chorea); (3) those that cause pain (for example, trigeminal neuralgia, postherpetic neuralgia, and migraine); and (4) those that cause recurrent disturbances of consciousness or neurological function, or both (for example, epilepsy and narcolepsy). Clearly, some patients will fall into more than one category. Thus a patient with Parkinson's disease may also show intellectual deterioration. Table 11.2 gives some rough figures for seven major neurological disorders in an average health district of 250 000 and in a group practice serving 10 000 people. These figures do not represent the whole picture, however, because of the very many neurological disorders that exist.

Practical implications of the epidemiological position

A few common disorders exist, such as stroke, Parkinson's disease, and migraine. There are also many uncommon disorders (such as muscular dystrophy, Huntington's chorea, myasthenia gravis, Friedreich's ataxia, cerebral tumour, spina bifida, cervical

Table 11.2 Seven common disabling neurological disorders

	Prevalence of disabilities	
	Per 10 000 (No)	Per 1/4 m (No)
Stroke	60 (36)	1500 (900)
Parkinson's disease	10 (15)	480 (360)
Multiple sclerosis	12 (9)	300 (225)
Motor neuron disease	1	14
Head injury	? 15	? (about 350)
Epilepsy	150 (50)*	3750 (1250)*
Alzheimer's disease and dementia	150	3750

*For epilepsy the figure in brackets is the number receiving anticonvulsant treatment.
The figures in this table are for an "average" health district of 250 000 and for a group practice serving 10 000 people, and are based on information collected by Wade and Langton Hewer.[1]

myelopathy, and peripheral neuropathy), which together affect many patients and generate a major workload.

In addition, there are more than 100 disabling neurological symptoms or problems such as spasticity, incontinence, sexual impotence, diplopia, and facial muscle weakness. The adverse effects of most neurological disorders can be ameliorated by appropriate treatment or management, which may include counselling and giving advice. This requires considerable expertise, however, and necessitates ready access to the appropriate services.

Most neurological disorders can be managed within a patient's immediate locality. Some, however, require expertise at supra-district or national level. These include those that present particularly difficult diagnostic problems and rare disorders for which there is unlikely to be local expertise and which require advice and support (such as hereditary ataxias and uncommon muscle disease).

There are also patients who present with particularly difficult symptomatic problems, such as refractory epilepsy (including those requiring surgery) or severe spasticity or unusual involuntary movements.

The ready availability of expertise is an essential element of neurological provision, and it is most important that this should not be restricted by geographical or financial reasons. The ability to refer to appropriate centres elsewhere in the United Kingdom should be preserved.

287

It should be noted that neurological and non-neurological patients (such as those with rheumatoid arthritis or severe asthma) experience many of the same problems—for example, immobility, inappropriate housing, and limited educational opportunity.

Age and disability

It is important to note the age structure of the population under consideration. For practical purposes five groups may be identified.[2] The first contains children, the second disabled school leavers and young people, in which three arbitrary sub-groups may be identified—those with mainly physical problems, those with mainly learning difficulties, and those with mixed problems. There is little published epidemiological data. Chamberlain *et al* and current work in Bristol suggests that a population of 250 000 people will generate 30–40 disabled school leavers a year.[8] Of these, 10–15 will have mainly physical problems—about half will have spina bifida, about a quarter cerebral palsy, and the remaining quarter will have a wide range of conditions such as muscular dystrophy, hereditary ataxias, and epilepsy. Rheumatological, respiratory, and gastrointestinal problems account for a few children leaving school with major physical problems. Thomas *et al* found that communication skills, mobility, upper limb function, nutritional status, and skin care may all deteriorate after leaving school.[9] Such deterioration is likely to restrict the young person's independence but may well be largely preventable. Disabled young adults may also benefit from supervision of anticonvulsant medication, dental care, and many other topics, as well as counselling for themselves and their families.

The third group consists of people aged 25–54 who are developing families, jobs, and careers. This is the core of the "young disabled" group. Multiple sclerosis is responsible for nearly half the physically disabled people in this group. Most of the remainder who are severely disabled have neurological disorders. The fourth group consists of people aged 55–74—those reaching the end of employment and enjoying active retirement. Parkinson's disease, stroke, and dementia become increasingly important at this stage. The last group contains those aged 75 or more. About half of this group have disabilities—often due to multiple disorders.

Box 11.3   Some objectives of a specialist rehabilitation service

- Support or advice for general practitioners
- Assessment and reassessment at intervals
- Surveillance of at risk groups—for example, those with rapidly progressing motor neuron disease
- Control of symptoms such as severe spasticity, dysphagia, or incontinence
- Provision of information to patients, carers, and professional staff
- Education for professional staff and others

Stroke becomes increasingly important as a cause of disability with rising age. Parkinson's disease and Alzheimer's disease are further important causes.

Rehabilitation services

Rehabilitation is now recognised as a specific medical speciality. There are about 42 full time consultants in rehabilitation and a further 20 part time appointments. At the moment few health districts have access to specialist rehabilitation expertise, but this situation is gradually improving. A recent joint working party of the Association of British Neurologists, the Neuroconcern Group of Medical Charities, and the British Society for Rehabilitation Medicine has recommended that there should be a consultant in rehabilitation medicine for every 200 000 of the population.[10] At the moment, there is one such consultant for about 1·2 million people. A recent analysis of workload shows that the vast majority of clinical work undertaken by consultants in rehabilitation concerns patients with neurological disorders (Ward AR. Personal communication, 1994). Box 11.3 lists some objectives of a specialist rehabilitation service.

The shortage of neurologists has already been pointed out. Specific neurological expertise is clearly in short supply (see appendix 2) and most neurologists are currently unable to devote a major amount of their time to disability and its management. Many hospital patients with neurological disease are looked after by general physicians and geriatricians (appendix 3 and table 11.3).

Table 11.3 Total discharges of patients with one of six neurological disorders, and deaths by specialty, from hospital beds in England and Wales during 24 months 1988–90

| | Total No | % Occupying beds of specialties of: | | | Comment |
		Neurology	General medicine	Geriatrics	
Stroke	185 130	3	38	43	General practice 7% Neurosurgery 7%
Head injury	163 661	<1	<1	<1	General surgery 27% Accident and emergency 22% Trauma or orthopaedics 28% Paediatrics 9%
Anterior horn cell disease	4 428	39	22	14	Miscellaneous 15%
Multiple sclerosis	21 593	43	23	8	
Epilepsy	63 431	8	47	9	Paediatrics 19%
Parkinson's disease	23 749	12	15	58	
Total	461 992				

Box 11.4   Some other services used by disabled persons

- Respite care
- Equipment (such as wheelchairs)
- Residential care
- Rehousing or housing alterations
- Help with everyday activities—such as, cleaning, shopping, and cooking
- Advice regarding finances and state allowances
- Advice regarding employment and recreation

Services for the neurologically disabled are thus clearly severely constrained by a shortage of senior staff in both clinical neurology and rehabilitation.

Rehabilitation is a complicated activity, and involves many different professional groupings, including social workers, nurses, and therapists. Box 11.3 lists what a specialist rehabilitation service might be able to offer. The members of such a service must be willing to collaborate fully with general practitioners and their teams.

Effective rehabilitation depends upon the existence of many different staff and services. In the British system care in the community is largely the responsibility of the social services, and not of the NHS. Voluntary organisations or charities are often able to provide advice, support, and information. Ensuring effective collaboration between these various organisations represents a considerable challenge.

The large number of disabling neurological symptoms or problems has already been mentioned. For example, spasticity can be one of the most difficult symptoms to control. It requires great expertise which may include the use of pumps delivering intrathecal baclofen or surgery, or both. Spasticity management tends to be focused increasingly in a few centres in the United Kingdom because of the breadth of experience required. Pain is another neurological symptom, and the local pain service may have to be asked to help in managing such problems as post-herpetic neuralgia, thalamic pain, and traction injuries of the brachial plexus. Ataxia and involuntary movements are another important group of neurological symptoms, and several special clinics have been set up in the United Kingdom.

Many neurological patients are liable to develop contractures and postural deformities. These can often be prevented, which will be one of the main objectives of the domiciliary physiotherapy and rehabilitation service. Chronic respiratory insufficiency occurs in several disorders, including motor neuron disease and high spinal cord lesions. In a few cases, providing some form of assisted ventilation in the patient's home may be appropriate, particularly at night. Dysphagia is common, particularly in motor neuron disease and in many stroke patients. Its careful assessment and management is a skilled exercise and may involve the use of alternative feeding techniques such as nasogastric tubes and percutaneous gastrostomy. Dysphagia, dysarthria, and dysphonia are all common sequelae of neurological disease, and ready access to the speech therapy services and to communication aids is essential. Urinary incontinence is another common disorder, particularly in patients with multiple sclerosis. Effective interventions include consultant urological advice, urodynamic assessment, and the deployment of nurse continence advisers. Sexual problems, particularly erectile incompetence, are common in neurological practice—particularly multiple sclerosis. Assessment, papaverine injections, and advice or counselling are all effective interventions, and this service should be available in each locality.

Clinics

Disability assessment and management takes time. Dealing with difficult rehabilitation problems in a routine neurology clinic usually proves difficult, if not impossible. Patients greatly dislike many elements of such clinics, including long waiting times, short consultation times, and being seen by inexperienced junior staff. The neurological charities have indicated that patients should expect a coordinated and patient centred approach, using a multidisciplinary team when appropriate.[11]

Disease specific clinics are being increasingly operated for patients with, for example, epilepsy, Parkinson's disease, and multiple sclerosis. So far, there has been little objective evaluation of such clinics. Some units are known to operate specific disability clinics.

There is also an increasing move towards using specialist staff to work with neurologists or rehabilitation specialists. These include a liaison nurse, a specialist social worker, a key worker, and a neurological physiotherapist. A specialist multidisciplinary team should be in a position to liaise between hospitals and the community—working with consultants and the general practitioners. In this way, it ought to be possible to provide improved care and support for patients with chronic neurological disease (an example would be the Romford project[11]).

Special units

Several special units or departments deal with chronic neurological disease in the United Kingdom.

Spinal injury

The spinal injury service is well developed in the United Kingdom thanks to the pioneering work of Sir Ludwig Guttmann and his colleagues. Eight spinal injury centres provide prolonged inpatient care and rehabilitation and a regular review thereafter. This service is to some extent a model—some of the elements could be replicated in other areas.

Head injury

Head injury services are, in contrast, poorly developed. There are a handful of special units, some of which deal with major behavioural disorders. Most patients are looked after without specialist involvement, however, and there has been widespread dissatisfaction with the quality of provision.

Epilepsy

Several inpatient units exist for patients with uncontrolled epilepsy, and a few centres provide surgery for intractable epilepsy.

APPENDICES

Appendix 11.1   UK national audit of the care of common neurological disorders by the services subcommittee of the Association of British Neurologists and the research unit of the Royal College of Physicians

Thirty four consultant neurologists, representing the various sorts of neurologist and all parts of the UK, collected data regarding all new patients (outpatient clinics, domiciliary visits, emergency admissions, and ward referrals) seen in a two week period in November, 1991.

Of 1620 patients seen, five disorders (epilepsy, syncope, migraine, other headache, and cerebrovascular disease), accounted for 45%, and the 16 most common neurological disorders accounted for 74%.

(1) Of the 1203 patients suffering from the 16 most common neurological disorders 61% had been referred by general practitioners and 39% by hospital specialists; 50% were seen in regional neurological centres, 49% in district general hospitals, and 1% on domiciliary visits; 80% were seen as outpatients, and 20% as emergency admissions or ward referrals. Their mean age was 45 years. The male:female ratio was 47:53.

(2) Of the 955 patients first seen in outpatients, 61% were discharged after one visit, 29% were requested to reattend, and 10% were admitted; 62% of the patients were seen within 10 weeks from the date of the referral letter.

(3) Of 248 patients first seen as inpatients, 33% were emergency admissions and 67% were ward referrals (of which 60% remained under the care of the referring team, only 7% being transferred to neurological beds).

(4) Of the 184 patients admitted to neurological beds (from outpatients, as emergencies, or as transferred ward referrals), the average length of stay was 6·5 days and in 161 instances (88%) the neurological bed was located in the regional neurological centre. The mean interval between outpatient attendance and admission, in patients admitted from outpatients, was 5·0 weeks.

(5) Epilepsy was the most common single neurological disorder, the most common condition for follow up arrangements to be made after the first outpatient attendance, and the most common cause for admission to a neurological bed.

(6) The rate of use of diagnostic investigation, ordered by neurologists, in each of the 16 most common neurological disorders has been established. This does not take into account investigations arranged before neurological consultation, which is particularly relevant in the case of ward referrals (166 (14%) of the 1203 patients). Computed tomography of the brain, electroencephalography, and electromyography or nerve conduction studies were the three most common investigations.

(7) The resource implications of running a neurological service to care for the most common neurological disorders can be deduced per 100 cases of each condition. This can be done reliably for the four most common disorders (epilepsy, migraine, other headache, and cerebrovascular disease other than transient ischaemic attacks), and fairly reliably for the five next most common disorders (syncope, transient ischaemic attack, cervical disc disease, peripheral nerve palsy, and possible or probable multiple sclerosis). This information is available in the form of the numbers of: new outpatient appointments, follow up outpatient appointments, admissions and length of stay, and investigations performed.

Appendix 11.2 The number and distribution of consultant neurologists in the United Kingdom

Information about the number and distribution of neurologists comes from two sources. The first is a study undertaken on behalf of the Association of British Neurologists in 1987.[12] The second is the *Annual Review of Medical Staffing Prospects in the National Health Service in England and Wales.*[13]

Actual number of neurologists

There were 178 neurologists in post in 1986 and 215 in 1991.[13] This gives an annual growth of seven posts (3·9%) on the 1986 figures. About 18% of consultant neurological time has been shown to be used for academic work or private practice, and is therefore not available to the NHS.[12] If the 18% figure is accepted then the number of whole time equivalent neurologists in the United Kingdom in 1991 is reduced to 176. If the population of the United Kingdom, which includes Great Britain and Northern Ireland, is assumed to be 56·78 million then 322 613 people were served by each whole time neurologist in 1991.

Recommended number of neurologists, and shortfall

The Association of British Neurologists has recommended that there should be one whole time equivalent neurologist per 200 000 of the population. If the British population of 56·78 million is assumed then 335 neurologists will be required to meet the target, assuming that the 18% for academic and private work is still correct. This means 120 new posts. If the annual growth rate of seven posts a year is continued the Association of British Neurologists' target will be reached by the year 2008. This projection assumes no population growth, however, and makes no allowance for any geographical inequality in the distribution of consultant posts.

Distribution of neurologists

A study in 1987 found that 22% of health districts in England and Wales had the services of a full time neurologist, but 19% of health districts had less than one neurological session each week, and in 14% no neurological clinic was held.[12] It seems clear, therefore, that there is an overall shortage of neurologists and that this position is compounded by unequal distribution. There are no up to date figures on the distribution of neurologists and, for example, the proportion of general hospitals that have an appreciable number of consultant neurological sessions is not known. A new review is required.

Appendix 11.3   Hospital resources

Neurological centres

The 1987 study identified 40 neurological or neurosurgical centres, which were in health districts containing 19% of the population; 56% of consultant sessions were allocated to these districts.[12] Such centres make important contributions to the diagnosis and acute management of neurological and neurosurgical patients, but probably provide little specific expertise in disability management. No detailed analyses of the work of neurological centres has been published, and there has been no evaluation of centre-based versus district-based provision.

General hospitals

The term district general hospital is now to some extent redundant after the recent NHS changes. This means that the previous study of neurological services cannot be repeated in the same way as before.[12] The term general hospital is now used instead of district general hospital. An unpublished study from Bristol identified 340 hospitals with more than 100 beds that accept unselected medical emergencies. The distribution of neurological sessions and beds in these hospitals is not known.

A study undertaken from Bristol (Langton Hewer R, Wood VA. Unpublished data, 1992) covering the years 1988–90 analysed inpatient data for all hospitals in England and Wales concerning six common neurological disorders. A total of 461 992 patients were identified as having been discharged from, or died in, the bed of one of three specialties. Table 11.3 gives the relevant information. The analysis shows that neurologists look after nearly half of some groups of patients, particularly those with anterior horn cell disease or multiple sclerosis, but only small proportions of patients with stroke, head injury, or epilepsy. Both general medicine and geriatrics feature prominently as specialties concerned with managing many neurological disorders, particularly stroke. Nearly 60% of patients in hospital with Parkinson's disease were looked after by geriatricians. This study gave no information about the number of inpatients who had been seen by consultant neurologists while in hospital. Furthermore, the reason that patients were in hospital was not known, but many were probably in for rehabilitation reasons. This study emphasises the need to analyse the use of hospital beds by neurological patients and other groups. It also seems clear that there is a need for specific neurological expertise in general hospitals.

Little published information exists relating to the disability profile of patients in general hospitals. Up to 20% of general medical beds, however, are known to be occupied by stroke patients. Some evidence exists that segregation of such patients into stroke wards may be beneficial (Langton Hewer R, Wood VA. Unpublished data, 1992), but there is no published information about how many already exist in England and Wales.

Resources and facilities

There are deficiencies in most of the facilities and resources available for patients with neurological disorders and for patients with neurological disability, as follows

- By international standards, there are very few neurologists in the United Kingdom. The target of the Association of British Neurologists of one full time neurologist per 200 000 of the population is likely to be reached by the year 2008 at the present rate of expansion
- The neurosciences centres need to be strengthened
- Some enhancement of neurological outpatient facilities is required. This will necessitate an increase in the number of neurologists and also full use of supporting staff such as specially trained nurses
- Access to high quality, modern, neurological investigation and treatment methods should be easier for the relatively few patients who need them
- Neurological disability is common. Many disabling problems can be eliminated, or at least ameliorated, but expertise is required. An increasing number of neurologists are developing particular skills in this area
- There are few consultants in rehabilitation medicine. More are needed
- General practitioners are in a key or pivotal position. Specialist neurological services should work closely with GPs and their teams
- The effective management of disability depends to a large extent on the existence of core services such as respite care and domiciliary treatment. These need to be augmented. The many staff who are involved in the care of neurologically disabled people need improved education

1 Wade DT, Langton Hewer R. Epidemiology of some neurological diseases. *Int Rehab Med* 1987;**8**:129–37.

2 Warren M. The prevalence of disability. *J R Coll Physicians Lond* 1989;**23**:171–5.

3 *The health of the nation.* Government White Paper, 1990. London: HMSO, 1990.

4 Department of Health. *The patient's charter.* London: HMSO, 1991.

5 Neurological Alliance. *Living with a neurological condition: standards of services for quality of life.* London: Neurological Alliance, 1992.

6 Neurology Working Group, Royal College of Physicians. Standards of care for patients with neurological disease. *J Roy Coll Phys* 1990;**24**:90–7.

7 *Policy statement on the number and distribution of consultants in adult neurology.* Association of British Neurologists. 1990.

8 Chamberlain MA, Guthrie S, Kettle M, Stowe J. An assessment of health and related needs of physically handicapped young adults. *Report to the Department of Health*, 1992.

8a Chamberlain MA. Effective health care: stroke rehabilitation. Leeds: University of Leeds, 1992.

9 Thomas AP, Bax MCO, Smyth DPL. *The health and social needs of young adults with physical disabilities.* Oxford: MacKeith Press, 1989.

10 Joint Working Party of the Association of British Neurologists, The Neuroconcern Group of Medical Charities, and the British Society for Rehabilitation Medicine. *Neurological Rehabilitation in the United Kingdom.* London: Neurological Alliance, 1992.

11 Neurological Alliance. *Neurological provision: key areas and targets.* Neurological Alliance. Response to *Health of the Nation* by 26 Neurological Charities. London: Neurological Alliance, 1991.

12 Langton Hewer R, Wood VA. Neurology in the United Kingdom. II. A Study of current neurological services for adults. *J Neurol Neurosurg Psychiatry* 1992;**55**(suppl):8–14.

13 Medical and dental staffing prospects for the NHS in England and Wales, 1991. *Health Trends* 1993;**25**:4–12.

12 Neurorehabilitation

D L McLELLAN

Introduction

Neurological conditions contribute to disability in 13% of disabled people living at home and 30% of disabled people living in residential institutions in the United Kingdom.[1] The increased proportion of people in institutions with neurological disability reflects the severe impact on daily life of conditions that affect the brain, bringing about a combination of impairment of physical function, cognitive function, and behaviour. In children, adults, and elderly people the impact of such combinations of impairment is much greater than would be anticipated from simply adding the scores of each component disability.[2]

The essence of rehabilitation is the acquisition of new knowledge and skills to achieve a lifestyle that is desired by the patient. The human qualities of resilience, courage, and determination are particularly relevant. As with any educational process, those who feel able psychologically to take responsibility for their day to day life, and are committed to achieving specific goals, tend to make the greatest progress. Natural recovery does not itself depend very much on such factors, but the biological processes of tissue repair and reorganisation of function do not realise their practical potential without considerable effort on the part of the disabled person.

Those wishing to help someone achieve rehabilitation must therefore spend a lot of time and effort in engaging the interest, conviction, and energies of the patient—much as a skilled teacher spurs students to a level of performance and self fulfilment that they would not otherwise have reached.

The term neurorehabilitation also implies, to some, the existence of additional mechanisms in the nervous system that could be manipulated from outside the patient. Drugs or surgery can be used to change pathology and augment function in many specialties of medicine, needing no effort from the patient apart from acquiescence in the treatment. The function of the nervous system may also be changed by the use of electrical stimulation applied to muscles, skin, nerves, or different parts of the central nervous system itself to suppress unwanted activity such as tremor, pain, or spasticity or to augment impaired function as in the electrical stimulation of muscle. The application of this range of technologies has been termed restorative neurology.

Some forms of physical therapy such as repeated stretching of spastic muscles may also affect CNS function in a helpful way, although the effects are usually short lived so repeated intervention is necessary. Most of the pharmacological methods used to alter bowel and bladder function, the perception of pain, the excitability of motor neurons, and so forth do not bring about a lasting change, but rather a temporary perturbation of function that is either helpful or unhelpful depending on the dose used and the objective of treatment. By contrast, the value of knowledge and skills that have been acquired by the patient is generally greater because these functions decay much more slowly, do not depend on continual intervention from outside, and are directly under the patient's control. Recent advances in the understanding of how neural networks operate in the cerebral cortex have given an impetus to clinical studies of mental rehearsal in improving subsequent performance in people who are physically constrained from undertaking exercise by the acute effects of an injury.[3]

Rehabilitation medicine thus has a different frame of reference from most traditional medical and surgical specialties. It overlaps most obviously with the specialist areas of learning disability, psychiatry, and rehabilitation of the elderly. Rehabilitation's frame of reference also encompasses education, physical and cognitive neuroscience, sociology, physical and psychological therapies, and bioengineering. Most medical practitioners have not received specific training in rehabilitation medicine and some may have difficulty in defining their role—or even feeling that they have a role at all—once their armamentarium of drugs and surgery has been deployed.

To help medical students build up a conceptual framework of rehabilitation, Paul Dieppe, Dean of Bristol University Medical School, has introduced the familiarly bucolic acronym PILS (box 12.1). Musculoskeletal function is covered by the acronym GALS (gait, arms, legs, spine). Students are taught to be able to comment

---

Box 12.1   PILS rehabilitation framework

- Prevention (of complications)
- Independence (acquisition of the capacity to undertake the basic activities of daily living and to make choices)
- Lifestyle (the ability to follow a lifestyle of the disabled person's choosing)
- Social support (which may need to be augmented if people are isolated or have impairments of communication, cognition or behaviour)

Box 12.2   The A to H of prevention

- Accidents (for example, falls due to impaired mobility, inappropriate techniques of transferring, inappropriate environment or equipment; injuries in the kitchen arising from perceptual inattention, ataxia, inappropriate equipment, lack of a sense of smell, etc)
- Broken skin (pressure sores)
- Contractures
- Diet (body weight, state of nutrition)
- Elimination (bladder and bowel)
- Fitness (for example, failure to achieve basic independence because of the combined effects of muscular weakness through disease and other neurological deficits)
- General Health, Grief, and Heartache (including physical pain and other "medical" consequences such as stress, anxiety, and depression as well as the impoverishment of personal and family life)

---

on any abnormality in these areas and to record normal function explicitly with a tick. Prevention has been memorably packaged by Christopher Ward, professor of rehabilitation medicine at the University of Nottingham, as the A to H of prevention (box 12.2). Achieving all this is a tall order, and it is immediately obvious that medical practitioners cannot possibly provide on their own the help that a disabled person needs—to be effective they have to function as members of a multiprofessional team. The parody figure of a post-Edwardian consultant, dominating his staff and attempting to educate his followers through fear and ridicule, is the antithesis of a successful practitioner of rehabilitation medicine.

This chapter is specifically concerned with the rehabilitation that can be achieved by people with neurological disabilities, and how this process is best facilitated. In practical terms, rehabilitation in hospital has an emphasis and set of imperatives that differ from those of rehabilitation at home. This is largely because most inpatient rehabilitation takes place during the initial phases of recovery after an acute onset of disability through disease or injury—for example, after a stroke, traumatic brain injury, attack of encephalitis, or spinal cord injury. Medical priorities tend to be relatively prominent at this stage because there are pathological and pathophysiological processes to be stabilised. The patient and family are often in a state of psychological shock, with little or no experience of the implications of disability and rehabilitation. "Natural" biological recovery is often occurring (or is fervently hoped for), and the patient may therefore have a confused picture of the relation between the effort he is expending and the changes concurrently taking place in his performance. Such bewilderment may be reinforced by confusion in the mind of the patient's medical practitioner. A discharge summary about a woman discharged from my own hospital after a stroke read: "The patient underwent a good spontaneous recovery with physiotherapy." Neither the patient nor the physiotherapist was amused.

The inpatient phase

The principal functions to be achieved in this phase are: (1) stabilisation of: the underlying medical condition, respiratory function, nutrition, and elimination; (2) establishment of effective communication and trust between the inpatient team on the one hand and the patient and close family members on the other; (3) shared understanding of previous interests, attributes, and lifestyle of the patient in order to set the rehabilitation objectives; (4) prediction of the probable time scale and extent of functional recovery; (5) agreement between all concerned about (a) the level of function that would be needed for the patient to return home, and (b) the degree of support that can realistically and appropriately be expected from the family; (6) regular and repeated exchange of information about the above issues and the type of procedures to be used in rehabilitation, including the prevention of complications;

(7) setting up an appropriate sequence of short term objectives, and implementing the treatment and education needed to achieve them; and (8) counselling and support of patients and relatives.

Stabilisation of basic functions

The priorities of stabilisation are to ensure an adequate intake of calories and protein. The biological processes of recovery are prejudiced by negative nitrogen balance,[4] and the first few weeks after an illness or injury is not usually the appropriate time to starve people who are overweight. Energy requirements are greatly increased by spasticity and rises in temperature, whether from intercurrent infection or hypothalamic disturbance. The effectiveness of absorption from the gastrointestinal tract is also impaired in people who are in the acute or postacute phase of an illness.[5a–5c]

Many neurological conditions cause difficulties in chewing and swallowing. Eating and drinking may therefore be difficult, uncomfortable, and frightening for patients whose limited capacities may fatigue rapidly and make oral feeding impracticable. Damage to the frontal lobes and hypothalamus (as after subarachnoid haemorrhage or traumatic brain injury) can cause disturbances of fluid balance and suppression of the desire to eat and drink, which a patient may be unable to overcome by voluntary effort—a sort of acute anorexia. These features can understandably be accentuated in some people by the effects of fear, stress, and discomfort.

Maintaining a good state of nutrition is vitally important. Sometimes it is self evident from the routine neurological examination that movement of the lips, tongue, palate, and epiglottis are too impaired for oral feeding to be safe. Where there is doubt, close observation of the patient's capacity to take a sip of water is helpful because in neurogenic dysphagia liquids are more difficult to swallow than solids. The consistency of food that is offered must be carefully controlled. Speech and language therapists who have been specifically trained in the assessment of oropharyngeal function and swallowing, and in the management of choking, are an important source of expertise to the patient and other members of the rehabilitation team.[6]

The widespread use of percutaneous endoscopic gastrostomy has revolutionised the feeding of people who are unable to swallow

305

safely. Even fine-bore nasogastric tubes are uncomfortable and often poorly tolerated by people who are frightened or confused, and do not provide such good protection against inhalation of foreign material and respiratory infection. All patients who are not being fed orally must be weighed weekly. For those who are being nursed in bed there are expensive devices that measure the weight of the bed with and without its occupant. If patients can be lifted by two nurses a cheaper alternative is for each nurse to stand on a weighing scale and record the combined increase in weight registered on the scales as the patient is lifted clear of the bed.

Continence

The initial management of incontinence or retention of urine in an acutely ill patient is often to insert an indwelling catheter. These are often left in situ for far too long. In males who are incontinent without retention, a condom drainage system is preferable. For people who in their confusion pull on their catheters or experience repeated urinary infections, it is usually better to remove the catheter and to resort to appropriate forms of padding. Repeated and frequent checks by staff are then needed to ensure timely changes of padding, clothing, and bedding.

The return or retraining of bladder function after spinal cord injury is more predictable, and formal protocols are often used.[7] Considerable technical advances have been achieved in the use of implanted electrical stimulators to confer continence, erection, and seminal emission in people with paraplegia and complete lack of sensation below a spinal cord lesion.[8a-8d] Training in the voluntary control of urinary incontinence cannot begin until the indwelling catheter has been removed. The usual approach is to invite the patient to empty the bladder at two hour intervals. Once limited tolerance is established the intervals can be gradually increased. Nocturnal incontinence may continue for some time after daytime continence has been established. Continence of faeces is usually acquired first, the initial aim being to achieve evacuation at predictable times.

Communication

The first priority is for the patient to be able to signal basic needs or states of mind (such as thirst, pain, or other forms of distress) and preferences—at its simplest, to indicate "yes" or "no".

This task is most difficult when the level of consciousness is impaired or there are pronounced impairments of cognitive function and language. In these circumstances very careful observation is needed. Wide-angle lens video recording systems can be useful in identifying interactions between patients and their environments. Such recordings help provide evidence of the level of awareness, something of the content of consciousness, and the presence of perceptual difficulties such as visual inattention. They can also provide clues about the most appropriate input to use in a system of communication—for example, whether visual or auditory stimuli are eliciting the greater response—and whether the subject is capable of reliable motor responses that could be used to activate electronic switches.

People who know the patient well can often tell a great deal from their facial expression. When relatives and staff disagree about a patient's responses the passage of time usually shows that the family was right (the main exception being the patient who remains in a persistent vegetative state for six months or more after the event).

Formal assessment of treatment by speech and language therapists is an essential resource in the management of people with communication difficulties.[9a 9b] The therapists will advise on the selection of communication aids and electronic switchgear appropriate for individual patients with dysarthria or anarthria. People with dysphasia may find signing systems such as Bliss Symbols, Macaton, or Amerind, very difficult to use. Treating people with dysphasia involves time-consuming work on generating the confidence to attempt interaction with others and educating and training family members.

Apart from the basic requirements of making day to day choices, patients may need to communicate or simply to express emotions and fears. Arts-related therapies such as art or music therapy may be particularly valuable for people with aphasia or cognitive impairment or who, for other reasons, are unable to express or resolve disabling emotions. These therapies do of course require sufficient motor function for the patient to participate in the relevant medium, but with advances in technology such as "Soundbeam" even very restricted or poorly controlled movements can be harnessed to generate a wide range of sounds over which the subject becomes able to develop an effective degree of control.[10]

> **Box 12.3   General principles governing the way in which staff should approach patients with reduced consciousness**
>
> - Assume that understanding is not impaired. Speak calmly and clearly using simple sentences and in a tone of voice appropriate for addressing a sentient adult
> - Avoid background noise and other distractions, including the need for the patient to interact with more than one person at a time
> - Before any procedure, explain by words and gesture what is going to be done and, for patients who show awareness, check that they are willing for the procedure to go ahead before starting it
> - People whose impairments are recent and severe often have a short attention span and fatigue rapidly. Make allowances for this and do not leave them in a noisy environment where frequent periods of rest are impossible
> - The position and comfort of patients is vitally important. Whenever possible they should be comfortably seated in an upright position, supported as necessary, at the same eye level as the person communicating with them

Basic activities of daily living: the interaction of motor, sensory, and cognitive functions

Often considered the province of occupational therapists, basic activities require additional help from rehabilitation nurses and clinical psychologists. Skills to be acquired at this stage are those of washing, grooming (shaving, making up, etc), dressing and undressing, and guiding food and drink to the mouth. Patients must be able to turn over or adjust their position in bed to avoid the need for being turned at regular intervals. Transferring—the ability to move oneself between chair, bed, wheelchair, and toilet—is a basic set of skills that are crucial for independence.

The nature of the therapy given depends on how these basic functions are impeded. Weakness demands the use of exercises to build up strength and the use of specialised equipment to allow function to be achieved with reduced strength. If family members plan to help in, for example, transferring they have to be trained in the appropriate methods so that transfers are completed safely without injuring the carer. Carers must also be educated to assess what patients are capable of doing for themselves and not to disempower them by providing unnecessary help.

Sensory loss and impairment of vision may create obvious barriers for which specific training is needed. Perceptual disorders (such as sensory or visual inattention, disorders of spatial awareness, and sensory or visual agnosia) can prove difficult to circumvent because patients whose non-dominant occipitoparietal areas are damaged may lose awareness of part of space or part of the body and have little or no sense that anything is amiss. They can become very angry and frustrated if their attention is repeatedly drawn to deficits that they are unable to perceive. The best strategy is to supplement repeated explanation by building up a systematic approach to each task, using cognitive signposting, planning, and prompting until patients have learnt the appropriate sequence of functions and the ability to monitor their performances.

Basic activities become even more difficult to learn if there are coexisting impairments of frontal lobe function such as attention, planning, sequencing, and self-initiation of activity. In these circumstances, one helpful approach is to divide a task into a sequence of consecutive components or segments, helping the patient until the beginning of the final segment and, when that one has been learnt, progressively withdrawing help segment by segment ("backward chaining") until the whole task has been learnt. "Forward chaining" is sometimes a more appropriate alternative, but backward training has the advantage that a reward, in the form of successful completion of the task, is delivered at each trial. A quiet environment, no distractions, a clear and calm approach, and the avoidance of fatigue are important environmental ingredients in undertaking this training successfully.

Patients with amnesia may not remember previous treatment sessions but can nevertheless acquire new knowledge and skills by the process of "procedural learning" in which proficiency is gradually acquired by repetition even though the patient cannot recall to consciousness the fact that training has been given. Recently it has been realised that an "errorless learning" approach can accelerate procedural learning in patients with amnesia.[11] If they attempt to learn by trial and error, as each error is made it lowers the threshold for making the same error next time. Having no conscious memory of the previous mistake, the patient has no cognitive signpost to warn of a trap and falls into it with increasing alacrity each time—learning to make the error, rather than to follow the desired path. By continued supervision, prompting, and guidance, errors can be avoided from the outset and the patient protected from learning them.

These approaches require a sound practical grasp of the basis of cognitive psychology and are very labour intensive, usually requiring one-to-one input by an experienced professional.

Mobility, spasticity, and the prevention of deformities

A basic principle of managing people with impaired voluntary movement is that each joint should be put through a full range of movement several times in every 24 hour period to prevent progressive loss of range in the joint due to a combination of reduced compliance of the joint capsule and contractures of the muscles. This is a skilled task, for which physiotherapists and rehabilitation nurses are specifically trained. Excessive force can damage the soft tissues and may lead to subluxation of the joint, an increased risk of joint pain, and possibly to myositis ossificans.

Contractures can start to be clinically detectable in paralysed patients after as little as one week, especially if severe spasticity is keeping a joint in a static position at one end of its range throughout each 24 hours. The amount of time that a flexed muscle needs to be stretched to its full length to avoid contracture is not known. For ambulant children with spastic cerebral palsy, six hours' stretch per 24 hours is sufficient to prevent contracture at the ankle joint.[12] For a severely spastic immobile patient recovering from a head injury, however, more than 12 hours in 24 hours is required.[13] It may be necessary to encase the limb in plaster and remove, reposition, and replace the plaster each week. Sometimes the strength of involuntary contracture is so great that splints and plasters cause damage to the soft tissues. If this seems likely, nerve or muscle blocks with alcohol or phenol or infiltration of the relevant muscle with botulinum toxin should be considered.[14] These measures are much better than inflicting excessively painful stretches on the patient or allowing contractures to develop.

If contractures do develop, they can cause a great deal of discomfort and travail to the patient later in recovery, requiring further surgery and admission to hospital. The most common sites are the ankles, knees, hips, shoulders, wrists, and fingers, but any muscle group in the body can be affected.

Spasticity

Spasticity is an inappropriate and excessive involuntary contraction of skeletal muscles occurring in association with an upper motor neuron syndrome. Passive stretch responses are characteristically increased, the resistance increasing with velocity of stretch. It also increases with the degree of stretch in flexor muscles, but decreases in the outer ranges of stretch of extensor muscles (the clasp knife response). Increased muscle activation at rest and during stretch impedes positioning and the prevention of contractures. Spastic muscles are not necessarily activated when they are stretched during the process of voluntary movement, however, because the mechanism of reciprocal inhibition of antagonist muscles may be unimpaired, especially in mild or moderate spasticity. Even in severe spasticity, restraint of voluntary movement by spastic antagonist muscles is more likely to occur as part of a spastic synergy (a stereotyped pattern of activation and antagonism) occurring equally strongly in isotonic and isometric conditions. Antispastic medication such as baclofen can reduce spastic stretch responses, and also the frequency and intensity of involuntary spasms, without affecting the pattern of activation during voluntary movements. Better functional results may be obtained from focal nerve or muscle blocks, although it is not yet clear whether continuing suppression can be maintained for more than about three years by these means.[15]

There is good evidence that periods of prolonged stretch (20 to 30 minutes) of a spastic muscle or muscle group can in some subjects lead to a reduction in resting tone and an improvement in voluntary function lasting six to eight hours. Such physiotherapy needs ideally to be given daily or twice a day.[16]

Many experienced physiotherapists believe that spasticity can be reduced by careful training, and in particular by insisting that voluntary limb and trunk movements approach a "normal" configuration as closely as possible and by avoiding excessive effort that could intensify the degree of spasticity or give rise to spasm as the movement proceeds. Thus patients recovering from stroke may be discouraged from walking (even though they have recovered the ability to do so) until they are able to re-learn a pattern of movement that approaches the non-impaired state more closely. Though there is little scientific evidence to support this strategy, there is none to refute it. These approaches have given rise to many interesting theories and observations that call out for further research.

Remobilisation of a severely impaired person is a time-consuming process requiring a skilled physiotherapist and the resources of a small gymnasium. Severely disabled patients may need work by two or three therapists together. A common strategy is to encourage the reacquisition of control of absolute postural proximal girdle musculature, moving on to the reacquisition of sitting balance, standing, standing balance, walking over smooth ground, and finally walking on rough ground and ascending and descending stairs.[17]

Wheelchairs, special seating, and orthoses

Essential resources exist for optimum motor function in many neurologically disabled people. Service standards appropriate to the United Kingdom have recently been published by the Amputee Medical Rehabilitation Society and the Royal College of Physicians.[18]

Mobility is needed within the home, in its immediate environment, and further afield. Maintaining the ability to stand and walk is important physically and psychologically, but so is the need to get about and participate in social life and work with the minimum of unnecessary energy expenditure, discomfort, or risk. Wheelchairs may be needed on a temporary basis—for example, by those recovering from a stroke or a relapse of multiple sclerosis. Other people, such as adolescents with four-limb cerebral palsy entering the "growth spurt" or adults with motor neuron disease, may come to depend upon them increasingly. Accurate identification of the problems to be solved by a wheelchair is essential for its successful provision; delays in provision are very demoralising for the patient.

Neurological conditions call for careful correlations between (a) the need to provide a comfortable seating position that provides support and discourages deformity, and (b) the weight and dimensions of the chair. Many patients have established or intermittent weakness of the arms (which are needed to push) and hands (which are needed to grip the propulsion rim). The location of the patient's centre of gravity relative to the rear axle is crucial—directly over the axle allows for optimum propulsive efficiency (provided that the height above it is appropriate for

312

Box 12.4   Four key questions to be considered in relation to wheelchair provision

1 How will the patient get into and out of the chair?
2 How strong are the patient's arms and hands? Over what terrain and for what purposes will the chair be used? Who will be providing the propulsive force?
3 Are there difficulties with trunk control or support?
4 Are there any cognitive or psychological factors that could restrict the selection or use of the chair?

---

extensor thrust from the arms to be delivered tangentially to the rim) but gives greater risk of instability and overturning. The location of the axle in the vertical and anteroposterior planes must be checked for each patient and revised if, for example, a new cushion is provided that changes the previous relation.

Special seating needs (such as a moulded insert or matrix seating) usually imply impaired arm function, and the additional weight entailed may predicate an electrically driven wheelchair. Technology exists to allow powered wheelchairs to be controlled by the occupant or an assistant. The combination of computerisation and voice recognition and spatial scanning systems implies greatly enhanced possibilities for independent control in the future, even for those with cognitive impairments who cannot at present be protected against collisions with their surroundings.

For full postural control, seating may have to be specifically shaped to contain the patient comfortably if deformity is already present and to prevent deterioration. All skin contact points must be considered carefully to ensure that undue pressures are not applied. It is important to remember that people may have other chairs they wish to sit in at home, which may need adaptation. Some plastic moulded seating systems allow for an insert shaped to the patient to move with the patient into a range of different chairs throughout the day. In practice this is easier to contrive for children because they can be carried more easily. Many people are understandably reluctant to use equipment that looks institutional or clinical in the familiar surroundings of their own home.

Regarding the control of sitting posture, the key element to get right is the position of the pelvis and thighs, for they provide the basis of support for the trunk. After this, the most difficult area to

313

cater for is the head, especially for those with weakness or involuntary movements of the neck. The head needs to be upright for optimum social interaction and for feeding. Collars are not tolerated well, especially when involuntary movements are taking place, because they are hot and restrictive, chafe the skin, and prevent full opening of the mouth. A head band linked flexibly to a point of attachment above and behind the head is much more useful, although such arrangements restrict the number of different places or chairs in which a person can sit.

A final point to note is that many neurological patients are put to totally unnecessary discomfort and inconvenience because basic wheelchair monitoring has not been done: the most frequent failures are footrests, which should be at the right height and angle; cushions, which should be in good condition and provide effective distribution of weight-bearing; and tyres, which should be kept fully inflated. Flat tyres can increase the energy costs of propulsion by 50%.

Orthoses

Orthoses are externally applied devices that constrain the movement of a body segment or provide it with support. They are more difficult to fit and are less well tolerated in conditions of increased tone or involuntary movements than in flaccid weakness. Successful use of orthoses requires a precise biomechanical objective to have been agreed, a skilled orthotist to ensure that it actually performs its function and fits the patient without damaging soft tissues or taking up too much space, and commitment (preferably enthusiastic) from the patient.

Orthoses may be fixed (like a cock-up splint for the wrist), have restricted flexibility (as in bespoke footwear or support collars) or moderate flexibility (one piece polypropylene ankle and foot orthoses for flaccid foot drop), or be dynamic (specifically allowing movement in certain planes for a specific purpose). Dynamic orthoses range from simple finger-extension springs or hinged ankle and foot orthoses to more complex devices. An example of the latter is the orthosis that enables the digits to be mechanically brought into opposition by dorsiflexion of the wrist, enabling a pinch grip to be achieved by people with flaccid weakness.

Patients often prefer to manage without wearing an orthosis by using trick movements or adapting their surroundings (for example their kitchen and bathroom equipment). The responsibility of rehabilitation professionals is to ensure that appropriate bio-mechanical solutions are offered to patients, together with training in their use, so that they can make informed choices as to whether to use them or not. Their underprovision in the United Kingdom also reflects the fact that the current standard of medical prescription and commercial manufacture of orthoses for neurological patients is generally poor.

Disturbances of behaviour

Disturbances of behaviour can rarely be explained solely by the pattern of physical damage inflicted on the brain. It is wise to assume that disturbed behaviour is primarily the response of the individual to unpleasant or unwanted aspects of his or her environment, including the behaviour of other people. Disturbed behaviour is best regarded as a preventable complication, and prevention is both better and considerably easier than cure.

It is helpful to think of disturbed behaviour in two broad categories—excesses (behaviours that occur too often) and deficits (those that occur less often than is necessary for social and functional independence). Obviously it is important to try to understand the behaviour in the context of the patient's experience of becoming disabled and expectations for the future. The patient's previous pattern of response to stress and adversity, experience of authority and institutions, self-image and hopes for the future, and understanding of the current situation must be understood.

This said, behaviour disturbances are much more common in people with organic cognitive impairment, especially when there are disorders of memory, language, and frontal lobe functions such as attention, concentration, learning, sequencing, judgement, and self-control of emotions.[19] Explaining the nature of these invisible deficits is time-consuming and difficult, but it pays dividends in helping the patient and family understand the reasons for their frustrations and day to day difficulties, and then to make a start on working round them. In support of this approach and running concurrently with it, measures based on associative learning techniques are effective in reinforcing wanted behaviours and suppressing unwanted ones. In most clinical rehabilitation units, reinforcement techniques are easier to apply and ethically more acceptable than punishment and aversive stimuli. Undesirable behaviours can, however, be decreased by differential reinforcement of other behaviours, of incompatible behaviours, and of low rates of the unwanted behaviour. Recent work suggests that the effectiveness of these approaches can be strengthened by training the patient to monitor the occurrence of their own unwanted behaviours.[20]

It is often more difficult to induce desirable behaviours in people with low levels of arousal combined with impaired attention, initiation, and memory. In common clinical parlance, this situation is referred to as lack of drive, or lack of motivation. These terms are imprecise, and their use may obscure the real reason for such behaviour and the optimum strategy for preventing it.

In general, neurorehabilitation for disturbances of behaviour in the United Kingdom appears to be less coherently and effectively practised than the rehabilitation for physical consequences of neurological disease. This may be partly because the presence of behaviour problems goes undetected. A study in which individualised information packs were drawn up by therapists and given to families of people discharged from hospital after a stroke found that the packs were helpful in explaining to relatives the nature and management of physical problems but were criticised for failing to pay close enough regard to disturbances of cognition and behaviour, which tended to cause more problems at home.[22]

Aggressiveness and violence

Aggressiveness and violence tends to be seen most frequently in people recovering from diffuse brain injury associated with trauma, subarachnoid haemorrhage, or hypoxia, but it can also occur in other conditions. One recent study comparing the outcome of patients six to 12 months after discharge from hospital found that people who displayed physical violence towards members of hospital staff while inpatients were more likely to do so after returning home.[21] This likelihood was, however, three times greater in those who had been discharged direct from surgical wards than in those with similar patterns and severities of injury who had spent some time in a rehabilitation unit before discharge. In both groups, violent behaviour was associated with impaired memory and high level language disorders. This suggests that some at least of the aggressive behaviour occurring after head injury could be prevented by the avoidance of frustrating situations combined with cognitive counselling, without having to resort to more complex methods of behaviour modification.

Predicting the outcome and setting the goals and objectives

Short term objectives can be set up from the outset. As soon as a consensus has been reached about the level of function and community resources required to enable the patient to return home, negotiations must be started with the community-based teams. Even when communications are good, it is difficult to avoid delays or premature discharge. Discharge home too early restricts the intensity and effectiveness of therapy that can be given and places undue strain on families. Too great a delay in discharge from hospital is demoralising for the patient and family, and this may adversely affect progress after discharge home.

Community phase of rehabilitation and maintenance of function

The above principles apply equally to community rehabilitation, but the setting and day to day objectives are different.

There are three broad categories of disabled adults living at home or in non-hospital settings.

Young adults in transition

Disabled young people entering adult life often have disabilities dating from before birth or from early childhood. Their identity is therefore as a person who has always been functionally different from most other people. Their education has often been restricted or interrupted by the effects of their disability and attempts to treat their underlying disease. Their social experiences and confidence may also have been restricted and they may rely heavily on the support of their parents or other adults both physically and psychologically. At the same time, the specialist umbrella provided by paediatric services is closed as they leave school and the youngsters have to learn to negotiate their follow up in the more fragmented adult medical services. Many drop out and develop preventable complications.[23]

Adults discharged from hospital after sudden onset of disability

For some, the period during which further recovery occurs is relatively short. For example, most survivors of stroke show little change after six to nine months.[24a 24b] At the other end of the scale, after traumatic brain injury, performance often continues to improve for three to five years, and continuing evidence of cognitive improvement can be detected as long as 10 years after the injury.[25a 25b]

After patients are discharged from hospital, they and their families are faced with further readjustment and challenges in the form of social reintegration. The course of these adjustments can be particularly complex in conditions such as traumatic brain injury, where the social challenges to be overcome continue to change as the patient's basic capacities gradually improve. Once such experiences start to lead to frustration, aggression, or withdrawal the patient's social and even physical performance can decline, and regular monitoring is needed to help negotiate solutions to the various new problems as they emerge. The aims for rehabilitation are then: (a) preservation and development of personal independence; (b) preparation for employment and negotiation with the employers of patients whose jobs are still open; (c) establishing the means of communication, mobility, and transport needed for participation in community life; and (d) personal development and recreation.

Adults with established disability that is static or deteriorating

The causes of static conditions include previous spinal cord injury or stroke. Deteriorating impairment is a feature in people with multiple sclerosis, Parkinson's disease, motor neuron disease, and neurodegenerative diseases. All these people are at risk of avoidable complications as listed above and should be offered regular monitoring. For some, skills and functions that have been acquired can only be maintained by constant practice and "maintenance" therapy. This is difficult to obtain because of the inadequate number of therapists available to deliver it and the difficulty of measuring outcome in the absence of precise methods of predicting what will happen if no therapy is given. Nevertheless it is very discouraging for people to have to suffer a loss of mobility or an increase in the extent of their contractures between each burst of maintenance therapy.

Organisation and management of rehabilitation in the community

Current rehabilitation services are fragmented and many do not have the human resources to provide the service required. The person who has a problem with mobility that needs the help of only a physiotherapist may do well. Paradoxically, someone with a complex combination of cognitive, physical, and behavioural problems faces far more difficulty—not only because their impairments are more extensive but also because the relevant therapy and other help is provided by separate groups of people working to different guidelines. Probably the two most important factors are: (1) the presence of a named individual manager responsible for rehabilitation services in a locality; (2) the ability to identify a named individual professional who will maintain contact and take personal professional responsibility for the nature of the package provided. It is possible to identify appropriate targets and indicators for rehabilitation services, but collecting the data systematically enough is difficult because services are so fragmented and general practitioners may not have the skills to do so effectively.[26]

Clinical audit of hospital and community rehabilitation

Clinical audit in rehabilitation is both easier and more difficult than in traditional neurology. It is easier because the clinical team meets regularly for discussion and records the discussion, so that regular opportunities exist for reviewing objectives and progress and reflecting on both. It is more difficult because the range of objectives is much greater and also highly specific to an individual's personal characteristics, disabilities, and social situation.

Moreover, few hospitals at present have more than one rehabilitation team able to cope with the range of neurological disorders, and many hospitals have none at all. Because audit requires mutual reviews between at least two people from different services, there are often considerable logistical difficulties in effecting a meeting between two or more rehabilitation teams for audit purposes. It is never possible for all team members to participate because of the need to maintain a clinical service. This can be countered by ensuring that a rota of attendance by all team members (including the most junior ones) is observed. A more obdurate problem is that there is no tradition yet in the United Kingdom for permitting time "off piste" and travelling expenses for nurses and therapists. Until this is formally embraced by management and the necessary resources are provided, clinical audit for many teams will continue to be partial in both senses of the word.

The two principle objectives of audit are to optimise the effectiveness and competence of the service. The most important test of effectiveness is the outcome for patients and their families. It is also helpful to audit timeliness and efficiency, for which links need to be made between the outcomes attained and the resources available. The basic structure of audit is the same as in other topics of clinical practice. Data are collected as an indicator of the quality of activity; unsatisfactory results are discussed so that a better standard can be set. The changes needed to achieve the standard are identified, the changes are implemented, and relevant new data collected until the next review when it is tested against the standard (the audit cycle).

Outcome measures

Generic outcome measures such as the Barthel scale, the functional independence measure scale, and activities of daily living scale are often used to chart progress. It is certainly helpful for a rehabilitation team to collect comprehensive data about its patients using validated and reliable scales. This enables each patient's location in the range of different types and levels of disability to be logged, and comparisons to be made between the nature of patients' problems and the outcomes achieved in different rehabilitation units. Regular reassessment enables the trajectory of progress to be fed back to the team in the form of bar charts or graphs for each patient.

Whether the outcome scales used are fully relevant to the patient's particular problems and the therapy that is being given is another matter. To ascertain this, it is helpful to record both the current outcome and the anticipated outcome on each occasion that the patient is assessed. Anticipated outcome can relate either to the long term realistically hoped-for outcome or to a medium term outcome such as the level of performance to be achieved to be able to leave hospital. In this way it is possible to check retrospectively whether the team's expectations are realistic and accurate, or in other words whether the performance meets the goal because a legitimate goal has been scored or because the team has moved the goal posts. Even this is unlikely to be enough, because many worthwhile and time-consuming objectives cannot be captured on such generic scales.

The individual goal-setting and review that takes place at the regular team metings must be recorded accurately. Each time a new goal is set, its precise formulation must be agreed by the team in terms that enable everyone (including the patient) to know whether it has been met. For example, "improve standing balance" is a poor formulation because no-one can be certain when the goal is achieved. "To stand for one minute with support, to be achieved by the next but one team meeting" is better. These goals can be related to the patients' therapy and activity timetables to check on the time and resources expended. It is important to record whether the goal was met on time and if it was not, to give the reasons for not attaining it. The inventory currently used in Southampton for this is a modification of the one introduced by Alan Thompson's team at the neurorehabilitation unit at Queen's Square, London (see box 12.5).

A further opportunity provided by this system is for the percentage of goals reached on time, and the relative frequency of reasons for failure, themselves to be audited. Though this gives good data for auditing the efficiency of goal-setting, in our experience the team adjusts its expectations according to the patient's potential and the resources available. About 70–80% of the goals set in the manner described above are achieved irrespective of staff shortages. A higher percentage than this probably indicates that the goals that have been set are insufficiently challenging; too low a percentage is demoralising both for the patient and for the team. Clearly the absolute on generic outcome measures and predictions must come into the equation when evaluating the effectiveness of the service.

The views of patients and relatives or informal carers are also of great importance and should be collected on a regular basis for audit purposes. When attempting to ascertain their degree of satisfaction, it is important to formulate the questions that are posed so as to be able to distinguish between satisfaction with the overall outcome ("But I am still disabled!") and salient aspects of the service being provided.

321

Box 12.5   Coding system for reasons of non-achievement of specific rehabilitation goals by dates set

Patient or condition
001   Patient cognitive difficulties
002   Patient behavioural difficulties
003   Activity tolerance reduced
004   Medication problem (eg toxicity, side effect, etc)
005   Intercurrent illness
006   Pressure area concern
007   Tone problem
008   Coordination problem
009   Patient mood disturbance
010   Neurological improvement
011   Neurological deterioration
012   Cognitive improvement
013   Pain
014   Accident

Patient and carer
020   Patient not available on the unit
021   Patient readmitted to acute unit
022   Patient declines treatment
023   Patient disagrees with goals
024   Carer disagrees with goals
025   Carers unavailable
026   Patient keen
027   Patient reluctant
028   Patient afraid
029   Appointment with carer not made

Therapist nurse or clinician
030   Appointment changed
031   Planned meeting cancelled
032   Await other consultation which has been requested
033   Await other consultation because referral not been made
034   Goal considered inappropriate
035   Assessment unavailable (eg test result missing)
036   Extra therapy given
037   Equipment being adapted
038   Over-optimistic time period
039   Over-cautious time scale for goal
071   Time became available for therapist to work on goal
072   Insufficient communication between team/staff and family/carers
073   Team member forgot to do task

continued overleaf

Box 12.5   Coding system for reasons of non-achievement of specific rehabilitation goals by dates set—*continued*

External system
060   Alternative accommodation unavailable
061   Adaptations incomplete
062   Home care not available yet
063   Transfer to other hospital or ward delayed
064   Transport delay
065   Community care assessment delayed
066   Unavailability of equipment (hoists, ramps, rails, etc)
068   Funding difficulties

Rehabilitation unit systems
040   Staff on annual leave
041   Staff on sick leave
042   Staff on study leave
043   Staff not available for other reason
044   Equipment unavailable (eg hoist unsuitable)
045   Department closed
046   Inadequate information from other units/wards
047   Early discharge (with discussion prior to leaving)
048   Early discharge against medical advice
049   Lack of ward clerk (eg photocopying, notes, etc)
050   Insufficient professional time
051   Necessary skill unavailable
052   Goal set in therapists absence
053   Information lost
054   Lack of training
055   Insufficient communications between team members

Competence of rehabilitation teams

The professional competence of the rehabilitation team as a whole can be assessed using the above approach but this leaves open the matter of the professional competence of individual members of the team. In general terms, this should cover the technical aspects of the team member's performance in assessment, treatment, and effectiveness of communication with the patient, the patient's family, and other team members.

It is difficult but essential to deal effectively with any member of the team who is failing. Close liaison must be maintained between the team leader and the professional supervisor of the team member so that professional advice and support, training, or disciplinary action can be provided as appropriate.

Stress in team members

For team members there is often a considerable emotional and psychological toll in working with newly disabled people and their families through periods of deep personal crisis. Ways of recognising this that help team members understand their own involvement in psychological defences and transference probably offer the best defence against the consequences of unresolved stress—continuing stress and time off work for team members, and unintended abuse of withdrawal from patients. This tends to be dealt with more sophisticatedly and effectively in psychiatric or psychotherapeutic practice, where proactive psychological support for staff is seen as a means of ensuring good practice rather than a symbol of staff failure. Such approaches may have to be introduced obliquely as "staff continuing education and development" to avoid confronting too abruptly the need most of us have to believe that we are well and it is the patient and families who are not. This does pose barriers to effective practice in rehabilitation, but how best to audit them is not clear—at least to me. Employment of a fully accredited psychotherapist to assist rehabilitation medicine teams in their work, and staff time off with stress-related symptoms, would be simple process indicators.

Location and integration of rehabilitation

For the inpatient phase, a rehabilitation ward is essential, with enough space for therapeutic and leisure activities (involving family members or visitors also) and a liberal supply of single-room accommodation. Treatment should be delivered in the dose prescribed by the rehabilitation team with sufficient resources to cover staff holidays and weekends. No-one suggests that only two days' penicillin should be given to treat pneumonia or that treatment should be suspended when the pharmacist is on holiday, yet rehabilitation therapy is frequently restricted or interrupted through inadequate provision.[27] Rehabilitation teams need to be put together carefully, to meet regularly to discuss patients' progress and team needs, and to be led effectively. For inpatient teams this will usually fall to the consultant in rehabilitation medicine who will have been prepared for this task during specialist training. Clinical audit in this specialty needs to cover not only the progress of individual patients and the effectiveness of the team, but the contribution of individual members of the team.

For the community phase, things are more complex. Rehabilitation would theoretically always be achieved best in the location and context of the person's daily life—at home, at work, or out and about. However, the logistics and expense of the resources needed for acute or intensive early phase rehabilitation are such that effective inpatient facilities will be needed to serve each locality for the foreseeable future.

A range of different organisational models is currently being evaluated.[28] Many documents talk of seamless care, but this can happen only when the various professionals and others actually meet each other regularly and work together.[29] Current structures of management often militate against this, different managers being responsible for each profession and located in different hospitals, NHS trusts, community services, and so forth. Integration with the voluntary sector is an unsolved challenge at the moment—volunteers very often end up carrying the can while being isolated operationally from the statutory services.

Conclusion

This chapter attempts to give an overview of neurorehabilitation and to indicate how it relates to acute neurology and to other rehabilitation services. It is an exciting topic wide open for research and for new and more effective methods of improving performance. Developments in specialties as different as neurobiology, cognitive neuroscience and learning theory, and biomechanics, have the potential to transform the options open to disabled people.

At the same time, political and social influences are changing the way that non-disabled people regard disability. Removal of the barriers set up and manned by so called normal people would have an equally profound effect on the quality of life of those with neurological disability.

Management of neurorehabilitation

- The essence of rehabilitation is the acquisition and use of new knowledge and skills to achieve a lifestyle that is desired by the disabled person. It is basically an educational process supplemented by psychological, physical, and medical therapies and the provision of appropriate equipment
- Education and support may also be needed for other members of the patient's family
- Disability may occur as a result of sudden injury or illness, such as stroke, traumatic brain injury, encephalitis, or spinal cord injury. The patient is usually admitted to hospital and medical and surgical stabilisation, psychological adjustment, and rehabilitation have to take place concurrently. The aim is to establish a long term rehabilitation plan, to equip the patient and family for return home (in most cases), and to implement discharge home
- More detailed priorities during the hospital phase are: appropriate nutrition, establishing effective communication with the patient, assessing the person's attributes and impairments, and training in the daily activities needed for physical and psychological independence
- Many disabled people living at home acquired their disabilities at birth or gradually during their adult life. Objectives are to help them to acquire the knowledge and skills needed for adult independence and participation in society. Therapy to improve basic functions is directed towards particular contexts, with liaison with employers, educational and recreational establishments, driving schools, etc
- Teenagers disabled since birth or early childhood whose education and expectations have been restricted may have developed strong patterns of physical and psychological dependence on their families or adults in general. The transition to adult independence is complex and difficult and there is a greatly increased risk of medical complications occurring because of failure to maintain contact with services
- Both hospital and community rehabilitation have prevention of complications as an important general goal. These may be physical (for example, accidental injury, contractures, pressure sores, obesity or undernourishment, urinary tract infections, damage); psychological (stress, anxiety, depression, lack of confidence and self esteem); or social (isolation, underachievement in educational and social activities)

continued overleaf

Management of neurorehabilitation—*continued*

- Rehabilitation requires effective teamwork and the expertise of many professions to provide optimum results in difficult cases. Teams must be built up, educated, nurtured, and well led, and must meet frequently. A named manager should be responsible for the rehabilitation service as a whole, and a named clinical professional worker or social worker for coordinating and monitoring the effects of the programme on each patient. For hospital inpatients the team leader should be a consultant, and for non-elderly adults this will usually be a consultant in rehabilitation medicine
- The scientific basis of rehabilitation overlaps with medical sciences; educational theory; the neurobiology of skill acquisition, cognition, and motor control; psychotherapies; and social science

1 Martin J, Meltzer H, Elliot D. *The prevalence of disability among adults.* London: HMSO, 1988. (OPCS surveys of disability in Great Britain: report 1).

2 Hirst M. *Moving on: transfer of young people with disabilities to adult services.* York: University of York, Department of Social Administration and Social Work and Social Policy Research Unit, 1984.

3 Jeannerod M. The representing brain: neural correlates of motor intention and imagery. *Behaviour and Brain Sciences* 1994;**17**:187–245.

4 Young B, Ott L, Twyman D, *et al.* The effect of nutritional support on outcome from severe head injury. *J Neurosurg* 1987;**67**:668–76.

5a Clifton GL, Robertson CS, Grossman RG, *et al.* The metabolic response to severe head injury. *J Neurosurg* 1984;**60**:687–95.

5b Gaddisserex P, Ward JD, Young HF, Becker D. Nutrition and a neurosurgical patient. *J Neurosurg* 1984;**60**:219–32.

5c Twyman DL, Young AB, Ott L, *et al.* High protein enteral feeding: a means of achieving positive nitrogen balance in head injured patients. *Journal of Parenteral and Enteral Nutrition* 1985;**9**:679–84.

6 Whitaker J, Romer JA. The assessment and management of neurogenic swallowing disorders. In: Greenwood R, Barnes MP, McMillan T, Ward CD, eds. *Neurological rehabilitation.* London: Churchill Livingstone, 1993;327–34.

7 Grundy D, Russell J, Swain A. *ABC of spinal cord injury.* 1st ed. London: BMJ, 1990.

8a Brindley GS, Rushton DN. Long term follow up of patients with sacral anterior root stimulator implants. *Paraplegia* 1990;**28**:469–75.

8b Brindley GS, Sauerwein D, Hendry WF. Hypo-gastric plexus stimulators for obtaining semen from paraplegic men. *Br J Urol* 1989;**64**:72–7.

8c Brindley GS, Scott GI, Hendry WF. Vas canulation with implanted sperm reservoirs for obstructive azoospermia or ejaculatory failure. *Br J Urol* 1986;**58**:721–3.

8d Brindley GS, Polkey CE, Rushton DN, Cardozo L. Sacral anterior root stimulator for bladder control in paraplegia: the first 50 cases. *J Neurol Neurosurg Psychiatry* 1986;**49**:1104–14.

9a Enderby PM. Dysarthria. In: Greenwood R, Barnes MP, McMillan T, Ward CD, eds. *Neurological rehabilitation.* London: Churchill Livingstone, 1993;335–42.

9b Byng S, Jones EV. Cognitive neuropsychological approach to acquired language disorders. In: Greenwood R, Barnes MP, McMillan T, Ward CD, eds. *Neurological rehabilitation.* London: Churchill Livingstone, 1993;343–54.

10 Swingler T. *The Soundbeam manual.* 3rd ed. Norwich: Tim Swingler, 1984:1–57. (Tim Swingler, 463 Earlham Road, Norwich NR4 7HL (01603 507788). Video also available.

11 Wilson BA, Baddeley A, Evans J, Shiel A. Errorless learning in the rehabilitation of memory impaired people. *Neuropsychological Rehabilitation* 1994;**4**:307–26.

12 Tardieu C, Lespargot A, Tabary C, Bret ND. For how long must the soleus muscle be stretched each day to prevent contracture? *Dev Med Child Neurol* 1988;**30**:3.

13 Melville H. *The prevention of contractures in elbow flexors and calf muscles after severe head injury.* (MPhil thesis). Southampton: University of Southampton, 1994.

14 Skiel DA, Barnes MP. The local treatment of spasticity. *Clinical Rehabilitation* 1994;**8**: 240–6.

15 Barnes MP, McLellan DL, Sutton RA. Spasticity. In: Greenwood R, Barnes MP, McMillan T, Ward CD, eds. *Neurological rehabilitation.* London: Churchill Livingstone, 1993:161–72.

16 Odeen I. Reduction of muscular hypertone by long-term muscle stretch. *Scand J Rehabil Med* 1981;**13**:93–9.

17 Davis PM. Toward attaining independent walking: preparation and facilitation. In: *Starting again. Early rehabilitation after traumatic brain injury or other severe lesion.* London: Springer, 1994:382–433.

18 *Physical disability in 1986 and beyond.* London: Royal College of Physicians, Vol 20, no 3, 1986:160–94.

19 Newcombe F. Frontal lobe disorders. In: *Starting again. Early rehabilitation after traumatic brain injury or other severe lesion.* London: Springer, 1993:377–88.

20 Alderman N. *Maximising the learning potential of brain injured patients.* (PhD thesis). Southampton: Univ of Southampton, 1995.

21 Watson M, Horn S, Wilson BA, Shiel A, McLellan DL. The application of a paired comparisons technique to identify sequence of recovery after severe head injury. *Neuropsychological Rehabilitation* (in press).

22 Pain HSB, McLellan DL. The use of individualised booklets after stroke. *Clinical Rehabilitation* 1990;**4**:265–72.

23 Bax M, Smyth D, Thomas A. Health care of physically handicapped young adults. *BMJ* 1988;**290**:1153–5.

24a Wade DT, Wood VA, Langton Hewer R. Recovery after stroke—the first three months. *J Neurol Neurosurg Psychiatry* 1985;**48**:7–13.

24b Wade DT, Langton Hewer R. Functional abilities after stroke: measurement, natural history and prognosis. *J Neurol Neurosurg Psychiatry* 1987;**50**:177–82.

25a Wilson BA, Davidoff J. Partial recovery of visual object agnosia: 10 year follow up. *Cortex* 1993;**29**:529–42.

25b Wilson BA. *Life after brain injury: long term outcome of 101 people seen for rehabilitation 5–10 years earlier.* (Meeting proceedings). Australian Society for the Treatment of Brain Injury, 1995 (in press).

26 McLellan DL. The feasibility of indicators and targets for rehabilitation services. *Clinical Rehabilitation* 1992;**6**:55–66.

27 Hanspal R, Wright M, Procter D, Peggs S, Whitaker J, McLellan DL. Failure to deliver the formal therapy prescribed in an NHS rehabilitation unit. *Clinical Rehabilitation* 1994; **8**:161–5.

28 *Report of the Brain Injury Rehabilitation Conference* (Peterborough, March 1994). Department of Health, 1994:1–23. (F 66/003 1911 IP 5K).

29 Matsusaka N, Hamamura A, Fujita M. Linkage among medicine, health and welfare in community care—from viewpoint of investigation of care services offered to clients. *Japanese Journal of Rehabilitation Medicine* 1994;**31**:988–9.

Index

Also from the BMJ Publishing Group

NEUROLOGICAL EMERGENCIES

Edited by Richard Hughes

This practical guide to the most common neurological conditions likely to present as emergencies is written by a group of eminent neurologists from Britain and the United States. Thirteen chapters, including coma, head injury, stroke, visual failure, epilepsy, and acute confusional state, provide the non-specialist with the most up to date information on diagnosis and management.

ISBN 0 7279 0756 5   350 pages   1994

For further details of this book and our full range of titles write to Marketing Department, BMJ Publishing Group, BMA House, Tavistock Square, London WC1H 9JR or telephone 0171 383 6541.